# Computer-Assisted Planning in Craniofacial Surgery

# Computer-Assisted Planning in Craniofacial Surgery

**Amir H. Dorafshar**
MD, FACS
The John W. Curtin Professor and Chair of Plastic and Reconstructive Surgery
Rush University Medical Center
Chicago, Illinois
USA

**Joseph Lopez**
MD, MBA
Chief of Pediatric Head and Neck Surgery
Department of Children's Surgery
AdventHealth for Children
Orlando, Florida
USA

**Russell R. Reid**
MD, PhD
Bernard G. Sarnat Professor of Surgery and Craniofacial Research
Section of Plastic Surgery
University of Chicago Medicine
Chicago, Illinois
USA

ELSEVIER

Elsevier
1600 John F. Kennedy Blvd.
Ste 1800
Philadelphia, PA 19103-2899

COMPUTER-ASSISTED PLANNING IN CRANIOFACIAL SURGERY ISBN: 978-0-323-82668-6


*Content Strategist:* Lauren Boyle
*Content Development Specialist:* Kayla Jarman
*Publishing Services Manager:* Shereen Jameel
*Project Manager:* Maria Shalini
*Desiner:* Bridget Hoette

Printed in India

Last digit is the print number: 9 8 7 6 5 4 3 2 1

# Contributors

**Julio Acero,** MD, DMD, PhD, FDSRCS, FEBOMFS
Full Professor
Surgery
Alcala University
Madrid
Spain
Department Head
Oral and Maxillofacial Surgery
Ramon y Cajal University Hospital
Madrid
Spain

**Jennifer N. Akin,** MD
Resident
Plastic and Reconstructive Surgery
University of Texas Medical Branch
Galveston, Texas
USA

**Andre Alcon,** MD
Fellow
Hansjorg Wyss Department of Plastic Surgery
NYU Langone Medical Center
New York, New York
USA

**Lee WT Alkureishi,** MD
Assistant Professor of Surgery
Plastic, Reconstructive and Cosmetic Surgery
University of Illinois Chicago
Chicago, Illinois
USA

**Amir Aminzada,** MD
Resident Physician
Department of Surgery, Division of Plastic and Reconstructive Surgery
Saint Louis University School of Medicine
St. Louis, Missouri
USA

**Eduardo Arias,** BFA, MSc, CCA
Clinical Anaplastologist
Plastic Surgery
University of Illinois Chicago
Chicago, Illinois
USA

**Sydney H. Arnold,** MD
Resident
Plastic and Reconstructive Surgery
Rush University Medical Center
Chicago, Illinois
USA

**Anna R. Carlson,** MD
Fellow in Craniofacial Surgery
Plastic Surgery
The Children's Hospital of Philadelphia
Philadelphia, Pennsylvania
USA

**Brendan J. Cronin,** BA, MD
Resident Physician
Division of Plastic and Reconstructive Surgery
University of California Los Angeles
David Geffen School of Medicine
Los Angeles, California
USA

**Edward Davidson,** MD
Associate Professor
Department of Plastic Surgery
Case Western Reserve University School of Medicine Department of Plastic Surgery
Cleveland, Ohio
USA

**Patricia de Leyva,** MD, PhD
Oral and Maxillofacial Surgeon
Oral and Maxillofacial Surgery
Ramón y Cajal University Hospital
Madrid
Spain

**Amir H. Dorafshar,** MD, FACS
The John W. Curtin Professor and Chair of Plastic and Reconstructive Surgery
Rush University Medical Center
Chicago, Illinois
USA

**Mark Egbert,** DDS
Chief of Pediatric Oral and Maxillofacial Surgery
Seattle Children's Hospital
Seattle, Washington
USA
Associate Professor
Oral and Maxillofacial Surgery
University of Washington
Seattle, Washington
USA

**Roberto L. Flores,** MD
Joseph G. McCarthy Associate Professor of Reconstructive Plastic Surgery
Hansjorg Wyss Department of Plastic Surgery
NYU Langone Health
New York, New York
USA

**Christopher R. Forrest,** MD, MSc, FRCS(C), FACS
Chief, Division of Plastic and Reconstructive Surgery
Surgery
The Hospital for Sick Children
Toronto, Ontario
Canada
Chair, Division of Plastic and Reconstructive Surgery
Surgery
University of Toronto
Toronto, Ontario
Canada

**Mickey Gideon, MD**
Professor
Director of Pediatric Neurosurgery
Department of Neurosurgery
Soroka Medical Center
Be'er Sheva
Israel

**Warren Grayson, BSc, PhD**
Professor
Biomedical Engineering
Johns Hopkins University
Baltimore, Maryland
USA

**Thomas Haglund, MS BME, BS BME**
Sr. Biomedical Engineer
Heart Institute
Nicklaus Children's Health System
Hollywood, Florida
USA

**Jeffrey A. Hammoudeh, MD, DDS, FACS**
Professor
Associate Chief
Plastic and Maxillofacial Surgery
University of Southern California,
Children's Hospital Los Angeles
Los Angeles, California
USA

**Kelly A. Harmon, BS**
Medical Student
Surgery, Division of Plastic and
Reconstructive Surgery
Rush University Medical Center
Chicago, Illinois
USA

**David Hirsch, DDS, MD**
Professor
Chairman of Dental Medicine
Zucker School of Medicine at Hofstra/
Northwell
Hempstead, New York
USA

**Richard A. Hopper, MD, MS**
Chief
Division of Craniofacial and Plastic
Surgery
Seattle Children's Hospital
Seattle, Washington
USA
Surgical Director
Craniofacial Center
Seattle Children's Hospital
Seattle, Washington
USA
Marlys C. Larson Chair of Craniofacial
Surgery and Professor
Department of Surgery
University of Washington
Seattle, Washington
USA

**Tsung-yen Hsieh, MD**
Assistant Professor
Department of Otolaryngology – Head
and Neck Surgery, Division of Facial
Plastic and Reconstructive Surgery
University of Cincinnati College of
Medicine
Cincinnati, Ohio
USA

**Adam S. Jacobson, MD**
Director, Head and Neck Surgery
Department of Otolaryngology – Head
and Neck Surgery
New York University
New York, New York
USA

**Noor ul Owase Jeelani, BMed. Sci, BMBS, MRCS, MBA, MPhil, FRCS**
Professor
Department of Pediatric Neurosurgery
Great Ormond Street Hospital for
Children
London
UK

**Christian Jimenez, BS**
Resident
Division of Plastic and Reconstructive
Surgery
University of Southern California
Los Angeles, California
USA

**Chris Kalmar, MD, MBA**
Resident
Vanderbilt University Medical Center
Nashville, Tennessee
USA

**Hitesh Kapadia, DDS, PhD**
Chief of Craniofacial Orthodontics
Seattle Children's Hospital
Seattle, Washington
USA
Affiliated Assistant Professor
Orthodontics
University of Washington
Seattle, Washington
USA

**George Kokosis, MD**
Assistant Professor
Plastic Surgery
Rush University Medical Center
Chicago, Illinois
USA

**Katelyn Kondra, MD**
Resident
Division of Plastic and Reconstructive
Surgery
University of Southern California
Los Angeles, California
USA

**Dmitriy Kravchenko, DO, DMD, MPH**
Chief Resident
Oral and Maxillofacial Surgery
Yale School of Medicine
New Haven, Connecticut
USA

**Anand Raj Kumar, MD, FACS, FAAP**
Professor of Plastic and
Reconstructive Surgery
Plastic and Reconstructive Surgery
Mercer University School of Medicine
Savannah, Georgia
USA

**Justine C. Lee, MD, PhD**
Professor of Surgery
Division of Plastic and Reconstructive
Surgery
University of California Los Angeles
Los Angeles, California
USA

**Jamie P. Levine, MD**
Associate Professor
Plastic Surgery
NYU Langone Medical Center
New York, New York
USA
Chief of Microsurgery
New York, New York
USA

**Fan Liang, MD**
Assistant Professor
Department of Plastic and Reconstructive Surgery
Johns Hopkins University
Baltimore, Maryland
USA

**Christopher D. Lopez, MD**
Resident Physician
Plastic and Reconstructive Surgery
Johns Hopkins School of Medicine
Baltimore, Maryland
USA

**Joseph Lopez, MD, MBA**
Chief of Pediatric Head and Neck Surgery
Department of Children's Surgery
AdventHealth for Children
Orlando, Florida
USA

**Uma Maduekwe, MD**
Visiting Assistant Clinical Professor of Surgery
University of Illinois at Chicago
Chicago, Illinois
USA

**Paul N. Manson, MD**
Distinguished Service Professor
Plastic Surgery
Johns Hopkins University
Baltimore, Maryland
USA
Professor of Surgery
Maryland Shock Trauma Unit
University of Maryland
Baltimore, Maryland
USA

**Evan Matros, MD**
Associate Professor
Surgery – Plastics and Reconstruction
Memorial Sloan Kettering Cancer Center
New York, New York
USA

**Paul A. Mittermiller, MD**
Plastic Surgeon
Plastic Surgery
Private Practice, Los Angeles
California
USA

**Leila Musavi, MD**
Resident Physician
Division of Plastic and Reconstructive Surgery
University of California Los Angeles
Los Angeles, California
USA

**Harsh Patel, MD**
Resident
Division of Plastic and Reconstructive Surgery
University of California Los Angeles
Los Angeles, California
USA

**Pedro Salomao Piccinini, MD**
Clinical Instructor
Division of Plastic Surgery
University of Pennsylvania
Philadelphia, Pennsylvania
USA

**Dale Podolsky, BSc, BESc, MD, PhD, FRCSC**
Surgeon
Craniofacial Surgery
The Hospital for Sick Children
Toronto, Ontario
Canada

**Hannes Prescher, MD**
Resident
Surgery/Section of Plastic and Reconstructive Surgery
University of Chicago Medicine
Chicago, Illinois
USA

**Chad A. Purnell, MD**
Assistant Professor
Divisions of Plastic Surgery and Department of Neurosurgery
University of Illinois Chicago
Chicago, Illinois
USA
Craniofacial Surgeon
Plastic Surgery
Shriners Children's Chicago
Chicago, Illinois
USA

**Majeed Rana, MD**
Professor
Department for Oral and Maxillofacial Surgery
University Hospital Düsseldorf
Düsseldorf
Germany

**Nikesh Regmi, MSE**
Product Marketing Specialist
Surgical Planning – Design and Manufacturing
ImmersiveTouch Inc.
Chicago, Illinois
USA

**Russell R. Reid, MD, PhD**
Bernard G. Sarnat Professor of Surgery and Craniofacial Research
Section of Plastic Surgery
University of Chicago Medicine
Chicago, Illinois
USA

**David J. Reisberg, DDS, FACP, FAAMP**
Head, Dental Unit/Prosthodontics/Maxillofacial Prosthetics
The Craniofacial Center
The University of Illinois Hospital and Health Sciences System
Chicago, Illinois
USA
Professor
Department of Surgery
The University of Illinois College of Medicine
Chicago, Illinois
USA

**Idean Roohani, BS**
Plastic Surgery Research Fellow
Children's Hospital Los Angeles
Division of Plastic and Reconstructive Surgery
University of Southern California
Los Angeles, California
USA

**Tulsi Roy, MD, MSc**
Assistant Professor of Plastic Surgery
Department of Surgery
Rush University Medical Center
Chicago, Illinois
USA

**Michelle Seu, BA**
Research Fellow
Division of Plastic and Reconstructive Surgery
Rush University Medical Center
Chicago, Illinois
USA

**Farooq Shahzad, MBBS, MS, FACS, FAAP**
Assistant Professor
Plastic and Reconstructive Surgery Service
Memorial Sloan Kettering Cancer Center
New York, New York
USA
Assistant Professor
Weill Medical College of Cornell University
New York, New York
USA

**Pasha Shakoori, MD, DDS, MEd**
Resident
Division of Plastic and Reconstructive Surgery
University of Southern California
Los Angeles, California
USA

**Pradip R. Shetye, DDS, BDS, MDS,**
Associate Professor (Orthodontics)
Wyss Dept of Plastic Surgery
NYU Langone Health
New York, New York
USA
Director of Craniofacial Orthodontics
Wyss Dept of Plastic Surgery
NYU Langone Health
New York, New York
USA
Director of Craniofacial Orthodontic Fellowship
Wyss Dept of Plastic Surgery
NYU Langone Health
New York, New York
USA

**Eldad Silbertstein, MD**
Associate Professor
Department of Plastic Surgery
Soroka Medical Center
Be'er Sheva
Israel

**Amanda Silva, MD**
Assistant Professor
Plastic and Reconstructive Surgery
University of Kentucky
Lexington, Kentucky
USA

**Srujan Singh, Ph.D.**
Doctoral Researcher
Chemical and Biomolecular Engineering
Johns Hopkins University
Baltimore, Maryland
USA

**Akanksha Srivastava, BDS, MSc, MDSc, FACP, FRCD(C), FAAMP**
Maxillofacial Prosthodontist
Department of Surgery
University of Illinois at Chicago
Chicago, Illinois
USA

**David A. Staffenberg, MD**
Professor and Vice Chairman
Hansjorg Wyss Department of Plastic Surgery,
NYU Langone Medical Center
New York, New York
USA

**Eloise Stanton, BA**
Plastic Surgery Research Fellow
Keck School of Medicine
Children's Hospital Los Angeles
Division of Plastic and Reconstructive Surgery
University of Southern California
Los Angeles, California
USA

**Derek M. Steinbacher, MD, DMD, FACS, FRCS(Ed.)**
Professor of Plastic Surgery
Plastic Surgery, Oral/Maxillofacial
Yale New Haven Health
New Haven, Connecticut
USA

**Jordan P. Steinberg, MD, PhD, FACS, FAAP**
Surgical Director, Craniofacial Program
Plastic Surgery
Nicklaus Children's Hospital
Miami, Florida
USA
Clinical Associate Professor
Plastic Surgery
Florida International University Herbert Wertheim School of Medicine
Miami, Florida
USA
Voluntary Assistant Professor
Plastic Surgery
University of Miami Miller School of Medicine
Miami, Florida
USA

**Edward Bradley Strong, MD**
Professor and Vice Chairman
Otolaryngology
University of California, Davis School of Medicine
Sacramento, California
USA

**Srinivas M. Susarla,** MD, DMD, MPH
Associate Professor
Department of Surgery, Division of Plastic Surgery, and Department of Oral and Maxillofacial Surgery
University of Washington Medical Center
Seattle, Washington
USA
Chief, Division of Pediatric Oral and Maxillofacial Surgery
Craniofacial Center
Seattle Children's Hospital
Seattle, Washington
USA

**Jesse A. Taylor,** MD
Chief, Division of Plastic, Reconstructive, and Oral Surgery
Department of Surgery
Children's Hospital of Philadelphia
Gladwyne, Pennsylvania
USA

**Andrew Timberlake,** MD, PhD
Resident
Hansjorg Wyss Department of Plastic Surgery
NYU Langone Medical Center
New York, New York
USA

**Christina Tragos,** MD
Associate Professor
Plastic and Reconstructive Surgery
Rush University Medical Center
Chicago, Illinois
USA

**Mark M. Urata,** MD, DDS
Chief
Division of Plastic and Reconstructive Surgery
Keck School of Medicine of USC
Los Angeles, California
USA
Chair
Division of Oral and Maxillofacial Surgery
Ostrow School of Dentistry of USC
Los Angeles, California
USA
Associate Dean of Surgery and Hospital Affairs
Ostrow School of Dentistry of USC
Los Angeles, California
USA
Division Head
Division of Plastic and Maxillofacial Surgery
Children's Hospital Los Angeles
Los Angeles, California
USA

**Howard Wang,** MD
Assistant Professor
Pediatric Plastic and Reconstructive Surgery
Case Western Reserve University/ Rainbow Babies and Children's Hospital
Cleveland, Ohio
USA

**Max Wilkat,** MD, DMD
Maxillofacial Surgeon
Department for Oral and Plastic Maxillofacial Surgery
University Hospital Düsseldorf
Düsseldorf
Germany

**Erin M. Wolfe,** MD
Research Associate
Division of Plastic Surgery
Nicklaus Children's Hospital
Miami, Florida
USA

**S. Anthony Wolfe,** MD
Chief
Division of Plastic Surgery
Miami Children's Hospital
Miami, Florida
USA

**Erik M. Wolfswinkel,** MD
Assistant Professor
Division of Plastic and Reconstructive Surgery
Oregon Health and Science University
Portland, Oregon
USA

**Helen Xun,** MD
Integrated Plastic Surgery Resident
Surgery
Beth Israel Deaconess Medical Center
Boston, Massachusetts
USA

**Robin Yang,** DDS, MD
Assistant Professor
Department of Plastic and Reconstructive Surgery
Johns Hopkins University
Baltimore, Maryland
USA

**Pooja Yesantharao,** MD, MS
Resident Physician
Division of Plastic Surgery
Stanford
Palo Alto, California
USA

**Joshua Yoon,** MD
Research Fellow
Division of Plastic Reconstructive and Maxillofacial Surgery
R Adams Cowley Shock Trauma Center
Baltimore, Maryland
USA

**Yuxiao Zhou,** PhD
Assistant Professor
Department of Mechanical Engineering
Texas A&M University
College Station, Texas
USA

# Foreword

Computed tomography (CT) imaging with 2-dimensional (2D) and 3-dimensional (3D) CT scans – how they came to cause craniofacial surgery to employ computer-assisted surgical planning, models, surgical guides, and patient-specific implants in challenging and routine craniofacial surgery

Craniofacial imaging is a fast-growing field offering diagnostic analyses, anatomic orientation, individualized surgical planning, patient education and consent, virtual and physical simulation of results, 3D modeling, implant construction, and educational teaching in craniofacial surgery. The recent rapid expansion of possibilities and techniques across broad maxillofacial disciplines justifies a separate publication on the techniques, uses, expectations, and possibilities for future utilization, and to reveal augmented user opportunities.

It was not so many years ago that the treatment of craniofacial problems was "closed" with external fixation and external molding devices. Two world wars produced thousands of injuries whose open nature stimulated utilization of the wounds themselves for open definitive reduction. At first, surgical approaches were dictated by open-wound experience, cadaver dissections, and early surgery, but all inquiries were severely hindered by the limited bone and absent soft tissue definition provided by plain x-rays.

Slowly, knowledge of anatomy caused open approaches to be employed electively for traumatic and non-traumatic entities, including elective craniofacial surgery. Gilles[1,2,3] gained mastery from thousands of war injuries widely opened by ballistic or smaller wounds which were easily extended for regional visualization. Many were treated in the aftermath camps following the world wars in England, Baltimore's Fort McHenry, Pennsylvania's Valley Forge, and other centers, with the help of surgeons with injury experience from NYU and Boston plastic and oral/maxillofacial surgeons. They not only used that time to learn from the injuries, but also to learn from their unique camaraderie. The Valley Forge experience specifically created among surgeons a desire to return to their universities and form specialty specific learning groups (surgical divisions) such as plastic surgery. These groups created plastic surgery divisions within departments of surgery. Later, the pressure for increasingly specific anatomical expertise created the initial craniofacial subdisciplines of the time.

Historically, individuals with the genius to visualize 3D anatomy without the use of imaging, such as Leonardo da Vinci[4] ("The Orbit" in the Queen's Collection, London) and the early work of Paul Tessier,[5,6] were leaders because of their distinct and remarkably prescient perception. Neither of these men could rest until they had thoroughly explored cadavers and gained mastery of the anatomy. After the introduction of the CT scan in the 1980s, the marvelous ingenuity historically shared by such rare perceptive individuals would become available to anyone who had the ability to read an x-ray, gaining abundant information about both bone and soft tissue.

Open approaches to craniofacial trauma and elective surgery demanded better, more precise fixation: first, interfragment wires, then rigid fixation. Both techniques rapidly spread because open operations were more reliably stabilized. The rapid exchange of information among subdisciplines in craniofacial surgery frequently began with trauma open approaches and advanced rapidly to general stabilization principles. In Switzerland, the US, and then further afield, teaching courses in rigid fixation were financed through the sale of equipment by manufacturers. Specific specialty knowledge was rapidly homogenized by these courses, and popularized universally among all the disciplines operating within the face: oral and maxillofacial surgery, otolaryngology, ophthalmology, and plastic surgery. A nonreversible exchange and blending of specialty knowledge across disciplines occurred.

Besides open approaches, more imaging techniques were needed to guide and lead these advances. The 1980s provided the CT examination with the ability to radiologically visualize both bone and soft tissue anatomy without dissection or open exploration. Original 2D CT scans were soon augmented by 3D visualization, which provided panoramic symmetry comparisons in addition to the detail of axial, coronal, sagittal, and special CT slice sections. All disciplines rapidly incorporated these evaluations into the analysis and treatment of defects of the soft tissue and bone of the craniofacial region, congenital or acquired. The ability of CT scans to generate accurate volume calculations, and the addition of contrast and vascular imaging, further added to their usefulness. Postoperative imaging for result assessment followed.

The first uses of CT were in definition, anatomical classification, and treatment organization. CT classification yielded prioritization and order determination in treatment; these studies were closely followed by CT evaluation of postoperative results. At the University of Maryland Shock Trauma Unit, I was finishing a case of a zygoma open reduction next to my orthopedic colleague Andy Burgess, and stepped into the scrub hall where he was standing in a protective x-ray gown, shielding himself outside the room while they imaged an open tibia fracture reduction via a plain intraoperative x-ray. The use of intraoperative and postoperative result assessment was routine in orthopedic surgery, but not so in maxillofacial surgery at the time. "Why do you need an x-ray?" I queried, "when you have an open wound and are looking right at the fracture reduction?" Shortly thereafter he appeared in the recovery room with a radiograph, which showed a mistake, despite the view provided by the open reduction procedure. I then took my just-finished zygoma patient from the recovery room to the CT scanner, obtained a postop CT scan, and discovered a malreduction. Thereafter, postop CT scans were routine until intraop CT scans created the possibility of immediate intraoperative correction.

Today, CT for preoperative planning, intraoperative confirmation and postoperative analysis are here to stay, and represent the fundamental sequence of a planning, operative implementation, and evaluation process for all craniofacial surgery. CT imaging and planning techniques were rapidly incorporated first as an exercise for challenging cases: orbital reconstruction,[6] facial implants,[7] and cranioplasty.[8,9,10] Cleverly, cranial cases were imaged so that an implant could compensate for deficiencies of both bone and soft tissue by design of the bone implant alone.[11] Sargent and Day[12] characterized the composite experience as "analysis, virtual surgical planning (VSP) 3D modeling, 3D Custom and Patient Specific Implants (3D PSI) and recommended application to procedures where bone was insufficient, or such complexity existed that refinement of the operative plan in the physical environment was not possible despite the experience of the surgeon."[12]

In this text, we finally have a multidisciplinary collection, authored by a group of innovative first-users, who pioneered and advanced these techniques. This comprehensive volume is now available to benefit introductory, experienced, and potential users. Presented are state-of-the art skills in the use of preoperative evaluation, planning, and intraoperative correction of craniofacial problems of all kinds, supplemented by postoperative evaluation and value determination.[12] This text will aid the easy acquisition of refined skills which minimize the "learning curves and the problems of missed perceptions".[12]

The authors of the text form the ten years or more of advanced users; thus, they set the stage for teaching us these skills by providing established patterns of analysis derived from a decade of experience. They have been well chosen from across the craniofacial disciplines – each contributor focuses on a specific area of expertise. Every chapter is meant to be a detailed, valuable, and thorough perspective, emphasizing application of these techniques to a variety of fields. The 26 chapters cover the subjects of general workflow, general areas of interest, craniofacial syndromes, trauma of the orbit, maxilla, zygoma, and mandible, tumors, transgender affirmation, and finally, four on virtual reality, robots, biomaterials, and maxillary prostheses.

Many chapters conclude with recommendations for future development and areas for further research and exploration as well as how application could be improved. Negatives such as cost, infection/exposure of artificial material, and the inevitability of confronting disparity between the simulated and the operative result are explained. The chapters guide clinicians in cost-effective implant selection, the choice between "manufactured" vs "desktop" sources and suggest guidelines for PSI purchase. Finally, Guidelines for interactions with industry, and how to integrate 3D technologies in resident and fellow medical education, choice of biomaterials, and evaluation of outcomes are subjects managed within these chapters.

Inherent in these approaches are many opportunities for "teaching/planning of junior associates by simulation of complex portions of operations".[12] Finally, suggestions on where fields should progress, and what is further needed in clinical practice and research, are included.

We can only look forward to much more information as experience develops, which will guide us to better evaluations, analyses, and results, making our patients more satisfied, and our practices more successful. This is likely a field that will progress as fast as textbooks can keep up, if my guess is correct.

My sincere and grateful appreciation to all the authors, for their timely and relevant contributions to our learning and education.

**Paul N. Manson MD**
Distinguished Service Professor of Surgery,
Johns Hopkins School of Medicine
Professor, The University of Maryland Shock Trauma
Unit and the Department of Surgery

## References


1. Gilles HD, Millard DR. *Principles and Art of Plastic Surgery*, Vol I & II. Little Brown and Co., Boston, 1957.
2. Gilles HD. *Plastic Surgery of the Face (Based on Cases of War Injuries of the Face Including Burn Injuries, with Selected Illustrations)*. Henry Frowde, Oxford University Press, Houghton and Stoughton, London, 1920.
3. Fitz Harris L. *The Face Maker – A Visionary Surgeon's Battle to Mend the Disfigured Soldiers of World War I*. Farrar, Straus and Giroux, New York, 2022. ISBN 9780374282031.
4. Da Vinci L, Clayton M, Philo R. *Leonardo Da Vinci: The Anatomy of Man: Drawings from the Collection of Her Majesty the Queen*. The Museum of Fine Arts, Houston, Little Brown and Co., Boston, 1992:33 2A. ISBN 0821219162.
5. Tessier P, et al. *Plastic Surgery of the Orbit and Eyelids*. French Society of Ophthalmology, Jacques Rougier. Translated by SA Wolfe; MD Masson Pub., USA, 1981. ISBN: 0893520411.
6. Wolfe SA. *A Man from Héric: The Life and Work of Paul Tessier MD, father of Craniofacial Surgery*. Vol I & Vol II, Lulu.com, North Carolina, United States, July 15, 2011. ISBN 9781257782192; 978-1-257-782.
7. Gordon CR, Susarla SM, Yaremchuk MJ. Quantitative assessment of medial orbital fracture repair using computer-designed anatomical plates. *Plast Reconstr Surg*. 2012;130(5):698e-705e. PMID 23096623.
8. Yaremchuk M. *Atlas of Facial Implants*, 2nd Ed, Elsevier, New York, 2019. ISBN 9780323624763.
9. Belzberg M, et al. Cranioplasty outcomes from 500 consecutive neuroplastic surgery patients. *J Craniofacial Surg*. 2022;33(6):1648–54. PMID 29489570.
10. Wolff A, et al. Adult cranioplasty reconstruction with customized cranial implants: preferred technique, timing and biomaterials. *J Craniofacial Surg*. 2018:9(4):887–94. PMID 35245275.
11. Santiago GF, et al. Post-neurosurgical temporal deformities: various techniques for correction and associated complications. *J Craniofac Surg*. 2018;29(7):1723–9. PMID 29863558.
12. Day K, Gabrick K, Sargent L. *Application of computer technology in complex craniofacial reconstruction. Plast Reconstr Surg Glob Open*. 2018;6(3):e1655.

# Prologue

In less than a lifetime, a digital tsunami has shaped every facet of our personal and professional lives. The technology that fits in our palms (mobile phones) possesses over 1 million times more memory than the guidance computer that successfully landed the Apollo 11 spacecraft on the moon; other technology control self driving cars; and terms such as "artificial intelligence," "supercomputers," and "augmented reality" comprise daily parlance. Arguably, no field of surgery has embraced such technological advances as much as craniofacial surgery, which has rapidly evolved over the last two decades with the development of digital technology. During their careers the editors of this book have witnessed this amazing transformation firsthand and have been some of the early adopters of the application of computer-assisted design and computer-assisted manufacturing (CAD/CAM) to perform computer-assisted craniofacial surgery (CAS). Herein, three generations of craniofacial surgeons have helped to develop the concepts and ideas of this book. RRR was mentor to AHD who subsequently became mentor to JL.

The introduction of CAS into our careers has certainly improved the quality of care we deliver to our patients by allowing the time and comfort of planning craniofacial procedures virtually so that guides and designs could be developed for use intraoperatively, eliminating the stress of having to design these in real time. We have each authored several early manuscripts in the use of CAS for congenital differences and demonstrated how optimal clinical results could be attained with a shorter learning curve. But in our segregated penmanship, we recognized a greater void in the surgical literature: we "in silico" were working "in silo"; that is, we recognized that our great field could benefit from our collective experiences if we shared our best practices in an organized and lean manner. Thus, the birth of *Computer-Assisted Planning in Craniofacial Surgery*.

This book has brought together leaders in the field of craniofacial surgery from around the United States and the world to highlight the different applications of CAS in areas such as congenital differences, trauma, and cancer. The book has been designed to feature case illustrations, videos, and flow diagrams wherever possible to limit text length and improve readability and applicability to real-life clinical scenarios. The text was designed for the senior resident, fellow, or faculty member interested in craniofacial surgery from either neurological surgery, oral and maxillofacial surgery, otolaryngology, head and neck surgery, or plastic surgery disciplines. We hope that this is a useful guide to help the young surgeon or "well experienced" surgeon learn how to apply CAS to their practice and improve their clinical outcomes.

1. Kendall G. Would your mobile phone be powerful enough to get you to the moon? *The Conversation*, July 1, 2019. (https://theconversation.com/would-your-mobile-phone-be-powerful-enough-to-get-you-to-the-moon-115933)

# Contents

## Part 3: Future applications

# Video Contents

Chapter | 1 |

# The history of the computed tomography scan: how computer-assisted tomography changed craniofacial surgery, and use of computerized digital planning in patients with severe craniofacial congenital anomalies

Erin M. Wolfe, Pedro Salomao Piccinini, Thomas Haglund, Jordan P. Steinberg, S. Anthony Wolfe

CHAPTER OUTLINE



## History and introduction

Innovation in three-dimensional (3D)-scanning technology has now enabled all plastic surgeons to have a 3D scanner at their disposal for use in surgical planning. These developments began with innovation in the aviation industry, which translated to innovation in 3D imaging in surgical subspecialties such as craniofacial surgery. The father of craniofacial surgery, Dr. Paul Tessier, and Dr. David Hemmy, a neurosurgeon from Milwaukee, took note of such innovation. Hemmy took a sabbatical year in Adelaide, working with the General Electric (GE) laboratory to develop a functioning 3D scanner. The concept was born of the 3D scans used in the aviation industry to check jet engine rotors for defects. Dr. Hemmy became interested in developing 3D images from CT scans when he met Gabor Herman in 1978.[1] Herman was a mathematician who had been consulting with GE, and Hemmy had been supplying GE with patients for a prototype GE 8800 CT scanner. Together, Herman and

Hemmy realized the potential to relate multiple CT slices to each other to develop a 3D image. They proceeded to acquire studies on two patients. The raw data included large magnetic tapes comprising 10 to 15 CT slices which had to be processed overnight by a computer in a room cooled to 10° C. The next morning, the CT images had been related and 3D images were successfully displayed. This process was published by Hemmy and Gabor in 1979.[2] Hemmy and Gabor brought the concept of developing 3D images from multiple CT slices to radiologists, who quickly rejected it. Hemmy was not dissuaded by this reception, as he was interested in offering something new to the field of craniofacial surgery and sought out Dr. Paul Tessier to show him the utility of these images.

Dr. Tessier was very interested in the development of the 3D CT scans, becoming an "agitator" to push them into reality. According to Hemmy, it was immediately apparent that Tessier appreciated the utility of 3D CT images, and this began an obsession by Tessier to perfect imaging by his high standards. For Tessier, the true utility of 3D CT imaging lay not so much in the surgical planning aspect, but in having the tools to completely understand the anatomy of craniofacial deformities. This was the start of a lifelong working relationship between Tessier and Hemmy, the products of which led to innovation and advances in 3D CT imaging. Three-dimensional CT imaging changed craniofacial surgery, but craniofacial surgery also changed the course of 3D CT imaging.

In Video 1.1, we can see Dr. Paul Tessier, changing his scrub shirt and puffing on his morning cigar in the unisex locker room at Clinique Belvedere, musing on the use of x-rays and 3D imaging. He said he never looked at the x-rays before examining the patient, that he had a "3D scanner in his brain," and that he had done so many cases that he could envision pathology and outcomes as a 3D scanner and ultimately computerized digital planning could (Video 1.1).

Although Dr. Tessier never used 3D imaging in practice, he wrote an entire treatise on the topic, and was very interested in potential future applications of 3D imaging and modeling to craniofacial surgery.[1] Application of 3D printing to craniomaxillofacial surgery dates back to the early 1980s using computer numerically controlled milling machines based on CT scans and cutting geometric shapes in polyurethane or Styrofoam blocks. In their 1986 paper, "Three-Dimensional Imaging in Medicine," Hemmy and Tessier detail their opinions on the subject, which remain relevant today.[3] The discussion highlighted how in the near future, 3D imaging would be required for soft tissues as well as for bones. Without that, 3D was doomed to fail, becoming obsolete and forgotten, because of limited application, high cost, and subsequent "limited cost recovery." Another salient point was raised in the conclusion: "Three-dimensional imaging developed to a proper level of sophistication will no longer be just a gimmick but rather the most useful clinical tool for anatomic investigation of the living human organism."

Although computer-assisted planning is now readily available, elevated costs can make computerized digital planning (CDP) prohibitive. The process requires a clinical engineer or someone well trained in the functioning of computers, often one of the members of the surgical team, to perform, and there can be a significant learning curve in mastering the use of different software and equipment. However, CDP can be beneficial for a number of reasons: (1) more thorough and stepwise preoperative planning, allowing for "rehearsal" of a procedure; (2) potential decreased operative time, as less tweaking on-the-fly is necessary during surgery, which may lead to; (3) less cost and morbidity from long surgical times; (4) potential for better teaching and discussion with colleagues. CDP can be particularly useful to understand complex reconstructive surgery, especially when skeletal movements in multiple vectors are required, or when operations are planned for tumors or defects in anatomical regions that are hard to access.

Indications include oncologic resections, posttrauma reconstructions, congenital craniofacial deformities, and facial transplantation, as well as facial feminization procedures. The ability to discuss and envision different skin incisions and osteotomies preoperatively, as well as to obtain cutting guides and prefabricated plates, may be helpful to the novice and experienced surgeon alike. Importantly, cost is a significant consideration. Whether third-party companies are involved or one is to acquire 3D printing and scanning technology, cost-effectiveness of using CDP must be taken into consideration. Although preoperative costs may be higher, (because planning in advance may decrease operating room time and subsequent costs, as opposed to decision making on-the-fly) CDP may prove to be positive from a cost-benefit standpoint (i.e., if this reduces complications and/or the need for further operation/revision). Further studies comparing the costs of craniofacial reconstruction with or without CDP, as well as potential differences in outcomes, are still lacking.

## Clinical considerations

- Thorough preoperative physical exam and proper clinical photographs are fundamental for any craniofacial operation, but perhaps even more so when using CDP, when it can be easy to become sidetracked by the apparent facilitation offered by 3D printed or computerized models. CDP is not simply a "follow-the-dotted-line" approach to surgery, but rather a tool to enhance understanding, planning, and execution of complex procedures. Prior to evaluating the CDP, the surgeon should have their own visualization of the problem in their mind, as per Tessier. Excellent clinical photography is also important in patients with visible deformities as well as to plan skin incisions when necessary. Previous plates, incisions, ventriculoperitoneal shunts, tooth roots, and the position of the mental, inferior alveolar and infraorbital nerves must all be taken into consideration. We must remember that CDP is an adjunct and not the principal actor in the surgical process.

- Proper cephalometric studies and high-quality dental models are also fundamental; we have found that splints taken by our dental lab are often more faithful to the patient's true anatomy than those produced by the CDP process. Another aspect that holds true not only for cases involving CDP, but for any craniofacial case involving the teeth, is that there should always be a strong working relationship with the orthodontic team. Patients may require extra hooks placed prior to surgery to have more options for fixation of elastic bands or wires.
- CT-based measurements of bone thickness are useful in preoperative planning to ensure good bone purchase with skeletal fixation. This is especially important in patients with cranial defects or those who have previously undergone surgery with mesh reinforcement, in which case adjacent areas of bone should be sought for fixation. The second case example shown in this chapter, a patient with Pfeiffer syndrome, had titanium mesh in the skull as well as cranial bony defects. This is a problem for rigid external distraction (RED) fixation, which requires adequate bone thickness; the CDP demonstrating areas of thicker and thinner bone assists greatly in planning screw placement for the device, not only for safety but also to ensure a good bone anchor from which to distract.
- CDP has proven useful in cases of orthognathic surgery planning with some of the segmental osteotomies, or cases where movement will be in yaw, pitch, and rotation, such as with the first patient presented in this chapter, with unilateral condylar hyperplasia, whereas CDP is not necessary for more straightforward cases, (e.g., bilateral sagittal split osteotomy) and most cases of LeFort I maxillary advancement.
- Dental stability must be accounted for, as shown in Case example 3 illustrated in this chapter, a patient with multiple orofacial clefts; not only the areas of planned resection, but also adjacent teeth. Areas of concern can be better visualized, especially areas of required resection for bone movements, (i.e., retromolar/pterygoid region). This patient had significant dental root anomalies and additionally required multiple and complex segmental osteotomies with movement in X,Y and Z planes; there was a need to design them in such a way as to maintain a soft tissue pedicle for adequate vascularization.

The surgeon must also account for soft tissue restrictions which may lead to difficulty in plate fixation; although the placement of plates or screws on a preoperative model may look appropriate, it can sometimes be difficult to introduce a drill or screwdriver at the planned angle or location, and intraoperative adjustment may be necessary. It is important for the surgeon to realize, again, that CDP is the adjunct, not the main actor. For example, if a custom plate does not have a good fit, off-the-shelf plates or wire fixation may be necessary and should be planned for accordingly preoperatively. In the case of the patient with the oro-ocular cleft, for example, macrostomia facilitated intraoral access, but in other cases limited mouth opening can restrict access.

Mixed reality can allow one to understand intricate anatomical structures for surgical planning, with improved visuospatial perception owing to the examination of the anatomy from multiple angles (Figs. 1.1 and 1.2). Studies also show better memory recall compared to the traditional two-dimensional screen interface; indeed, virtual reality (VR) has been validated for studying temporal and skull base anatomy with good fidelity compared to cadavers.[4]

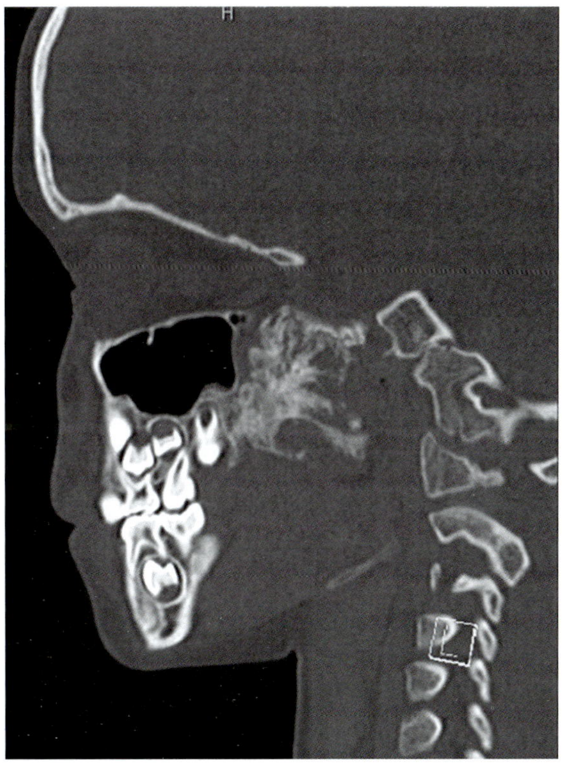


**Fig. 1.1** Sagittal section CT scan of a 6-year-old male with a large, calcified mass in left pterygomaxillary region.

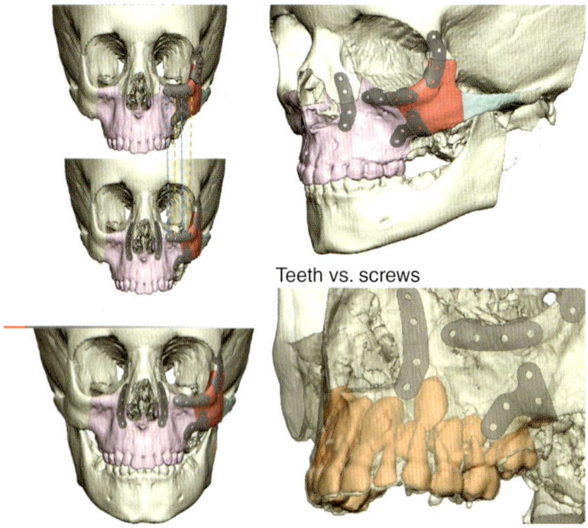


Fig. 1.2 A 6-year-old male patient with osteosarcoma of the left pterygomaxillary region. KLS Martin preoperative planning shows planned osteotomies and position of tooth roots in relation to plates/screws. Intraoperatively, we found that the LeFort osteotomy was not required, as access to the tumor was adequate through removal of the zygoma and zygomatic arch.

## Workflow for computer-assisted design/computer-assisted manufacturing (methods)

### Workflow for mixed reality surgical planning with in-house biomedical engineer

#### Three-dimensional reconstruction

3D models are generated from CT scans. To create virtual and 3D printed models of the patient's anatomy, SimpleWare by Synopsis (Mountain View, CA) is used; this is a commercially available 3D image processing and model generation program for creating 3D models from medical imaging. Segmentation is done using a threshold method where Hounsfield unit (HUs) values are chosen for each tissue type relevant to the case, shown in Fig. 1.3A. Any missing structures are painted-in manually and interpolated between slices. Excess surfaces are then removed via cutting tools and the models separated into individual 3D reconstructed surfaces for the skull, mandible, and vessels when appropriate, as seen in Fig. 1.3B. Surface corrections and cuts for tumor visibility are done in SimpleWare and then exported in 3D Manufacturing Format (3MF) for 3D printing and Standard Tessellation Language (STL) format for mixed reality. All segmentation is done by the biomedical engineer and verified by the plastic surgeon before finalizing each model. A diagram for the workflow can be seen in Fig. 1.3C.

#### Mixed reality and three-dimensional printing

The workflow for preparing models for 3D printing or mixed reality is identical, reinforcing the synergy of the two technologies. 3D models are a valuable tactile aid for surgical planning and visualization of the tumor, while mixed reality allows for on-the-fly edits to the 3D model in case a surgeon wants to alter their viewpoint of the model, or toggle the visibility of any part. In the case presented, 3D visualization of the model with and without the mandible was helpful, to better evaluate potential skin incisions and osteotomies required for optimally approaching this hard-to-reach tumor (Fig. 1.3D).

After 3D reconstruction is performed, models are deidentified and uploaded to the Virtual Surgical Intelligence (VSI) Apoqlar (Hamburg, Germany) Holomedicine program via web Application Programming Interface (API). The VSI Holomedicine application is installed on mixed reality HoloLens 2 devices (Microsoft, Redmond, WA). HoloLens technology has the ability to show a virtual model in the user's native surroundings. Additionally, the VSI application has a feature which enables multiple people to work on the same model in real time, called shared experience. Surgical planning sessions are held using the shared experience function of the software for review and surgical planning.

The in-house 3D models are printed on the J5 MediJet 3D printer (Stratasys Ltd., Eden Prairie, MN), (Fig. 1.3E). This is a PolyJet machine that prints 3D models using a photopolymer resin. The materials used for these prints are VeroCyan-Vivid, VeroYellow-Vivid, VeroMagenta-Vivid, DraftWhite, VeroUltraClear, and Support 710. Once printed they are cleaned and delivered to the surgeon, allowing them to directly draw and plan out incisions for the osteotomies, facilitating interspecialty discussion with neurosurgery and ENT colleagues.

### Workflow for computerized digital planning with third-party/external biomedical engineer (KLS Martin)

CDP planning begins with the patient consultation, when CT scans and dental models are ordered as indicated. An optional planning form may be completed to simplify the planning process. Data are then submitted directly to the KLS Martin IPS system, where a form is filled out online and a .zip file is uploaded with complete patient data. Physical dental models may be shipped separately. A data check is then performed where the data team confirms the quality of the data and requests either additional information, new

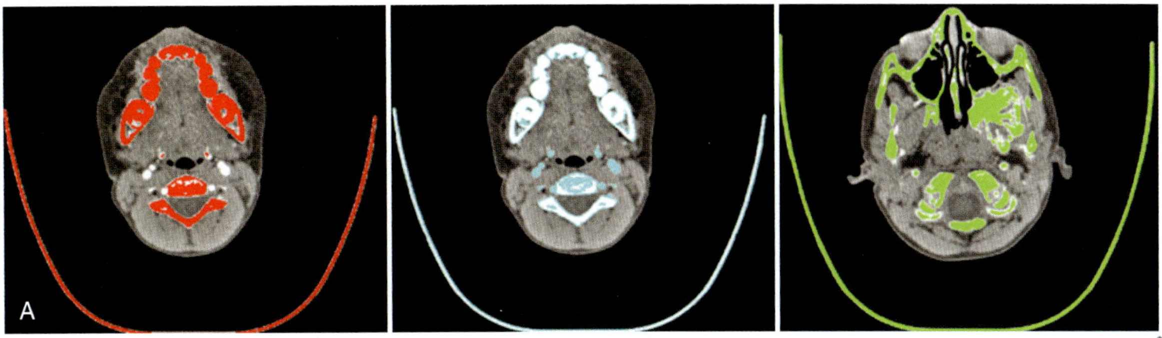


**Fig. 1.3A** Threshold for bone, 300–3000 Hounds units (Hus) *(left)*, vessels 160–400 HUs *(middle)*, and tumor 260–1500 HUs *(right)*.

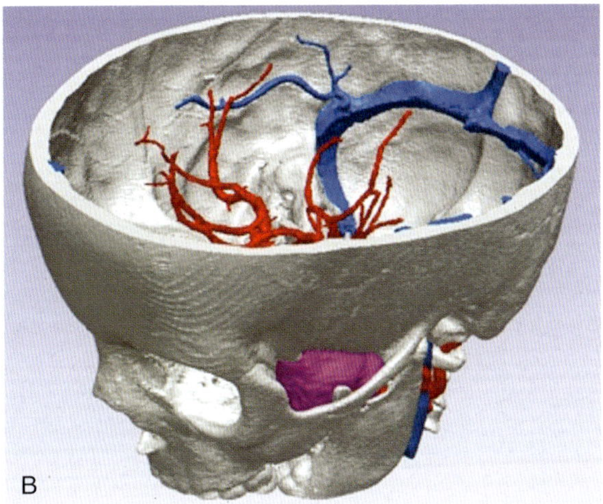


**Fig. 1.3B** Three-dimensional reconstruction of anatomy presurgery.

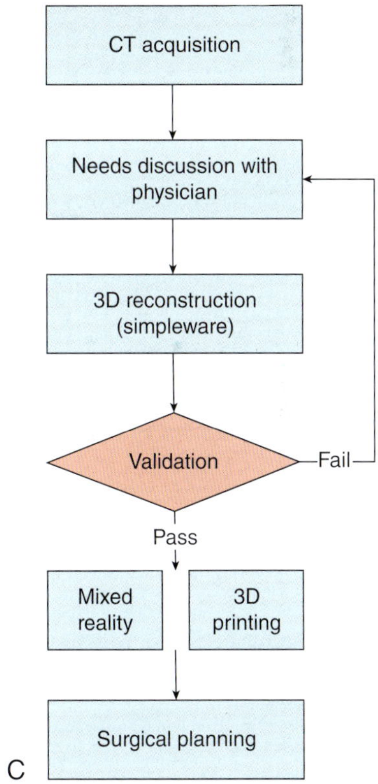


**Fig. 1.3C** Diagram of three-dimensional reconstruction workflow.

data, schedule planning, or no further actions until approval. A link is then provided to schedule a web meeting. Reports are sent outlining planned procedures and products. Products are then manufactured and shipped to the sales consultant or location of preference.

To create virtual and 3D printed models of the patient's anatomy, certain CT scan requirements must be met. Helical CT scans are recommended. The gantry must be oriented perpendicular to the occlusal plane and symmetrically with the midline. Original, uncompressed digital imaging and communications in medicine (DICOM) data must be submitted, and the data must not be reformatted or compressed. The smallest slice thickness/increment and pixel size possible should be used. Dental model requirements should also be followed. Dental models should include full dental arch and palate if palatal products are required. There should be no movement, distortion, or stitching errors. For segmental cases, preoperative dental models should be included. For intraoral scans, STL format should be used. However, 3Shape and iTero transmissions may also be used. For stone models, physical formats are preferred, although CT or intraoral scans may also be used. Minimal alginate should be used for physical models and there should be no distortion. However, CT or intraoral scans may also be used.

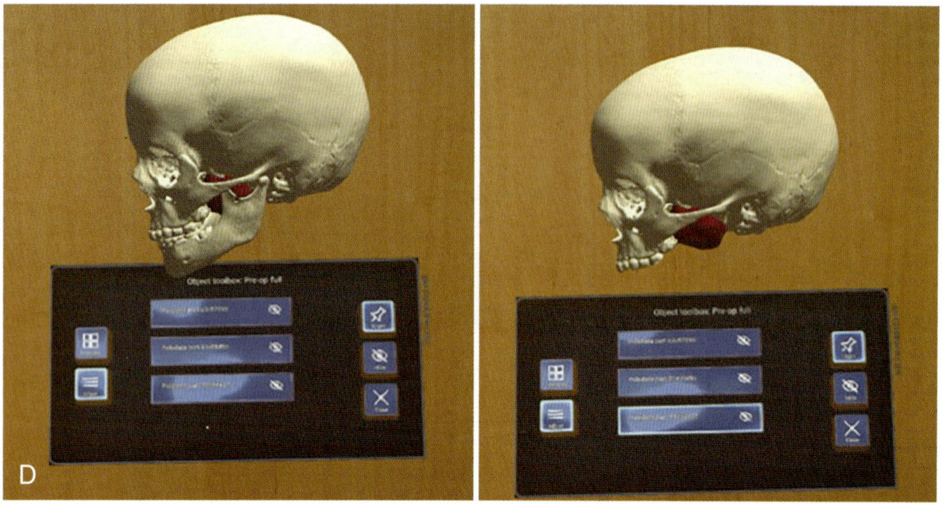

**Fig. 1.3D** A virtual model of the patient's anatomy with the jaw toggled on or off.

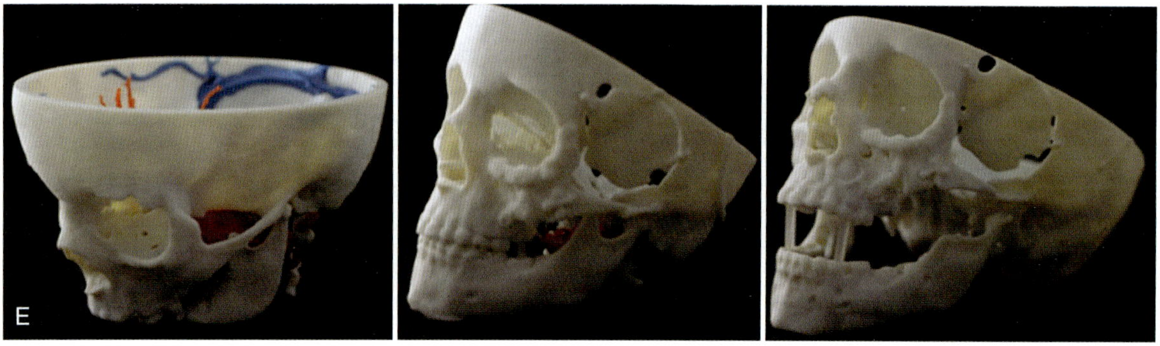

**Fig. 1.3E** Three-dimensional printed models of the patient's anatomy. Presurgical intervention *(left)*, after the initial operation *(middle)*, final result *(right)*.

## Computer-assisted design

Slides are provided with images of examples of cutting guides and splints developed via computer-aided design (CAD). A third party (KLS Martin) is consulted for development of computer-assisted designed tools such as splints and cutting guides that are used for the procedure. Planning sessions are used to elicit the craniofacial surgeon's input on the CAD process. Cutting guides and splints are utilized in some but not all patients who undergo surgical planning with CDP. Custom plates may also be used. However, they may sacrifice flexibility for precision. Although they are designed to precisely fit the anatomical area of interest, once manufactured, they may not always fit in reality and are not flexible. Cutting guides developed with CAD may be more useful than the custom plates themselves. We have found ourselves in situations where custom plates do not fit precisely, even though cutting guides may fit. In these cases, the use of off-the-shelf plates is warranted; even so, the cutting guides prove their utility in planning precise osteotomies.

## Computer-assisted manufacturing

Manufacturing of skull models is performed either with a third party (KLS Martin) during the CDP process and CAD process for development of custom plates, splints, and cuttingguides to be used intraoperatively, or in-house during the mixed reality planning process (Figs. 1.4, 1.5, 1.6). This is akin to Tessier's thinking in three dimensions about

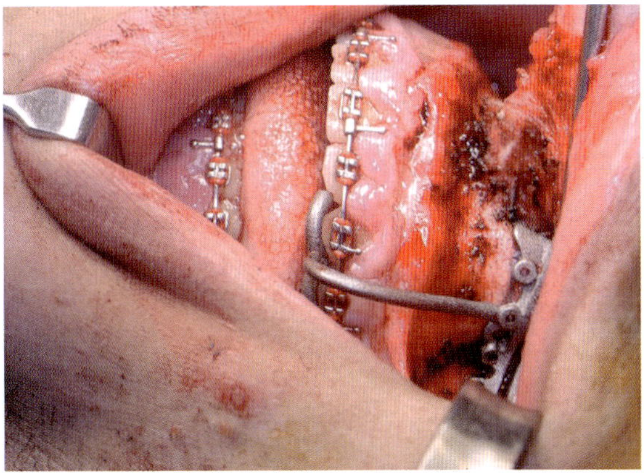

Fig. 1.4 Cutting guide in patient with condylar hyperplasia.

patients preoperatively; the major advantage is that it is possible to perform the planned osteotomies on the skull model, which greatly helps to visualize planned postoperative changes. If models are developed in-house, anatomical features are taken into account as segmentation is done using a threshold method where HU values are chosen for each tissue type relevant to the case. Missing structures are then added, excess surfaces are removed, and surface corrections and cuts may be performed, then exported in 3D.

For complex reconstructive cases, cutting guides created via computer-assisted manufacturing (CAM) are useful in planning osteotomies, especially when wedge osteotomies must be performed in order to correct maxillary cant (Fig. 1.4). We have found that cutting guides are almost uniformly quite predictable and precise, sitting flush with the planned osteotomy sites in most cases. However, due to the different resultant vectors of force due to soft tissue-bone interaction, many times the computer-manufactured plates do not sit snugly on the bone. While the preoperative precision that CAD/CAM offers is indubitable, it often occurs that there is something lost in translation; having more malleable custom plates, which may be bent and adapted to integrate with the actual intraoperative anatomy is a future helpful direction for the CAM process.

## Operative technique

Slides are provided giving an overview of the operative technique and the computer-assisted surgical plan, and pre-, intra-, and postoperative images are provided (ppt 1.1, Video 1.2). The cases include Case example 1 (Video 1.3), a patient with Pfeiffer syndrome, Case example 2 (Video 1.4), a patient with condylar hyperplasia, and Case example 3 (Video 1.5), a patient with multiple oral clefts. A narrated video of the operative technique is provided.

## Fidelity/verification

Our experience has been that for bone, fidelity is good, and plates often fit flush, although slight adjustments may be required. The fidelity for the dental models is not as accurate, which is one of the reasons why we believe a team approach along with an orthodontist is essential to

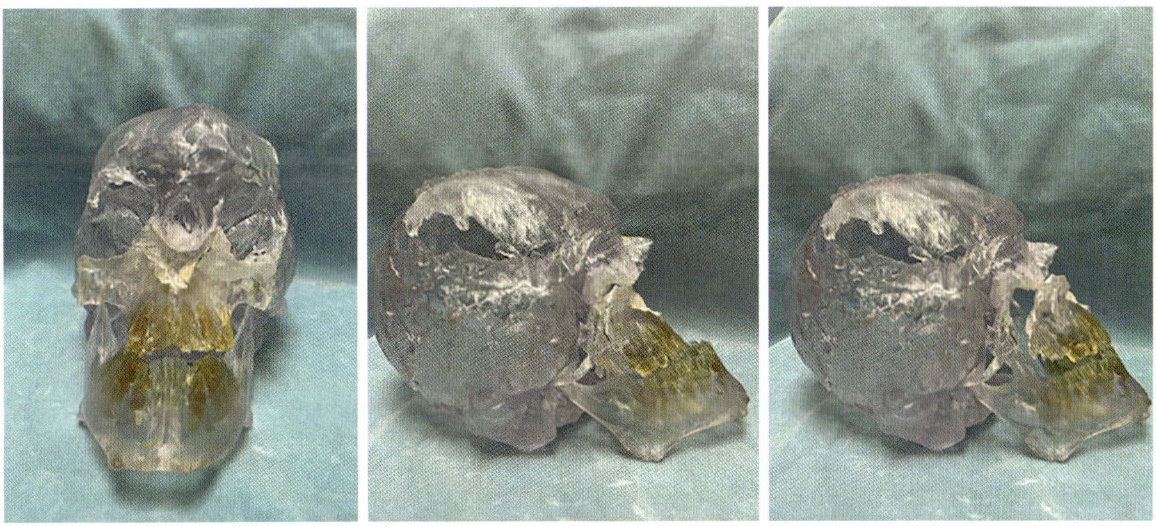

Fig. 1.5 Crystal skull model of patient with Pfeiffer syndrome.

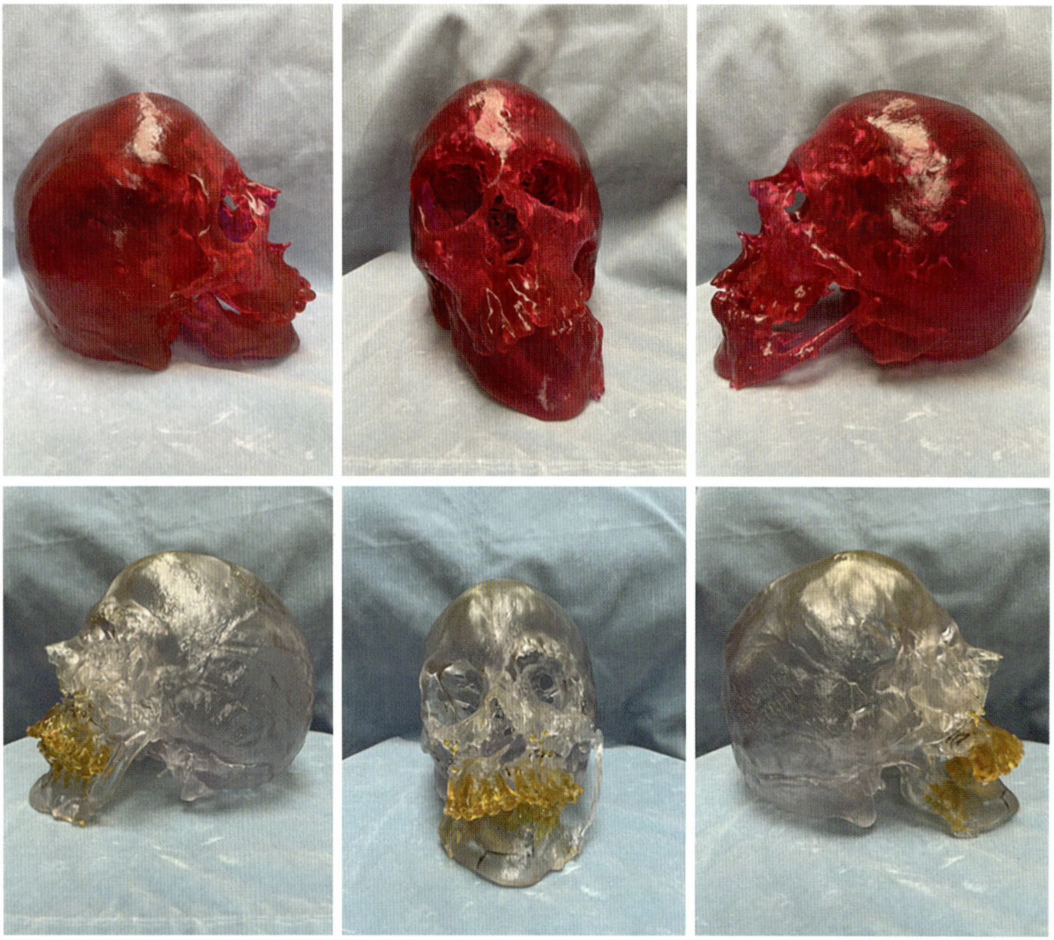

**Fig. 1.6** Crystal skull models of a patient with multiple oral clefts at two stages in the reconstructive process.

adequate surgical planning, and splints should also be made by the dental technician.

The ultimate test of fidelity is whether computer-assisted surgical plans and computer-manufactured appliances are accurate in three dimensions intraoperatively and postoperatively, comparing pre- and postoperative CT scans and CDP plans. We do not expect the computer-assisted surgical plan to be 100% faithful; rather, it serves to provide guidance in complex surgical cases. We assess accuracy with three approaches: assessment of the horizontal maxilla, assessment of the facial midline and whether it meets up with maxillary and mandibular midlines, and sagittal positioning. We use a 0.5- to 2-mm difference threshold for clinical relevance. At our institution, conformity of the computer-assisted surgical plan to the actual result is assessed via the following methods:

- Occlusion, cross bite, and whether patients require bone grafting to fill in any gaps are assessed in order to assess outcomes of the virtual planning in relation to the operative course and result.
- The intermediate splint is generally appropriate, but the final splint is frequently misaligned.
- Sometimes the plan may not work, which can be good or bad: In Case example 3, the virtual plan predicted poor occlusion, thus we had planned to place the patient in a headframe postoperatively. However, on the table, the patient had better occlusion than expected, obviating the need for a headframe and rigid external distraction.
- The splint can be assessed preoperatively or postoperatively. Prior to surgery, one can check whether the splint fits while adjusting the patient's mandible. The adequacy of splint fit can also be assessed postoperatively during follow-up visits.

- Postoperative CT scans can be compared to the final postoperative CDP plan to assess conformity and nonconformity of regions of interest.

Validation of the accuracy and conformity of CDP to actual postoperative results has been underemphasized in the literature, but this concept should not be overlooked in practice. It is important to note that true assessment of fidelity is difficult due to lack of a standardized assessment of reproducibility/accuracy. We agree with Gaber et al., in that at the start of operation, or when performing the first osteotomies, preoperative CDP/prefabricated cutting guides and plates are faithful to the patient's true anatomy, but once different surgical movements are done, other factors come into play like limits on soft tissue extensibility, tissue memory, other forces such as scar contractures and symmetry of muscle pull.[5]

Studies by Chen at al.[6] have shown that CDP and traditional surgical planning (TSP) techniques were similar in surgical accuracy for hard tissue in the sagittal plane, although the CDP technique was significantly more accurate in certain reference areas, especially in the anterior area of the maxilla. Both the CDP and TSP techniques had significantly better surgical accuracy for the maxilla than for the mandible. The CDP technique showed clinically significantly greater precision for soft tissue prediction in the sagittal plane. Patients who were treated via the CDP technique presented a more symmetrical frontal view, regardless of whether hard or soft tissue was involved. The CDP technique required more time for software planning, but it showed an advantage in time savings when considering the entire preoperative process. Accompanied by the use of an accurate computer-assisted splint, the CDP technique could effectively reduce the operative time.

## Pearls and pitfalls

- Dental models and intermediate splints made from CT scans are generally bulky and often imprecise, which underscores the importance of also having dental splints made by an orthodontist.
- CDP is useful for highly complex orthognathic cases in general, and in particular useful for visualizing procedures that are not performed often, such as condylar hyperplasia, Kufner procedure or segmental LeFort I (LFI). In addition to CDP planning session, performing cuts on the crystal skull models in advance of the procedure can be a useful supplement to the actual computer-assisted surgical plan.
- When there is potential for damage to adjacent areas such as the cranial base or nerves, CDP and cutting guides may help limit risks.
- One major pitfall is that one should not believe everything one sees: Just because something can be planned on a computer does not mean it will translate clinically. This is especially true when anticipating expected soft tissue movements.
- Adhering too much to the computer-assisted surgical plan may be detrimental to the planned outcome, i.e., if there are multiple small deviations in course, the end result may be "off" by a large amount.
- With complex patients, we often plan for multiple staged operations; this should be discussed with patients beforehand. CDP may sometimes give the illusion of being able to address all issues with a single operation, although this is not necessarily true for these patients with complex deformities, such as the patient with oro-ocular clefts.
- Having an in-house CDP program—cost permitting—is advantageous in that there is greater ease in discussing and adjusting plans with the engineering/CAD team. Future developments, such as software on the surgeon's computer or mixed reality using headsets or cell phone apps in which the surgeon can also manipulate images, will certainly be positive and lead to more widespread use of CDP.
- As we have encountered many times, the osseous advancement seen in CDP may be less than that seen intraoperatively, (i.e., CDP showing a 2-mm advancement, while real life advancement is 4 mm). In such cases, bone grafting may be necessary and the need for this should always be anticipated.
- CDP can be useful to assess and plan placement of screws and plates as well as areas of bone harvesting in relation to bony thickness, which is important in previously operated patients (trauma, previous bone harvest or mesh reconstruction).

## Outcomes/complications

The cases discussed in this chapter include one patient with a diagnosis of Pfeiffer syndrome, one patient with condylar hyperplasia, and one patient with multiple oral clefts. These were complex patients with congenital anomalies where CDP was utilized to visualize movements, solidify the clinical plan, and tailor the approach to each patient. We also have used CDP with success in other complex patients with diagnoses of complex maxillary deformity with open bite, where we performed a one-piece LFI and hemifacial microsomia.

Although outcomes have been overall good in this cohort of patients, complications/need for revision have included headframe infection in the patient with multiple oral clefts, pseudarthrosis in the Pfeiffer patient, and slight class II occlusion in the patient with condylar hyperplasia. Notably, we also experienced positive outcomes that were not anticipated from computer-assisted planning, such as getting the patient with multiple oral clefts into occlusion during the case, obviating the need for headframe usage.

The patient with multiple oral clefts is instructive because it points out the uncertainty of soft tissue movement. We were planning on distracting that segment of the maxilla in the first place because we thought that we would not be able to get the patient into occlusion and we wanted to get that segment into a better position postoperatively than what the plan showed. Through the use of distraction that segment of the maxilla could be moved without being devascularized. However, during the case we noted that it was possible to move the maxilla into the appropriate position and get the patient into occlusion, and we did not end up needing segmental distraction of the mandible. For the patient with condylar hyperplasia, postoperative occlusion was stable, and the maxilla had no further cant. Midlines lined up but there was a slight lateral crossbite in the right posterior quadrant. She was a 4-mm class II when she protruded her mandible to meet her upper teeth. This resulted from rotation around a pivot point of the left condyle as space was made by removal of a portion of the right. She ended up with excellent occlusion after orthodontics, with no occlusal cant and stable maxilla. The patient with Pfeiffer syndrome had a good outcome with a 20+-mm midface advancement following distraction. The patient had a pseudarthrosis of the maxilla postoperatively, which will require bone grafting. The patient's airway was significantly improved: preoperatively, a scope could not be passed through his nasal passages and he had no nasal airway because the maxilla was severely impacted posteriorly. The CDP enabled us to visualize the airway and the model allowed us to perform test osteotomies to further visualize the airway and surgical plan. However, the CDP did not anticipate significant beneficial soft tissue effects distinct from the bony planning that were encountered postoperatively. The patient had poor skin quality and laxity as a sequelae of the FGFR2 gene mutation associated with Pfeiffer syndrome. His midface advancement resulted in an "internal facelift" effect with substantial improvement in the appearance of his soft tissue postoperatively.

## Conclusion

The advent of computer-assisted surgical guides can improve the execution of craniofacial procedures, but ultimately, the results are dependent on the surgeon's ability to visualize the interplay between bone and soft tissue. This is the true holy grail and the next frontier in computerized digital planning, allowing the surgeon to see the final result of bone movements with skin and soft tissue overlays, although the estimated results are not always the same as the true movement. Often the soft tissue results are less dramatic than the actual bone movements. However, merely having an additional skin/soft tissue overlay is not as simple as it seems, as there are multiple forces and vectors in the soft tissue, including muscle, skin, and ligaments that often impede or reduce anticipated movements in planned advancements or setbacks.

Thirty-six years after Tessier and Hemmy's paper on 3D imaging for surgical planning, much has advanced, as anticipated, including higher resolution CT scans, improved computing power and decreased (although still significant) costs. However, the most important and useful tool that all craniofacial surgeons desire is still elusive: incorporating soft tissue results in planned skeletal movements. Once this barrier is overcome, CDP will truly become "the most useful clinical tool for anatomic investigation of the living human organism."[2]

## References

1. Hemmy DC. Docteur Paul Tessier, chirurgien plastique: a personal remembrance. *Ann Plast Surg*. 2011;67(6):S16-S24. doi:10.1097/SAP.0b013e31821835e0.
2. Hemmy DC, Herman GT, Millar EA, et al. Three-dimensional reconstruction of the spine and calvarium in children utilizing computer tomography. In: *Proceedings of the Second International Child Neurology Congress*. Blackwell Scientific; 1979:81.
3. Tessier P, Hemmy D. Three dimensional imaging in medicine. A critique by surgeons. *Scand J Plast Reconstr Surg*. 1986;20(1):3-11. doi:10.3109/02844318609006284.
4. Krokos E, Plaisant C, Varshney A. Virtual memory palaces: immersion aids recall. *Virtual Real*. 2019;23(1):1-15. Erratum: *Virtual Real*. 2019;23;17.
5. Gaber RM, Shaheen E, Falter B, et al. A systematic review to uncover a universal protocol for accuracy assessment of 3-dimensional virtually planned orthognathic surgery. *J Oral Maxillofac Surg*. 2017;75(11):2430-2440. doi:10.1016/j.joms.2017.05.025.
6. Chen Z, Mo S, Fan X, You Y, Ye G, Zhou N. A meta-analysis and systematic review comparing the effectiveness of traditional and virtual surgical planning for orthognathic surgery: based on randomized clinical trials. *J Oral Maxillofac Surg*. 2021;79(2):471.e1-471.e19. doi:10.1016/j.joms.2020.09.005.

Chapter | 2 |

# Computer-assisted design and computer-assisted manufacturing

*Helen Xun, Pooja Yesantharao, Chris Kalmar, Joseph Lopez*

**CHAPTER OUTLINE**



## Introduction

Computer-assisted design (CAD) and computer-assisted manufacturing (CAM) can play a unique role in craniofacial surgery because of the intricate three-dimensional (3D) anatomic considerations inherent to this field.[1] Through the use of CAD/CAM techniques, surgeons can uniquely plan for each patient's procedure by analyzing an unlimited number of iterations and options. By doing so, surgeons can optimize the surgical approach and create patient-specific, customized cutting guides, splints, anatomical models, and implants. Ultimately, using CAD/CAM preoperatively can help to reduce the amount of intraoperative trial and error necessary, to help minimize operative time and maximize patient outcomes both with regard to the craniofacial reconstruction itself and any potential associated donor sites. Especially in increasingly complex cases, CAD/CAM techniques can have enormous benefit in ensuring patient aesthetic and functional outcomes after correction of craniofacial defects.[2]

Since the advent of CAD/CAM techniques in craniofacial surgery, a number of technological advancements have helped to improve and streamline the CAD/CAM workflow specifically in the context of craniofacial surgery.[3] These include enhanced resolution and image quality of computed tomographic imaging and other radiographic techniques, allowing for the creation of more accurate 3D virtual models and patient-specific implants.[3] In addition, novel surgical simulation software packages allow surgeons to virtually manipulate patient anatomy on a 3D plane, and novel manufacturing techniques have allowed for the creation of enhanced 3D models, splints, cutting guides, and patient-specific implants.

Overall, CAD/CAM technology has been successfully implemented for diverse indications in craniofacial surgery, ranging from congenital reconstruction for syndromic conditions (Treacher Collins, Apert, Crouzon, etc.) to secondary maxillofacial trauma reconstruction in patients presenting with complex and/or severe deformities or defects. Though these technologies may increase the time and costs of preoperative planning, they have been demonstrated to result in savings in surgical time and surgical outcomes. Although further work is necessary to truly characterize the cost-utility of these technologies, they continue to represent the forefront of current trends in craniofacial surgery. Therefore, the craniofacial surgeon and trainees must become versatile in its utility to optimize patient clinical care. In this chapter, we will review general principles, definitions, and concepts necessary for the craniofacial surgeon and trainees to understand for the incorporation of this innovative technology in their clinical practice.

## Computer-assisted design

CAD involves the use of computer software to assist in the creation, modification, and optimization of a design. In the field of craniofacial surgery, CAD techniques use radiographic data to recreate digitized, manipulable models of patients' facial skeletal anatomy. This enables virtual preoperative surgical planning through the simulation of surgical procedures (e.g., osteotomies). CAD also allows for the design of patient-specific implants that can be integrated into the computer-assisted surgical plan.

There are a number of technical considerations when using CAD techniques in the context of craniofacial surgery, both with regard to the design process itself and the data acquisition necessary to inform the CAD/CAM process. Software packages used for CAD in craniofacial surgery include Mimics, 3-Matic (Materialize, Leuven, Belgium), and InVesalius (Renato Archer Center for Information Technology of the Ministry of Science and Technology, Campinas, Brazil).[4]

The complete workflow for CAD in craniofacial surgery is demonstrated in Fig. 2.1. The following sections will review important concepts and the steps necessary for CAD/CAM in the context of craniofacial surgery.

## Definitions

There are a number of critical considerations for CAD. Key definitions are as follows.

**Segmentation:** Image segmentation describes the process of partitioning a digital image into segments. Segmentation is important in digital image processing to locate objects and boundaries within the given image. Segmentation allows users to assign labels to groups of related pixels in an image, so as to simplify an image into more meaningful segments, which then facilitate image analysis. In craniofacial surgery, segmentation is used to convert two-dimensional slices of computed tomography (CT) image data into meaningful, three-dimensional virtual models.

**Analysis:** Image analysis in digital image processing for craniofacial surgery involves the process of extracting higher-level information from a given patient image. Analytic processes are facilitated by techniques such as image segmentation. The image analysis process depends on pattern recognition and signal processing to quantitatively and qualitatively characterize two-dimensional and three-dimensional medical images. For instance, in craniofacial surgery, finite element analysis methods can be used to design appropriate and robust osteosynthesis materials and implants using topology optimization.[5] Furthermore, these methods can be used to identify optimal locations for screws in maxillofacial surgery to optimize force distributions.

**Mirroring:** Image mirroring involves the transfer of a pixel or group of pixels across a pre-defined axis. Image mirroring is especially useful in CAD/CAM for craniofacial surgery, in order to achieve ideal symmetry and aesthetics.[6] In a patient image where the craniofacial defect is lateralized, image mirroring can be used to recreate the affected side using the normal, unaffected side. This technique has been demonstrated to be effective for reconstructing craniofacial defects.

**Fusion:** Image fusion is the process of consolidating the important features of multiple images into a single image, which is more informative and accurate than any single source information. The fused image therefore contains all the essential information. The purpose of image fusion is to streamline the amount of data available to facilitate image analysis. Image fusion is especially important in craniofacial surgery; none of the available craniofacial imaging techniques (e.g., computed tomography, magnetic resonance imaging, surface scanning, etc.) can capture facial soft tissues, the facial skeleton, and dentition with optimal quality.[7] Thus, image fusion can help to compile all of these soft tissue/skeletal layers from a variety of imaging techniques, in order to create a three-dimensional image that represents all of these anatomic elements.

**Execution:** In the process of computer-assisted surgical planning, virtual execution of surgical plans can allow surgeons to determine the optimal surgical approach.[8] During this process, surgeons can virtually carry out portions of the desired operation such as repositioning of osteotomy segments. In doing so, important clinical endpoints (e.g., occlusion) can be evaluated digitally to determine the relative efficacy of various surgical approaches. In this way, surgeons can optimize the surgical approach preoperatively to enhance the predictability of outcomes during the actual surgery itself.

**Verification:** CAD/CAM for computer-assisted surgical planning involves multiple checkpoints during the process to verify for accuracy.[9] This allows for any mistakes to be discovered preoperatively to maximize patient outcomes and minimize clinical time in the operating room itself. Verification can also be performed postoperatively to evaluate the fidelity of

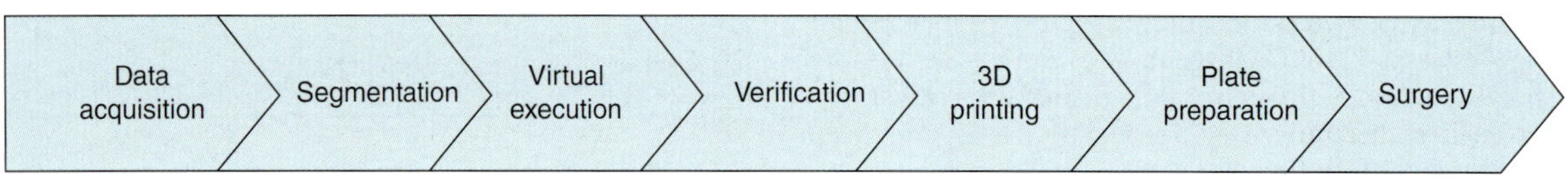


**Fig. 2.1** Computer-assisted design/computer-assisted manufacturing workflow.

the preoperative VSP: Virtual Surgical Planning is the use of computer program(s) to accurately perform or predict a procedure on a computer generated model. plan with the actual clinical result. In order to perform verification in the postoperative setting, repeat imaging after surgery is necessary.

## Data acquisition

The first step in the CAD process involves data acquisition. In the data acquisition step, patients' radiographic or magnetic resonance imaging (MRI) files are converted into mathematical and graphical models of the injured craniofacial anatomy using a CAD software package. These models are then used for surgical planning purposes.

Appropriate acquisition of radiographic patient data is necessary for optimal use of CAD/CAM-based surgical planning. To effectively use CAD techniques in craniofacial surgery, precise imaging of all relevant anatomy is critical. For computed tomography (CT) and cone-beam CT (CBCT) scans of maxillofacial/dental anatomy, for instance, a minimum of 1-mm section cuts are recommended.[9] If a flap is to be used, CT angiography may also become necessary to map out pedicle/perforator anatomy. Lastly, if dental information is required, high-resolution scanning of occlusal stone models (cut or uncut) or intraoral occlusal surface scanning may be necessary to improve the accuracy of dental anatomy data. For all these radiographic imaging data, it is important to ensure appropriate image-quality standards.

All CT, MRI, or scanning data used in CAD software packages require digital imaging and communications in medicine (DICOM) formatting. DICOM represents the international standard for medical images, detailing both appropriate image format as well as image quality. DICOM standards are typically implemented in all imaging and radiographic devices, so CT and MRI images acquired from most imaging devices are already in the DICOM format (".dicom" or ".dcm" file). This format ensures that high-quality patient images are retained.

One important consideration during the CAD workflow is data security and privacy. This is especially important when DICOM files linked to patient identifiers are used in external CAD software packages or if they are transferred to external groups for the design/manufacture of patient-specific implants/plates. Unlike other image formats, DICOM groups information into data sets, where the header typically contains patient information. In order to protect patient confidentiality, it is important to "anonymize" DICOM images by removing patient information from the DICOM header.[10] Software packages such as DicomWorks, ImageJ, D2P, and FP Image have the capability for image "anonymization," and can replace tags in the header with deidentified linkers so that patients' identities can be protected but their images can be linked to their clinical information.

## Computer-assisted manufacturing

CAM is the automation of manufacturing processes using software and computer-controlled machinery. Together, CAD/CAM describes the production process where designs created with CAD software are then transferred using the CAM input and output instructions to an automated manufacturing process.[11] In craniofacial surgery, CAD/CAM is useful in the production of patient models for surgical planning and education, and production of patient-specific implants, splints, or treatment and cutting guides.[12,13] Applications of CAD/CAM in craniofacial surgery have the potential to reduce operative time,[14-17] reduce the learning curve,[15] increase surgical precision,[15,16,18] and improve patient counseling.[18]

The workflow of CAD/CAM begins when a CAD file containing the model for production is imported into CAM software. The CAM software prepares the model for production, first by converting instructions for model production into language, such as G-code. G-code is the language used by computer numerical control (CNC) machines and contains instructions for model production. For example, the CAM software creates a toolpath for the model, and sets machine parameters. In addition, CAM software can also further optimize CAD files for production, including checking the model for any geometry errors, optimal production orientations, and generation of support structures. The machine is then able to use the language to transform raw materials to finished product.

Multidisciplinary teams and collaborations are critical for the successful realization of CAD/CAM. Typically, the team comprises the surgical team, biomedical engineers from the medical modeling company, and/or radiologists.[19] Patients must have high-resolution CT scans (1-mm cuts) of the operative area of interest timed with the workflow.[20] Timing of imaging must be close enough to the surgical date that the there are no significant changes in anatomy, but well ahead of time to allow for the CAD/CAM workflow. This is especially important in cases where soft tissue or skeletal anatomy is expected to change such as in the case of tumor progression. Often, multidisciplinary team meetings occur approximately 2 to 3 weeks prior to the scheduled case to provide adequate time for the biomedical engineers to model and/or produce the 3D models.[19]

Production modalities can be broadly categorized into additive manufacturing or subtractive manufacturing.

## Additive manufacturing (three-dimensional printing)

In general, additive manufacturing is when a model is built by adding layers of materials. It is largely dominated by 3D printing (3DP), and often the 3D printer can be linked directly to the software for model production. 3DP is the superior option for smaller, customized models with higher details and lower price points per model for small-volume production.[21] Simplification of supply chains and workflows with 3D printing allows for production flexibility, specializing in single-unit and low-volume production. However, additive manufacturing is often slower, and results in rough surfaces that often need to be post-processed by sanding or blowing.

In 3DP, the CAD file is transferred in a stereolithography (STL) file format to the CAM software that can directly communicate with the 3D printer to establish a production pathway. Most printers have their own proprietary CAM software that contains a slicing software. The slicing software converts the CAD file into coordinates and slices the model to determine layers of deposition for fabrication. The printer head is instructed to move along the X,Y plane to deposit a layer, and these layers are stacked along the Z-axis to produce the 3D model. Due to this layer-by-layer fabrication methodology, some models require the addition of support structures to prevent collapse of overhanging features (typically 40–45 degrees). Support structures can be generated in the CAM software and are removed during post-processing following production by clipping or sanding.

Due to the customizability of 3D printing, it often becomes the more economic option for production of patient-specific models, templates, and implants for craniofacial surgeons. For example, customized 3D printed biomaterial implants can be used for mandibular bone, and calvarial, maxillary, and nasal defects, and are commonly produced via laser printing or inkjet printing with hydroxyapatite ceramic, titanium metal, or synthetic polymers.[22]

The recent advent of commercial plug-and-play tabletop 3D printers has made it possible for craniofacial surgeons to 3DP in-house. In-house 3DP is approximately 20 times less expensive than outsourcing to third-party vendors.[23] Barring the learning curve, in-house 3DP may be a feasible option for production of models for education, providing the surgeon with more independence. However, in-house 3DP model production for direct patient use or clinical care still faces challenges in liability and regulatory pathways, with recommendations and regulations differing greatly from institution to institution.

A wide range of 3D printing techniques have thus far been developed, the most popular of which are described below.

**Fused filament fabrication (FFF):** Also known as fused deposition modeling (FDM), FFF 3D printing is the most classic 3D printing where material (known as filament) is extruded from a nozzle and deposited layer by layer to form the model. FFF printers are more common, cheaper, and relatively faster, and a broader range of materials/filaments are readily available. However, resolution may be limited in this production modality. There may be more post-deposition morphological warping, and FFF may be more sensitive to environmental factors such as humidity, temperature, and vibration. Factors to consider for FFF include the extruder temperature and diameter, number of nozzles, layer resolution, bed temperature, and infill of materials.

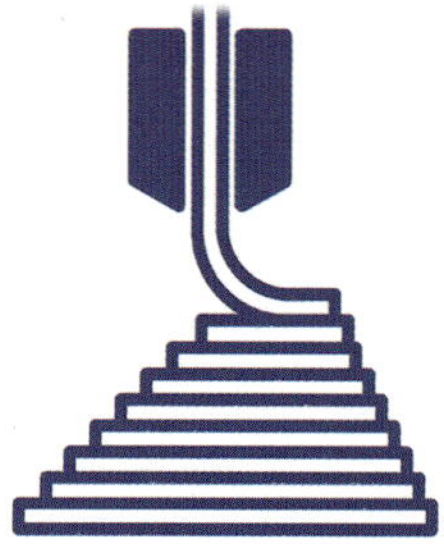

**Stereolithography (SLA):** SLA uses ultraviolet laser beams to cure liquid photopolymers, also known as resin, into solid layers. Due to the usage of laser beams, SLA is known for creating highly accurate, intricate, and precise models. However, the postprocessing is often more involved, including the need for multiple washes and additional postcure in an ultraviolet oven. The recent release of more biocompatible and diverse ranges of resins is quickly making SLA printing a preferred production modality for patient-specific models in craniofacial surgery.[24]

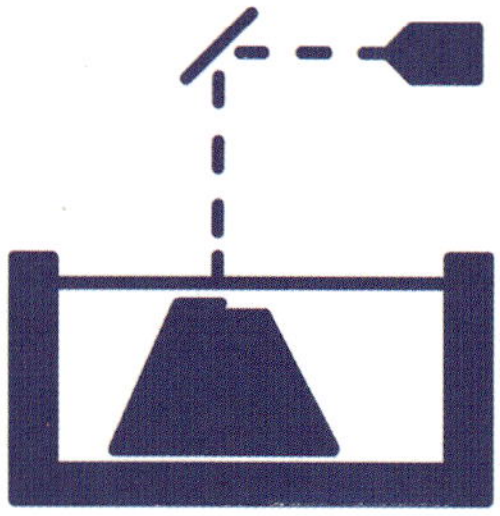

**Digital light processing (DLP):** Similar to SLA, DLP cures liquid photopolymers. However, instead of using ultraviolet light, DLP uses arc lamps, allowing resin to harden quicker for faster speed prints.

However, DLP cures complete layers, while SLA cures via a laser beam pathway. Consequently, DLP is of lower resolution.

**Inkjet printing:** Also known as binder jetting, inkjet printing uses a powder-based material (gypsum) and a bonding agent. The bonding agent is extruded as a liquid layer onto a powder bed; upon contact, the powder layer tightly adheres into a solid layer. Materials used for inkjet printing include ceramics, metals, and plastics, thus allowing production of medical-grade, biocompatible models. However, inkjet printing continues to be limited by resolution.

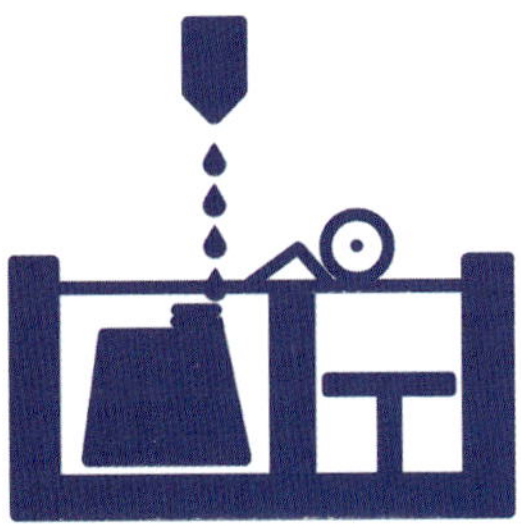

**Selective Laser Sintering (SLS):** In SLS, a $CO_2$ laser sinters (partially melts) powdered materials, fusing the powder together to form a solid layer. Generally laser sintering is used for metals, but it can also be used for ceramics, glass, and nylon. One benefit of SLS is that the structures are supported in the bed of powder, and therefore there is no need for supporting structures on the model. Additionally, the high level of accuracy and precision of SLS makes it an ideal production technique for preoperative planning.[25]

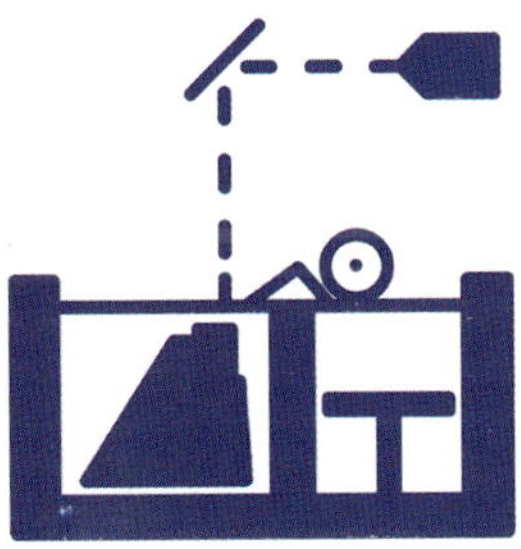

**Selective Laser Melting (SLM):** SLM uses high-powered laser beams to melt and fuse metallic powders together. SLM is stronger than SLS: while SLS sinters the metal together, SLM completely melts the powder, allowing full fusion and stronger layers. Although this is ideal for applications in aerospace industries, the increase in cost remains a barrier to entry for medical and craniofacial applications.

## Subtractive manufacturing

Subtractive manufacturing, or traditional manufacturing, is the creation of the model through removal of material from a starting block. It is ideal for larger parts, and higher volume production of clonal models, with lower production time.[21,26] However, it is challenged by the initial time, expertise, costs, and energy consumption required to establish the program and set up the production line.[21,27] While considered the conventional method of CAD/CAM, it is falling out of favor in light of recent advancements in additive manufacturing for the production of more precise, customized, and cost-effective models.[28,29]

Subtractive CAD/CAM utilizes computer numerically controlled (CNC) machining processes. Following CAD, the software encodes instructions to make the model communicate with power-driven tools to mold, machine (turn, drill, mill), or laser cut, the final model from a block of starting supplies.

**Turning:** Turning is a single-point tool, where the block is rotated, while the cutting tool moves linearly.

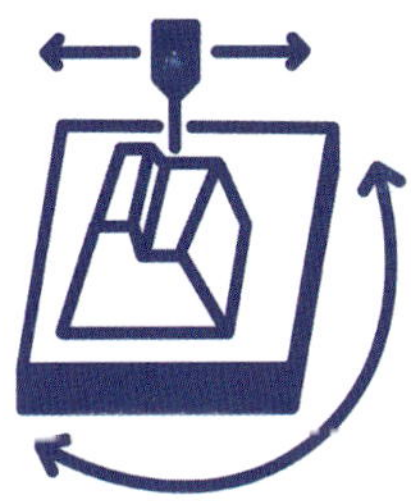

**Drilling:** A multipoint tool that uses a rotary tool with two or four helical cutting edges that creates round holes in the block.

**Milling:** A multipoint tool that rotates a cutting tool. Face milling creates flat surfaces and flat-bottomed cavities. Peripheral milling cuts threads and gear teeth. Milling is often used as a secondary process to create detailed features and finishing coats in already machined models.

**Molding:** Injection molding or casting is the pouring of materials in liquid form into a shape forming mold or cast; solidification of the liquid and removal from the mold or cast results in the final form. The mold or cast itself can be created from subtractive manufacturing. Injection molding occurs when the desired material is poured in liquid form under high pressures. Casting uses the force of gravity.

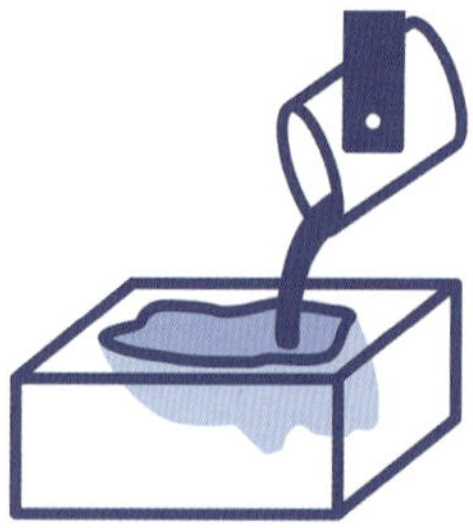

**Laser cutting:** Laser cutting is the use of high-powered lasers to melt, burn, or vaporize away materials. Laser cutting is precise and creates high-quality surface finishes.

## Future directions

Advancements in CAD/CAM and the rapid introduction of these new technologies in craniofacial surgery show their immense potential. However, given that CAD/CAM use in craniofacial surgery is still in its infancy, additional research and development is necessary to make CAD/CAM the inevitable standard of care in craniofacial surgery. First, additional research is required to clarify the values, benefits, and financial implications of CAD/CAM use in craniofacial surgery. Although numerous studies have already demonstrated its utility to improve the efficiency and efficacy of certain craniofacial procedures, further higher-level evidence studies will be required to prove its true utility. Second, further research is necessary to standardize CAD/CAM indications, protocols, and applications. Third, additional studies will be required to improve workflow optimization for modeling and production. The current workflow of imaging, design, and manufacturing often takes days to weeks, thus applications are often only reserved for elective surgeries. Optimization of the workflow includes improved imaging systems and software to generate CADs, and enhanced production lines to rapidly manufacture. Fourth, further work is necessary to optimize regulatory processes. This includes the development of more rigorous guidelines to protect patient information during the CAD/CAM workflow, and appropriate disposal of patient-specific models and/or implants. Nevertheless, the body of work to date is favorable toward the benefits of CAD/CAM in craniofacial surgery. These examples serve as exciting avenues to further advance CAD/CAM in craniofacial surgery and improve patient care and outcomes.

## References


1. Fisher M, Medina M, Bojovic B, Ahn E, Dorafshar AH. Indications for computer-aided design and manufacturing in congenital craniofacial reconstruction. *Craniomaxillofac Trauma Reconstr.* 2016;9(3):235-241. doi:10.1055/s-0036-1584391.
2. Jaffray DA, ed. *World Congress on Medical Physics and Biomedical Engineering, June 7-12, 2015, Toronto, Canada.* Vol. 51. Springer; 2015. Available at: https://link.springer.com/book/10.1007/978-3-319-19387-8.
3. Chim H, Wetjen N, Mardini S. Virtual surgical planning in craniofacial surgery. *Semin Plast Surg.* 2014;28(3):150-158. doi:10.1055/s-0034-1384811.
4. Numajiri T, Nakamura H, Sowa Y, Nishino K. Low-cost design and manufacturing of surgical guides for mandibular reconstruction using a fibula. *Plast Reconstr Surg Glob Open.* 2016;4(7):e805. doi:10.1097/GOX.0000000000000682.
5. Kraeima J, Glas HH, Merema BBJ, Vissink A, Spijkervet FKL, Witjes MJH. Three-dimensional virtual surgical planning in the oncologic treatment of the mandible. *Oral Dis.* 2021;27(1):14-20. doi:10.1111/odi.13631.
6. Jang WH, Lee JM, Jang S, Kim HD, Ahn KM, Lee JH. Mirror image based three-dimensional virtual surgical planning and three-dimensional printing guide system for the reconstruction of wide maxilla defect using the deep circumflex iliac artery free flap. *J Craniofac Surg.* 2019;30(6):1829-1832. doi:10.1097/SCS.0000000000005577.
7. Plooij JM, Maal TJ, Haers P, Borstlap WA, Kuijpers-Jagtman AM, Bergé SJ. Digital three-dimensional image fusion processes for planning and evaluating orthodontics

and orthognathic surgery. A systematic review. *Int J Oral Maxillofac Surg.* 2011;40(4): 341-352. doi:10.1016/j.ijom.2010.10.013.
8. Gandedkar N, Koo C, Chang C. Recent advances in orthognathic surgery diagnosis and management: 3D image acquisition, virtual surgical planning, rapid prototyping, and seamless surgical navigation. *J Contemp Orthod.* 2017;1:12-19.
9. Efanov JI, Roy AA, Huang KN, Borsuk DE. Virtual surgical planning: the pearls and pitfalls. *Plast Reconstr Surg Glob Open.* 2018;6(1):e1443. doi:10.1097/GOX.0000000000001443.
10. Varma DR. Managing DICOM images: tips and tricks for the radiologist. *Indian J Radiol Imaging.* 2012;22(1):4-13. doi:10.4103/0971-3026.95396.
11. Chatti S, Tolio T. *CIRP Encyclopedia of Production Engineering.* Springer Berlin Heidelberg; 2020. Available at: https://doi.org/10.1007/978-3-642-35950-7.
12. Pfaff MJ, Steinbacher DM. Plastic surgery applications using three-dimensional planning and computer-assisted design and manufacturing. *Plast Reconstr Surg.* 2016;137(3):603e-616e. doi:10.1097/01.prs.0000479970.22181.53.
13. Steinbacher DM. Three-dimensional analysis and surgical planning in craniomaxillofacial surgery. *J Oral Maxillofac Surg.* 2015;73(suppl 12):S40-S56. doi:10.1016/j.joms.2015.04.038.
14. Gray R, Gougoutas A, Nguyen V, Taylor J, Bastidas N. Use of three-dimensional, CAD/CAM-assisted, virtual surgical simulation and planning in the pediatric craniofacial population. *Int J Pediatr Otorhinolaryngol.* 2017;97:163-169.
15. Cho RS, Lopez J, Musavi L, et al. Computer-assisted design and manufacturing assists less experienced surgeons in achieving equivalent outcomes in cranial vault reconstruction. *J Craniofac Surg.* 2019;30(7): 2034-2038. doi:10.1097/SCS.0000000000005748.
16. Khechoyan DY, Saber NR, Burge J, et al. Surgical outcomes in craniosynostosis reconstruction: The use of prefabricated templates in cranial vault remodelling. *J Plast Reconstr Aesthet Surg.* 2014;67(1):9-16. doi:10.1016/j.bjps.2013.09.009.
17. Chang EI, Jenkins MP, Patel SA, Topham NS. Long-term operative outcomes of preoperative computed tomography-guided virtual surgical planning for osteocutaneous free flap mandible reconstruction. *Plast Reconstr Surg.* 2016;137(2): 619-623. doi:10.1097/01.prs.0000475796.61855.a7.
18. Mardini S, Alsubaie S, Cayci C, Chim H, Wetjen N. Three-dimensional preoperative virtual planning and template use for surgical correction of craniosynostosis. *J Plast Reconstr Aesthet Surg.* 2014;67(3):336-343. doi:10.1016/j.bjps.2013.11.004.
19. Shenaq DS, Matros E. Virtual planning and navigational technology in reconstructive surgery. *J Surg Oncol.* 2018;118(5):845-852. doi:10.1002/jso.25255.
20. Chang CC, Chiang HW. Three-dimensional image reconstructions of complex objects by an abrasive computed tomography apparatus. *Int J Adv Manuf Technol.* 2003;22(9): 708-712. doi:10.1007/s00170-003-1571-8.
21. Pereira T, Kennedy JV, Potgieter J. A comparison of traditional manufacturing vs additive manufacturing, the best method for the job. *Procedia Manuf.* 2019;30:11-18. doi:10.1016/j.promfg.2019.02.003.
22. Maroulakos M, Kamperos G, Tayebi L, Halazonetis D, Ren Y. Applications of 3D printing on craniofacial bone repair: a systematic review. *J Dent.* 2019;80:1-14. doi:10.1016/j.jdent.2018.11.004.
23. FormLabs. *Prototyping Medical Devices In-House with 3D Printing.* Available at: https://formlabs.com/blog/medical-device-prototyping-and-testing-in-house-using-3D-printing/.
24. Sinn DP, Cillo Jr JE, Miles BA. Stereolithography for craniofacial surgery. *J Craniofac Surg.* 2006;17(5):869-875. doi:10.1097/01.scs.0000230618.95012.1d.
25. Kaim A, Kirsch E, Alder P, Bucher P, Hammer B. Preoperative accuracy of selective laser sintering (SLS) in craniofacial 3D modeling: comparison with patient CT data. *Rofo.* 2009;181:644-651.
26. Van Noort R. The future of dental devices is digital. *Dent Mater.* 2012;28(1):3-12. doi:10.1016/j.dental.2011.10.014.
27. Watson JK, Taminger KMB. A decision-support model for selecting additive manufacturing versus subtractive manufacturing based on energy consumption. *J Clean Prod.* 2018;176:1316-1322. doi:10.1016/j.jclepro.2015.12.009.
28. Kim DY, Kim EB, Kim HY, Kim JH, Kim WC. Evaluation of marginal and internal gap of three-unit metal framework according to subtractive manufacturing and additive manufacturing of CAD/CAM systems. *J Adv Prosthodont.* 2017;9:463-469.
29. Roseti L, Parisi V, Petretta M, et al. Scaffolds for bone tissue engineering: state of the art and new perspectives. *Mater Sci Eng C Mater Biol Appl.* 2017;78: 1246-1262. doi:10.1016/j.msec.2017.05.017.

# Chapter 3

# Creating traumatic occlusal splints using computer-assisted design and computer-assisted manufacturing technology

*Joshua S. Yoon, Uma Maduekwe, Jordan P. Steinberg, Fan Liang*

CHAPTER OUTLINE



## Introduction

Complex maxillomandibular fractures can have devastating functional and aesthetic outcomes for patients. Traumatic occlusal splints can act as surgical guides for fracture reduction which can then serve as the foundation upon which the remainder of the face may be reconstructed.[1-5] The occlusal splint may be uniquely helpful in patients with extensive comminuted fractures and in those who are partially edentulous.[4-7] The use of these splints improves the accuracy of the bony alignment, decreases total treatment time due to improved stabilization and elimination of trial-and-error articulation on the day of surgery, and may reduce the need for subsequent surgeries for complications such as malocclusion.[3-5]

In patients with complex facial fractures involving the maxillomandibular unit, the fundamental objective should be to first establish the premorbid occlusion.[8-10] Once this has been established, the framework for the remainder of the surgery can be based around the reduced maxillomandibular region.[2] The reasons for this are twofold. Primarily, occlusion is important for aligning the physical components of the face: muscles of mastication, suprahyoid muscles, dentition, and the temporomandibular joint.[5,9] Proper occlusion will allow for optimal functional outcomes and allow the patient to remain pain free.[5] Malocclusion is a common complication of complex facial fracture reconstruction that results in functional impairment and abnormal cosmesis.[3,11-13] This functional impairment is a common cause for subsequent operations to correct the occlusal disharmony.[12,13] Secondarily, establishing premorbid occlusion can help to simplify the procedure in a patient who may have many fractured fragments.[2,4,5,8,9]

Traditionally, splint fabrication began by taking preoperative impressions from patients who had sustained complex facial fractures, from which dental casts were then made.[4-6] This is a laborious, time-consuming process requiring experience with obtaining dental impressions and creating plaster casts, which requires physical equipment and space in the form of a dental lab.[14,15] Once the impressions have set, surgeons take these casts and section them to replicate the fracture lines. From there, each tooth-bearing segment is repositioned to recreate the putative premorbid arch width, from the dental anatomy alone. Lastly, the casts are mounted on an articulator to establish the maxillomandibular relationship and used to fashion acrylic occlusal splints.

Such splints have gained popularity given their ability to facilitate the dental relationship quickly and accurately.[5,16] With the introduction of computer-assisted design/computer-assisted manufacturing (CAD/CAM) to medicine in the 1990s, the ability of physicians to develop rapid prototypes has grown exponentially.[16-19] In fact, computer-assisted surgical planning (CaSP) and three-dimensional (3D) printed splints have effectively replaced hand-designed splints for orthognathic cases. Several studies cite the improved efficacy, cost, and accuracy with CAD as compared to traditionally fabricated splints.[1,16-18] In these cases, computed tomography (CT) scans are combined with data from digitized dental casts or data obtained directly from intraoral digital scanners.[16-18] This is less commonly performed in the trauma setting due to difficulties in obtaining the impressions or digital scans of the teeth in hospitalized patients. By utilizing modern CAD/CAM technology, occlusal splints can be created with CT scans alone and without the need for additional dental data.

## Clinical considerations

Prior to pursuing facial reconstruction, all other life-threatening issues should be addressed first. Afterwards, a thorough physical exam should be performed and then followed up with a dedicated maxillofacial CT scan with slice thicknesses of 1.25 mm or less. The scan should include full imaging of the dental arch and palate with the gantry oriented perpendicular to the occlusal plane and symmetrically with midline. Previous case studies have established that, for facial trauma, the use of occlusal splints can effectively reduce operative time and offers surgical advantages such as improved accuracy.[1,16-18] This is particularly the case for complex, comminuted fracture patterns, because the splints allow for easier, more reliable alignment into class I occlusion for patients with multisegment maxillomandibular fractures (MMF) and partially edentulous cases with considerable savings in intraoperative time.

The accuracy of the model will be heavily influenced by the quality of the scan, thus higher resolution scans will produce the most optimal models. CT scans of 1.25 mm or smaller slice thickness provide adequate resolution for model creation. Dental detail can be enhanced, as in elective orthognathic cases, with the inclusion of dental casts or digital intraoral scans. However, if dental details are not enhanced, we have found that by making small allowances or offsets up to 1 mm to the cuspal grooves, splints of sufficient fidelity can be made from the thin-cut CT maxillofacial scans alone; when these splints are used in the context of virtually designed fracture reduction models and other adjuncts, anatomic restoration can be achieved, and premorbid occlusion adequately reattained. Furthermore, the combination of MMF with plate and screw fixation can help to secure additional accuracy, particularly in cases of significant comminution when bone stock may be inadequate for rigid plate fixation.

The creation of these occlusal splints is facilitated by third-party vendors. With widespread internet availability and the ability of vendors to expeditiously mail the finalized products, the only limiting factor in taking advantage of this technology would be the availability of high-resolution imaging, which is essential for creation of the model. Thus, this technology should be accessible to almost everyone who requires it. A commonly used vendor for the creation of these splints is the Individual Patient Solutions (IPS) division of the KLS Martin® Group (Jacksonville, Florida).

## Workflow for computer-assisted design/computer-assisted manufacturing (methods)

| | |
|---|---|
| **Perform** | Perform physical exam and obtain maxillofacial CT scan |
| **Convert** | Convert CT scan to digital imaging and communications in medicine (DICOM) file |
| **Send** | Send DICOM file to third party vendor for model engineering, virtual fracture reduction, and splint creation |
| **Meet** | Meet with engineers to review virtual model, anatomic reduction, and virtual splint customization |
| **Finalize** | Finalize splint, 3D print, and utilize intraoperatively |

**ppt 3.1** Workflow to create virtual occlusal splint from patient maxillofacial computed tomography scan.

## Computer-assisted design

### Design planning

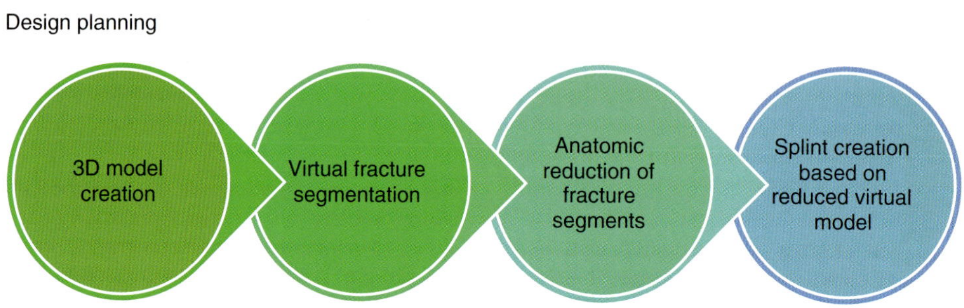


**ppt 3.2** Design planning steps to create a virtual model for a patient-specific occlusal splint.

## Anatomical design

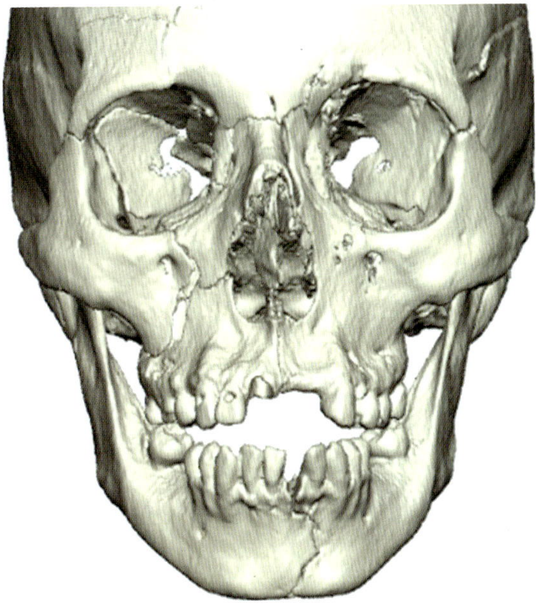

**Fig. 3.1** Three-dimensional rendering of the entire facial skeleton from index computed tomography scan.

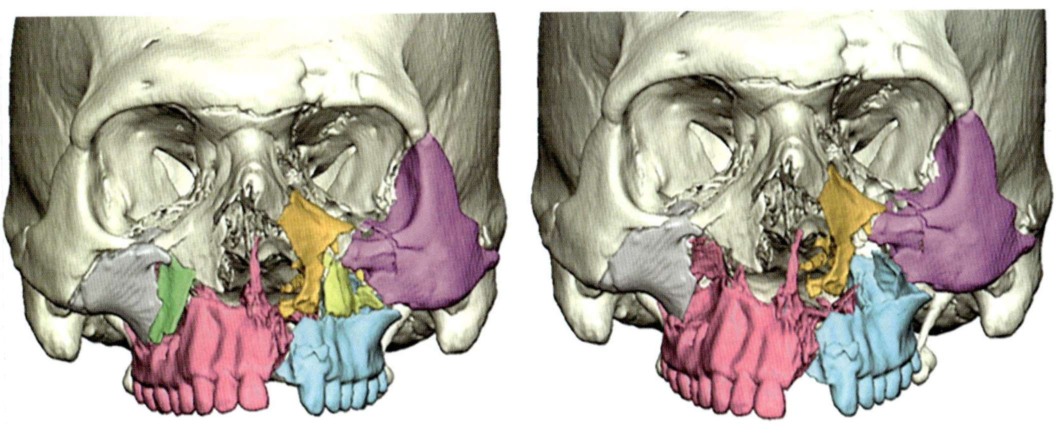

**Fig. 3.2** Virtual segmentation and reduction of maxillary fractures. Reduced fractured segments are color coded.

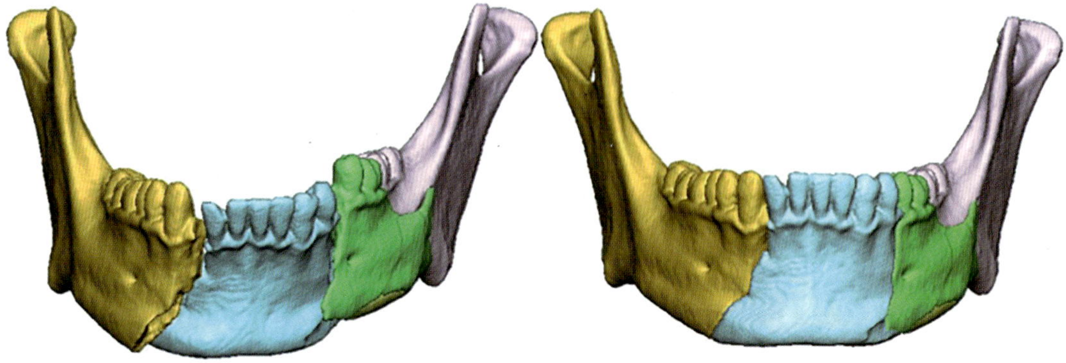

Fig. 3.3 Virtual segmentation and reduction of mandibular fractures. Reduced fractured segments are color coded.

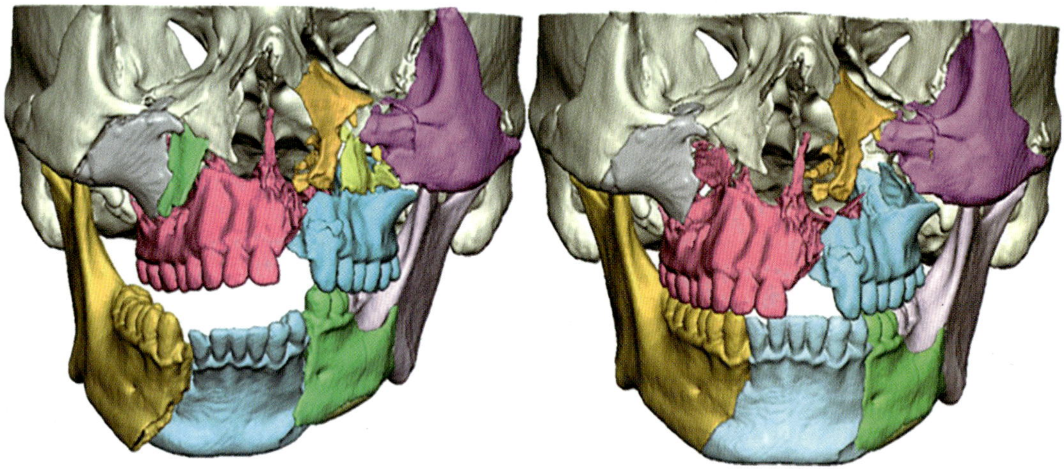

Fig. 3.4 Composite virtually segmented and reduced model with reduction and realignment into projected occlusion.

## Computer-assisted manufacturing

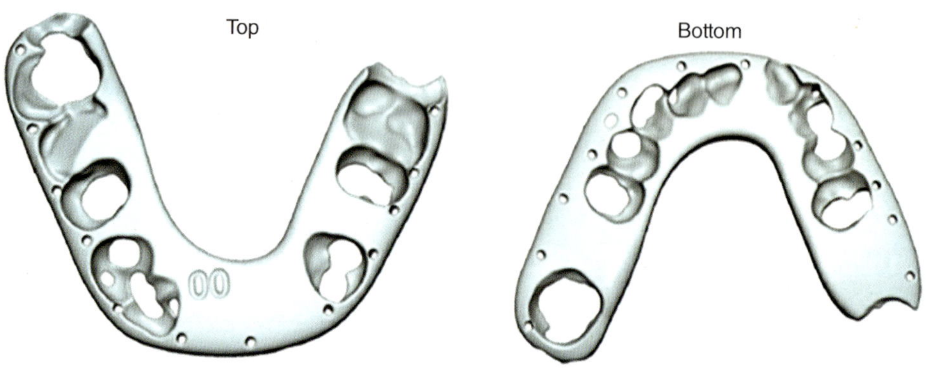


Fig. 3.5 Virtually created patient-specific wafer occlusal splint including areas of offsets in the cuspal grooves.

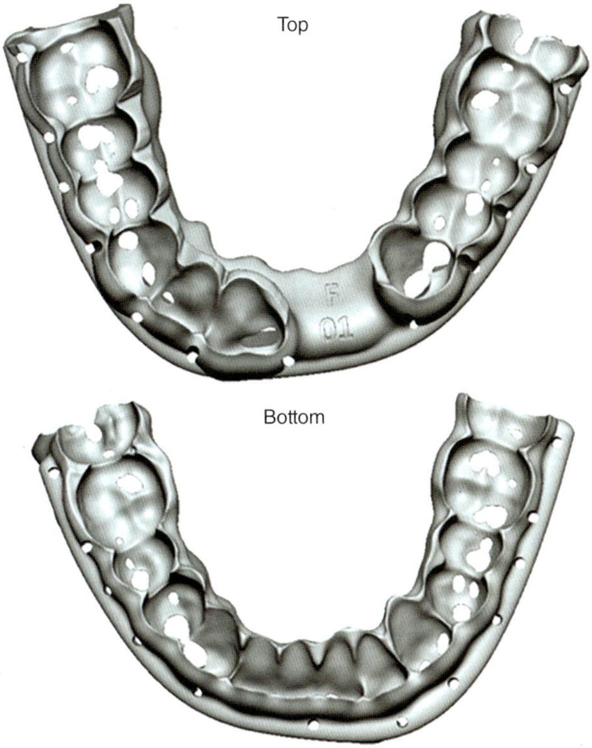


**Fig. 3.6** Virtually created patient-specific clear aligner splints including areas of offsets in the cuspal grooves.

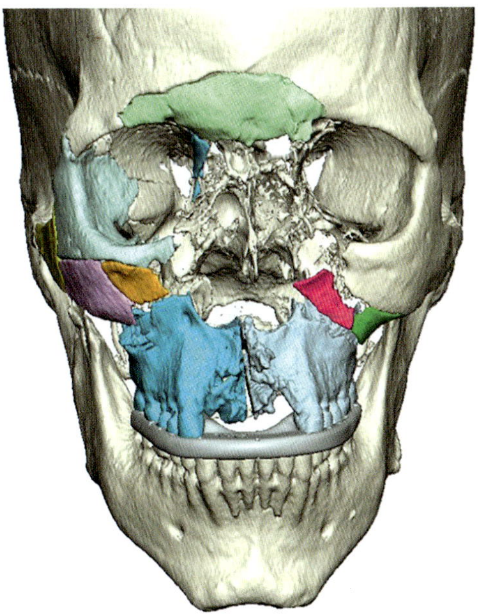

**Fig. 3.7** Frontal view of virtually reduced model with patient-specific wafer occlusal splint.

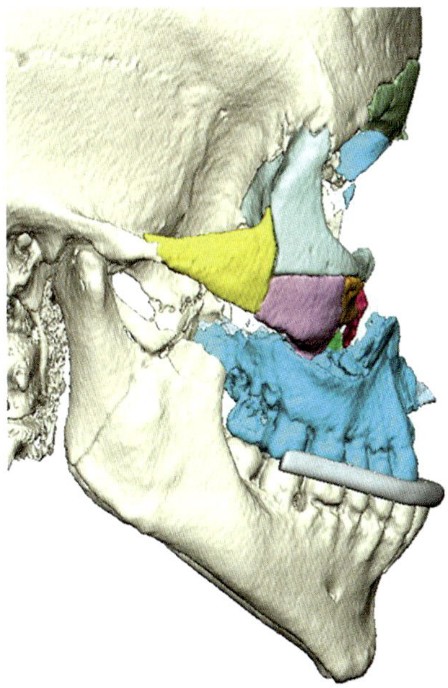

**Fig. 3.8** Sagittal view of virtually reduced model with patient-specific wafer occlusal splint.

## Operative technique

### Steps of the procedure

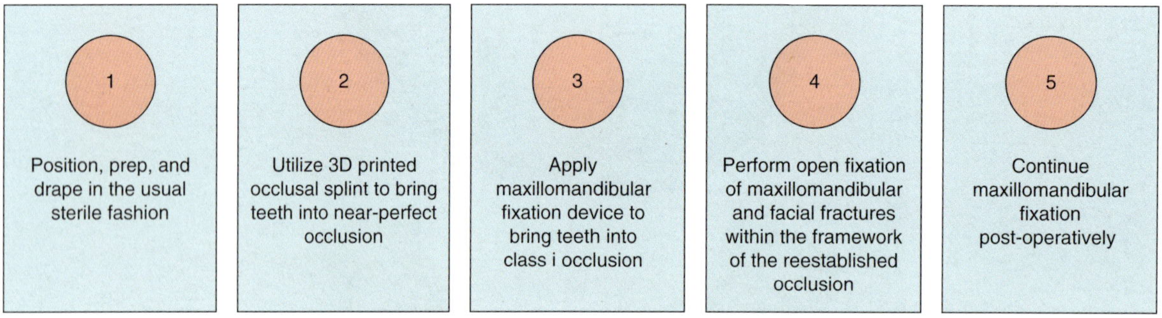


**ppt 3.3** General procedural steps for intraoperative application of three-dimensional printed occlusal splint.

### Clinical Cases

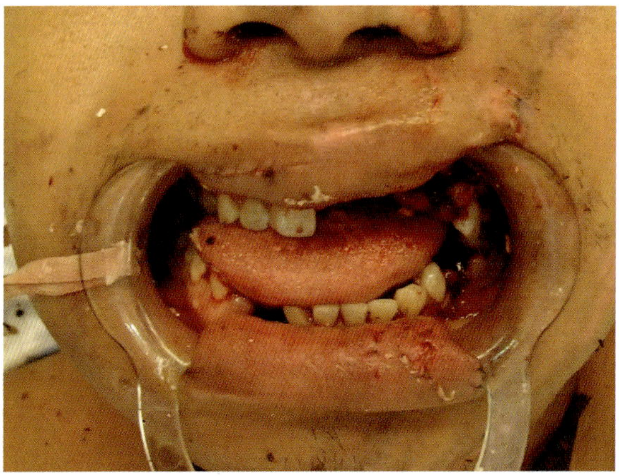

**Fig. 3.9** Intraoperative view of 22-year-old male assaulted by wooden plank and sustaining bilateral LeFort II fractures with a LeFort I component, partial sagittal palatal fracture, left ZMC fracture, left NOE fracture, bilateral parasymphyseal mandibular fractures with resulting tripartite segmentation of the jaw, left oblique ridge region with additional sagittal split-type mandibular fracture, and avulsions of teeth #9 and #10. *NOE,* Naso-orbito-ethmoidal; *ZMC* zygomaticomaxillary complex.

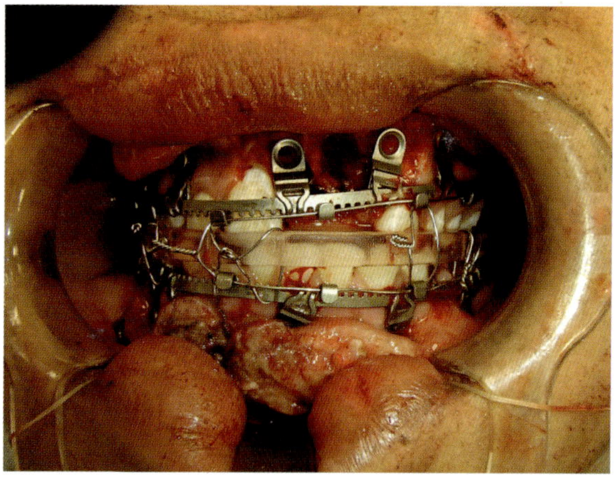

**Fig. 3.10** Intraoperative view· after application of three-dimensional printed wafer occlusal splint and maxillomandibular fixation device.

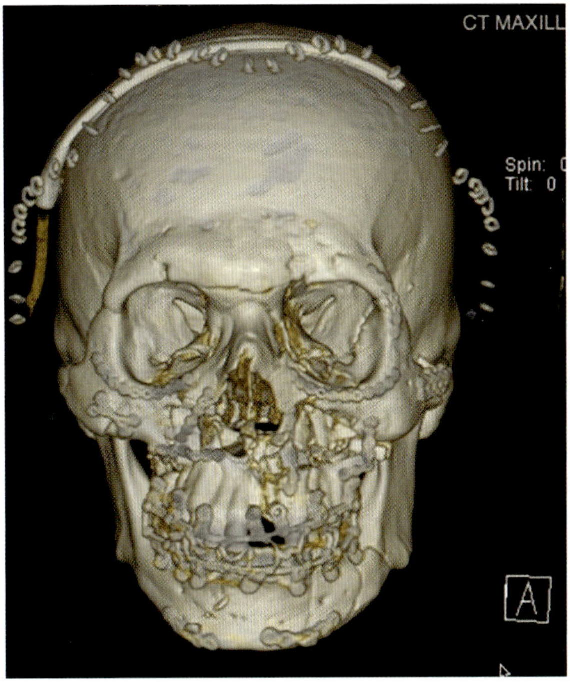


**Fig. 3.11** Postoperative computed tomography scan with continued three-dimensional printed occlusal splint and maxillomandibular fixation.

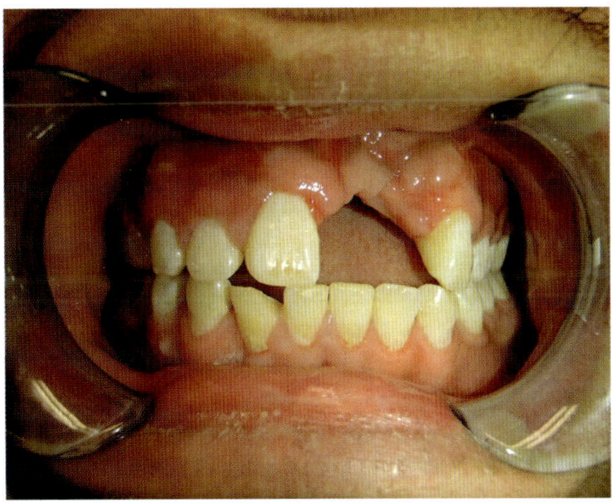

**Fig. 3.12** Follow-up photo at 6-week outpatient clinic visit.

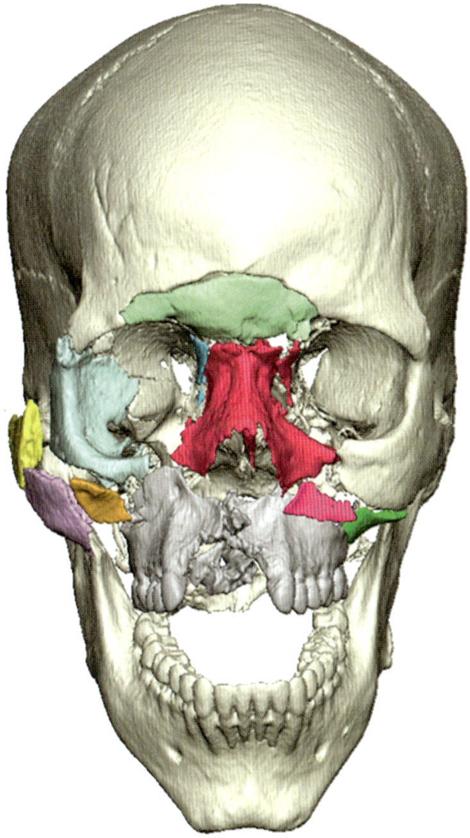

**Fig. 3.13** Preoperative virtual model with color-coded segments of fractures areas for a 50-year-old male assaulted with a wooden plank sustaining anterior and posterior table frontal sinus, bilateral NOE, right comminuted, right-sided LeFort III, left-sided LeFort II, bilateral LeFort I, palatal, right mandibular ramus, and right mandibular coronoid fractures. *NOE,* Naso-orbito-ethmoidal; *ZMC* zygomaticomaxillary complex.

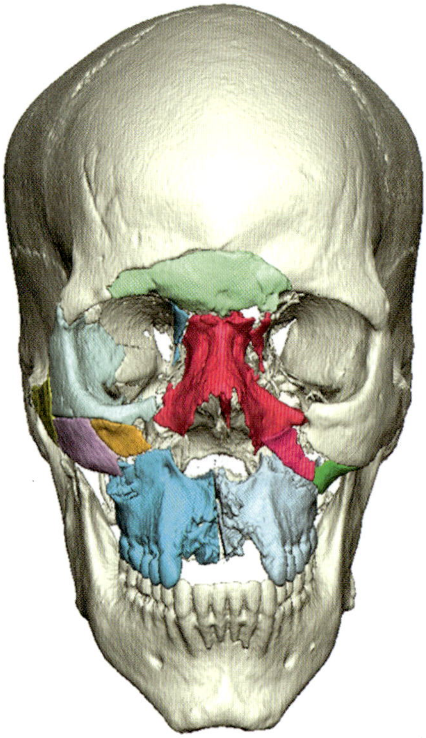

Fig. 3.14 Virtually reduced model with patient in projected class I occlusion.

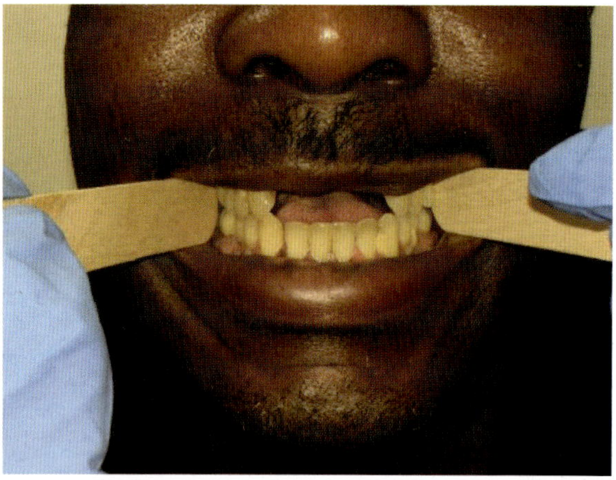

Fig. 3.16 Occlusal view at the outpatient follow-up appointment 8-weeks postoperatively.

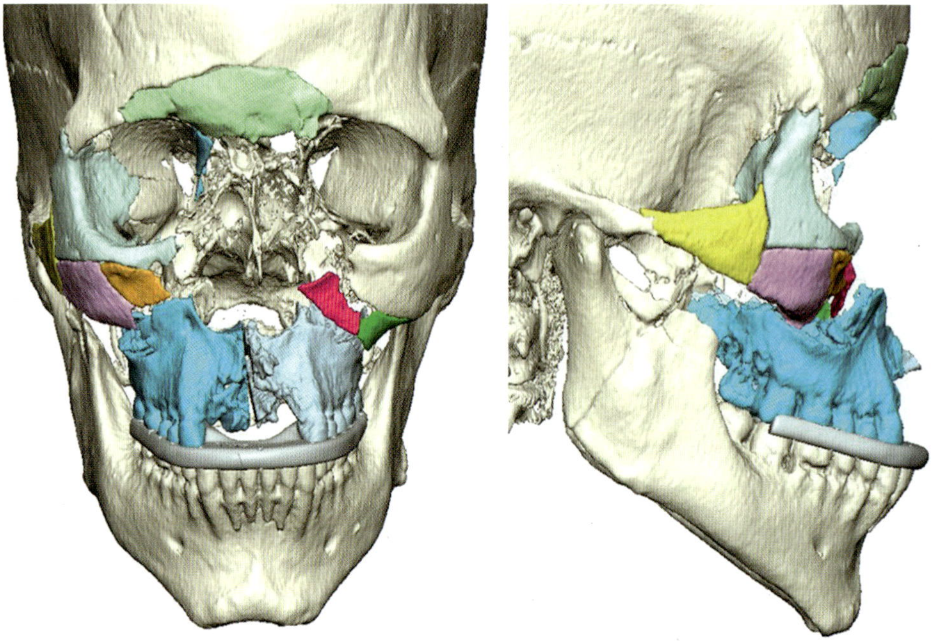

Fig. 3.15 Virtually reduced models with application of wafer occlusal splints in class I occlusion.

## Fidelity/verification

As mentioned previously, implementing offsets into the dental cusps will allow adequate compensation for the lack of dental granularity; however, this comes at a cost. The offsets in these virtually created splints provide the space for sub-centimeter movement, which may make establishing class I occlusion suboptimal. Thus, these occlusal splints should be used in conjunction with MMF, and given the extent of the fractures in this patient population, these patients will naturally require MMF postoperatively for stability. The occlusal splints should be utilized to help guide the dentition into near-perfect occlusion and then class I occlusion is established with the application of MMF. Postoperatively, these patients will undergo a CT scan to ensure proper skeletal realignment. At subsequent clinic visits, the splint and MMF will be assessed to ensure that proper occlusion is still maintained, during which adjustments can be made to the MMF if needed.

## Pearls and pitfalls

- High-quality maxillofacial CT scans with thicknesses less than 1.25 mm need to be utilized to create models of sufficient accuracy.
- All 3D models, virtually reduced images, and virtual splint characteristics and projected fit should be evaluated by the attending surgeon for all cases.
- 1-mm offsets should be built into the cuspal grooves to account for the lack of dental detail from CT scans.
- Splints created with only CT scans should be used in conjunction with MMF to ensure class I occlusion is established.

## Outcomes/complications

Traditionally, acrylic occlusal splints have been produced by taking dental impressions. The process was therefore sometimes difficult in partially edentulous patients or those with limited mouth opening.[20] Within a trauma setting, airway considerations and concomitant soft tissue and dentoalveolar trauma may prohibit surgeons from taking impressions. Additionally, the need for other equipment (e.g., intraoral scanner for digital "impressions") or supplies (alginate materials, lab space) and complications such as aspiration of materials and/or prolongation of operative time may lead to underutilization of occlusal splints in the management of jaw fractures.[20] With the advent of fine-cut CT scans and virtual planning technology, the technique of splint-guided fracture reduction and stabilization can now be more easily employed. The virtual planning has the benefit of restoring occlusion in the context of the remainder of the craniomaxillofacial skeleton, with appropriate alignment not only of the dental cusps, but also the transverse arch dimensions and alveolar segment torque. Prior techniques involving handmade acrylic splints are subject to errors in transverse arch dimensions and segmental torque, potentially resulting in residual or recurrent malocclusion.

Previous literature has indicated a precedent for virtually created splints in both orthognathic surgery and trauma craniofacial reconstruction. Adolphs and colleagues demonstrated that virtual splint generation produces clinically equivalent splints to splints made by conventional dental impressions in orthognathic surgery.[20] Kongsong successfully applied computer-assisted surgical planning for surgical splint fabrication in traumatic comminuted maxillomandibular fractures in three patients without the use of impressions or intraoral scans. Results indicated stable and repeatable occlusion with uneventful postoperative recoveries.[21] All of their patients underwent closed reduction with virtually created lingual splints with arch bars. This contrasted with the approach of Yoon and colleagues, who successfully utilized open reduction/internal fixation as well as hybrid arch bars or intermaxillary fixation (IMF) screws in a series of three patients.[1]

## Conclusion

In the treatment of complex facial fractures, occlusal splints can be a useful adjunct in the operative reduction and fixation of the fractures and reestablishment of premorbid occlusion: However, obtaining dental impressions to create traditional occlusal splints may not be feasible given the patient's condition and associated complications. With the advent of virtual preoperative surgical planning via 3D modeling and 3D printing, these occlusal splints can be created expeditiously using a high-quality maxillofacial CT scan without strict need for dental impressions.

## Take-home points

- This approach allows for the creation of occlusal splints in clinical situations where obtaining dental impressions may be difficult or not feasible.
- Occlusal splints can help improve operating room efficiency by providing efficient occlusal realignment in complex facial trauma reconstruction and help maintain stability postoperatively.

- Patient-specific occlusal splints utilizing only CT data are commercially available and accessible as they can be collaboratively made offsite/virtually by third-party vendors.
- When creating these occlusal splints with only CT imaging, offsets should be built into the cuspal grooves to account for the lack of fine dental detail in CT scans.
- These occlusal splints should be used in conjunction with maxillomandibular fixation to achieve optimal occlusion as the built-in occlusal splint offsets will bring the patient into near-perfect occlusion.

## References


1. Yoon J, Lock I, Fan CK, et al. Many moving pieces: virtual preoperative surgical planning for traumatic occlusal splints. *J Craniofac Surg*. 2022;33(4):1037-1041. doi:10.1097/SCS.0000000000008282.
2. Jack JM, Stewart DH, Rinker BD, et al. Modern surgical treatment of complex facial fractures: a 6-year review. *J Craniofac Surg*. 2005;16(4):726-731. doi:10.1097/01.scs.0000168766.33238.22.
3. Konaş E, Tunçbilek G, Kayikçioğlu A, et al. Splint-assisted reduction of comminuted or complex maxillofacial fractures. *J Craniofac Surg*. 2011;22(4):1471-1475. doi:10.1097/SCS.0b013e31821d193b.
4. Cohen SR, Leonard DK, Markowitz BL, et al. Acrylic splints for dental alignment in complex facial injuries. *Ann Plast Surg*. 1993;31(5):406-412. doi:10.1097/00000637-199311000-00004.
5. Chidyllo SA, Jacobs JS. Applications of dental splints with regard to modern techniques of rigid fixation. *J Craniofac Surg*. 1994;5(2):136-141. doi:10.1097/00001665-199405000-00020.
6. Jackson MJ, Wetmore SJ. Surgical prosthetic splints as an adjunct in treating facial fractures. *Arch Otolaryngol*. 1980;106(1):25-30. doi:10.1001/archotol.1980.00790250027006.
7. Sahand S, Saeedeh k, Elahe T, et al. A conservative method for treating severely displaced pediatric mandibular fractures: an effective alternative technique. *J Dent Mater Tech*. 2016;5(2):53-58.
8. Ellis E III, Miles BA. Fractures of the mandible: a technical perspective. *Plast Reconstr Surg*. 2007;120(7 suppl 2):76S-89S. doi:10.1097/01.prs.0000260721.74357.e7.
9. Stacey DH, Doyle JF, Mount DL, et al. Management of mandible fractures. *Plast Reconstr Surg*. 2006;117(3):48e-60e. doi:10.1097/01.prs.0000209392.85221.0b.
10. El-Anwar MW, Sayed El-Ahl MA, Amer HS. Open reduction and internal fixation of mandibular fracture without rigid maxillomandibular fixation. *Int Arch Otorhinolaryngol*. 2015;19(4):314-318. doi:10.1055/s-0035-1549154.
11. Afzelius LE, Rosén C. Facial fractures. A review of 368 cases. *Int J Oral Surg*. 1980;9(1):25-32. doi:10.1016/s0300-9785(80)80003-2.
12. Laine P, Kontio R, Salo A, et al. Secondary correction of malocclusion after treatment of maxillofacial trauma. *J Oral Maxillofac Surg*. 2004;62(10):1312-1320. doi:10.1016/j.joms.2004.02.014.
13. Steidler NE, Cook RM, Reade PC. Residual complications in patients with major middle third facial fractures. *Int J Oral Surg*. 1980;9(4):259-266. doi:10.1016/s0300-9785(80)80032-9.
14. Mühlemann S, Kraus RD, Hämmerle CHF, et al. Is the use of digital technologies for the fabrication of implant-supported reconstructions more efficient and/or more effective than conventional techniques: a systematic review. *Clin Oral Implants Res*. 2018;29(suppl 18):184-195. doi:10.1111/clr.13300.
15. Leberfinger AN, Jones CM, Mackay DR, et al. Computer-aided design and manufacture of intraoral splints: a potential role in cleft care. *J Surg Res*. 2021;261:173-178. doi:10.1016/j.jss.2020.11.085.
16. Choi JW, Kim N. Clinical application of three-dimensional printing technology in craniofacial plastic surgery. *Arch Plast Surg*. 2015;42(3):267-277. doi:10.5999/aps.2015.42.3.267. Erratum in: Arch Plast Surg. 2015;42(4):513.
17. Metzger MC, Hohlweg-Majert B, Schwarz U, et al. Manufacturing splints for orthognathic surgery using a three-dimensional printer. *Oral Surg Oral Med Oral Pathol Oral Radiol Endod*. 2008;105(2):e1-e7. doi:10.1016/j.tripleo.2007.07.040.
18. Kang SH, Kim MK, Kim BC, et al. Orthognathic Y-splint: a CAD/CAM-engineered maxillary repositioning wafer assembly. *Br J Oral Maxillofac Surg*. 2014;52(7):667-679. doi:10.1016/j.bjoms.2014.01.023.
19. Elegbede A, Diaconu SC, McNichols CHL, et al. Office-based three-dimensional printing workflow for craniomaxillofacial

fracture repair. *J Craniofac Surg*. 2018;29(5):e440-e444. doi:10.1097/SCS.0000000000004460.

20. Adolphs N, Liu W, Keeve E, et al. RapidSplint: virtual splint generation for orthognathic surgery – results of a pilot series. *Comput Aided Surg*. 2014;19(1-3):20-28. doi:10.3109/10929088.2014.887778.

21. Kongsong W, Sittitavornwong S. Utilization of virtual surgical planning for surgical splint-assisted comminuted maxillomandibular fracture reduction and/or fixation. *Craniomaxillofac Trauma Reconstr*. 2020;13(4):334-341. doi:10.1177/1943387520948677.

Chapter | 4 |

# Computer-assisted maxillofacial reconstruction

*Tsung-yen Hsieh, Edward Bradley Strong*

CHAPTER OUTLINE



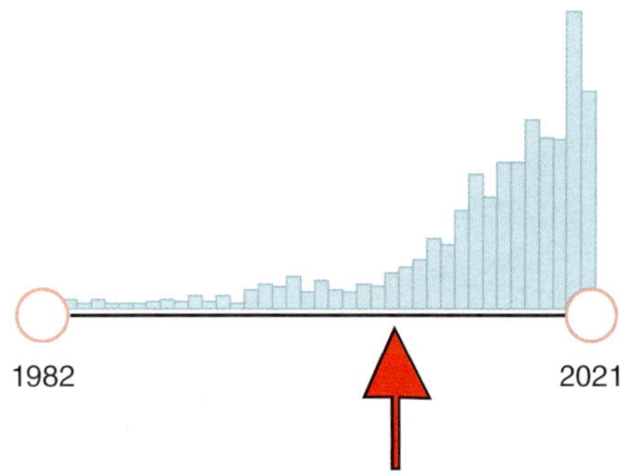


**Fig. 4.1** Publications found in PubMed search from query for "Computer-aided surgery", available by year from 1982 to 2021 with an exponential growth curve starting in 2006.

## Introduction

A comprehensive maxillofacial computer-assisted surgical workflow can be divided into three areas: 1) presurgical planning, 2) surgical execution, and 3) anatomic verification. Historically, ***presurgical planning*** has been a function of the surgeon's spatial cognition abilities, ***surgical execution*** was heavily dependent on surgeon experience, and ***intraoperative verification*** tools to confirm the surgical reconstruction were nonexistent. Advances in computer-assisted surgery (CAS) have resulted in a paradigm shift in each of these areas. A PubMed literature search starting in 1982 reveals fewer than 10 CAS publications per year, with an exponential growth curve starting in 2006 (Fig. 4.1). Since 2017 there has been an average of 131 publications per year looking at CAS applications. Computer-assisted planning software uses computed tomography (CT) or magnetic resonance imaging (MRI) data to generate representative three-dimensional (3D) objects that can be used for presurgical planning.[1,2] Virtual environments (augmented, virtual, and mixed reality) can be used to better visualize, understand, and communicate a computer-assisted surgical plan.[3-5] Additive manufacturing is commonly used to fabricate surgical models, guides and implants, which can guide an accurate surgical repair even with limited visualization.[6] Finally, intraoperative navigation and intraoperative imaging can be used to confirm the accuracy of the repair prior to leaving the operating room.[7,8] The authors will describe their current CAS workflow for maxillofacial reconstruction (Fig. 4.2).

## Presurgical planning

Computer-assisted surgical planning can be an extremely valuable tool for both young and experienced surgeons. It

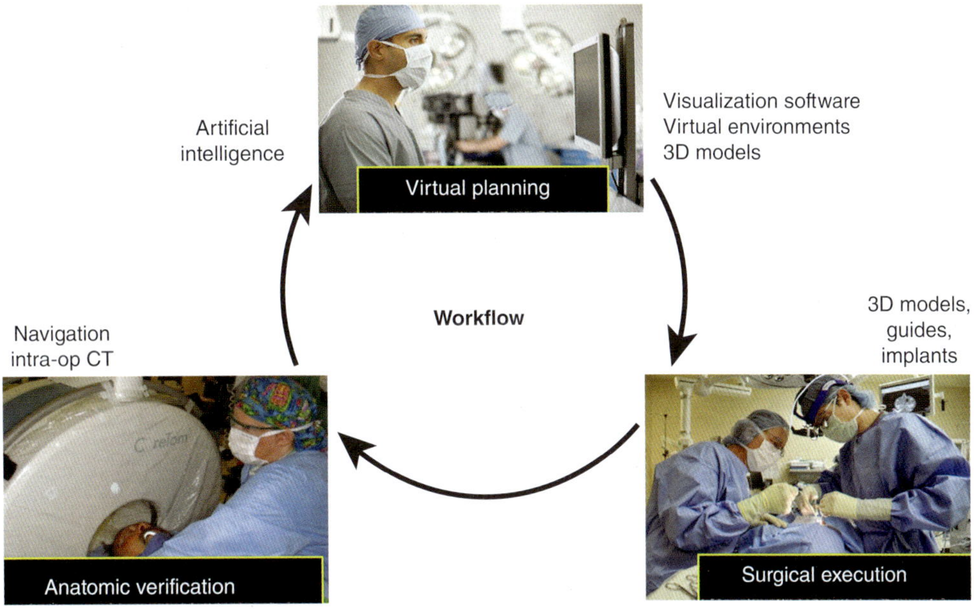


Fig. 4.2 CAS workflow divided into three phases: virtual planning, surgical execution, and anatomic verification. Each phase of the workflow can incorporate multiple technologies. *CAS*, Computer-assisted surgery

allows the surgeon to plan a surgical procedure, in a virtual environment, prior to surgical execution. Computer-assisted planning software imports digital imaging and communications in medicine (DICOM) data (from CT and MRI scanners). The software can be proprietary or open source. Proprietary software applications are highly varied; some offer broad bone and soft tissue planning capabilities, while others are limited to one anatomic region (e.g., facial skeleton) or procedure type (e.g., dental implants). The cost of proprietary software is highly variable, but most vendors use a subscription model necessitating an ongoing funding stream. Open source software can be downloaded for free. These applications are often less refined, rarely automated, less stable, have no technical support, and lack US Food and Drug Administration (FDA) approval. Consequently, open-source, computer-assisted planning software packages are more commonly used for research applications as opposed to clinical applications.

## Computer-assisted planning software functionality

Common computer-assisted planning software functions include segmentation, analysis, mirroring, and image fusion.

**Segmentation:** Segmentation procedures are used to separate virtual objects. Some examples might include separating the skin envelope from the facial skeleton (Fig. 4.3), or the right and left halves of the skull (Fig. 4.4). "Manual segmentation" requires selection of individual CT slices, which are then added to generate a volume. This is extremely time consuming and clinically impractical. Therefore, software manufacturers have developed "auto-segmentation" atlases that rapidly segment selected anatomy to facilitate presurgical planning in a timely fashion.

**Analysis:** Once segmentation is complete, properties of individual objects can be assessed. For example, preinjury orbital volumes (Fig. 4.5) and measurement of anatomic distances (Fig. 4.6).

**Mirroring:** Unilateral asymmetries lend themselves to segmentation and mirroring of normal anatomy to replace injured anatomy (Fig. 4.7).

**Object fusion:** Object fusion is useful (particularly after mirroring) to generate a final surgical plan (Fig. 4.7).

**Data set fusion:** Fusion of two data sets (CT, MRI, or one of each) can assist with presurgical, intraoperative, and postoperative analysis (Fig. 4.8).

## Computer-assisted planning software workflows

There are two common workflows for planning and fabrication of surgical tools: 1) surgeon-based and 2) industry-based. ***Surgeon-based*** workflows require the

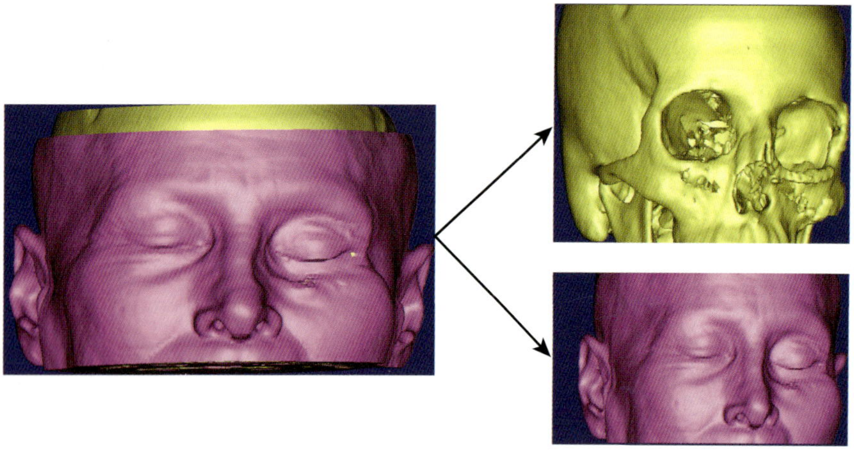

**Fig. 4.3** Bone and soft tissue segmentation.

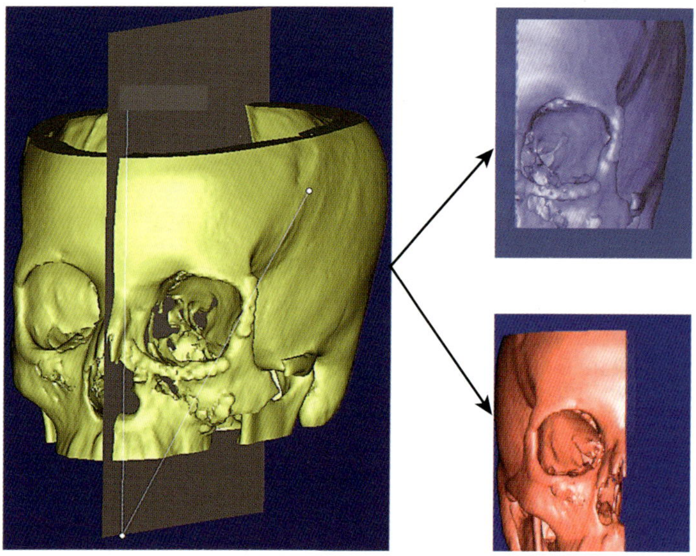

**Fig. 4.4** Segmentation of the left and right side of the facial skeleton.

surgeon to purchase and learn the computer-assisted planning software. Although the upfront cost and time commitment to learn the software are higher, the surgeon has ongoing access for planning and analysis, even if fabrication of models, guides, or implants are not necessary. Unfortunately, third-party reimbursement mechanisms for computer-assisted planning software is limited; therefore, the surgeon-based workflows are often only available to academic institutions and cosmetic practices. The industry-based workflow requires no financial investment. Planning is performed on a case-by-case basis in collaboration with an engineer via web conferencing. The industry partner pays for the software and manpower with the sale of models, guides, and implants. While this limits surgeon time and expense, it also restricts computer-assisted analysis to only those patients who will require fabrication of surgical tools.

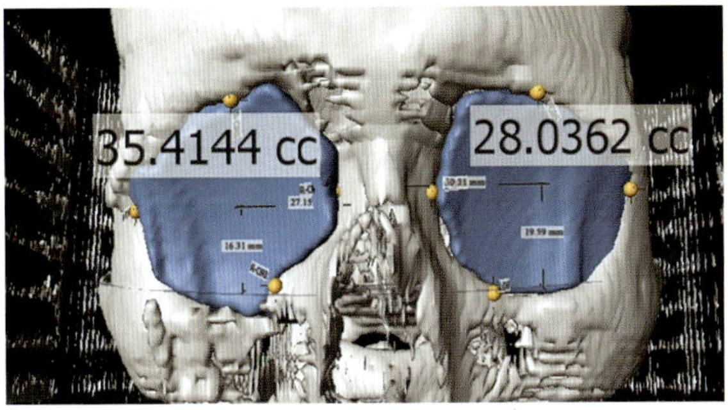


**Fig. 4.5** Orbital volume assessment using computer-assisted surgical planning. (Credit: Maxillo Software, Stratovan Corporation, USA)

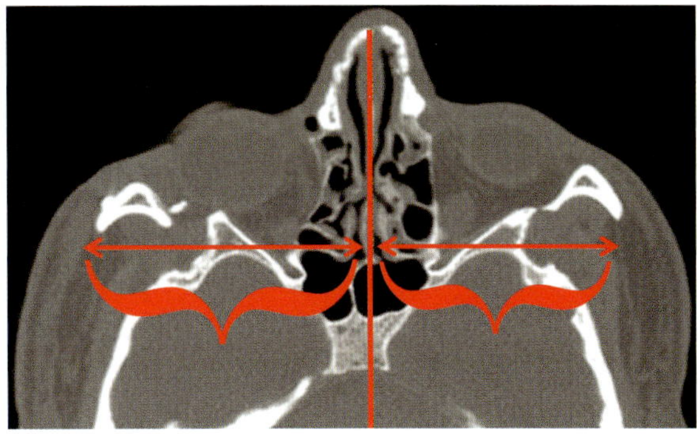

**Fig. 4.6** Illustration of virtual anatomic distance measurements being used to evaluate zygoma fracture displacement.

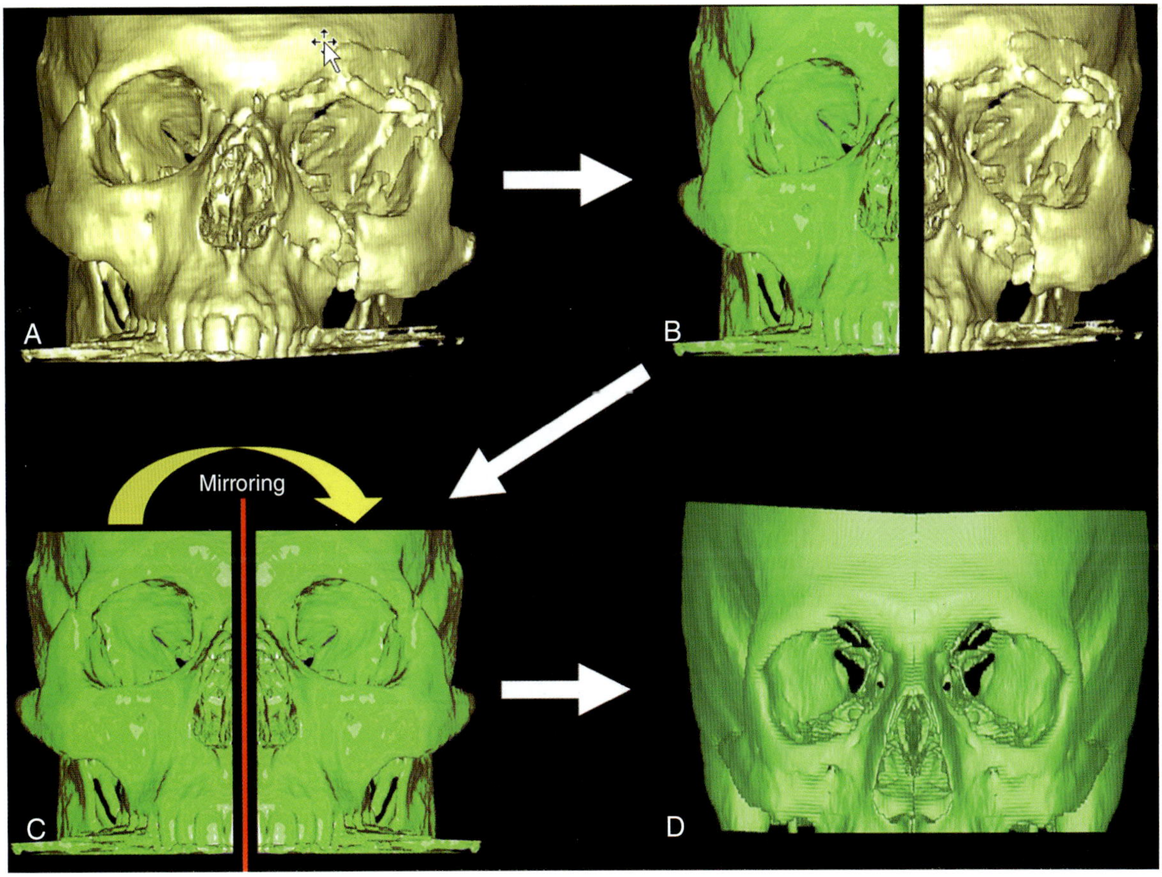


**Fig. 4.7** Example of mirroring process in computer-assisted surgical planning. The patient has a unilateral zygomaticomaxillary fracture (A). The normal side is segmented (B), mirrored to the contralateral side (C), and fused to generate a surgical plan (D).

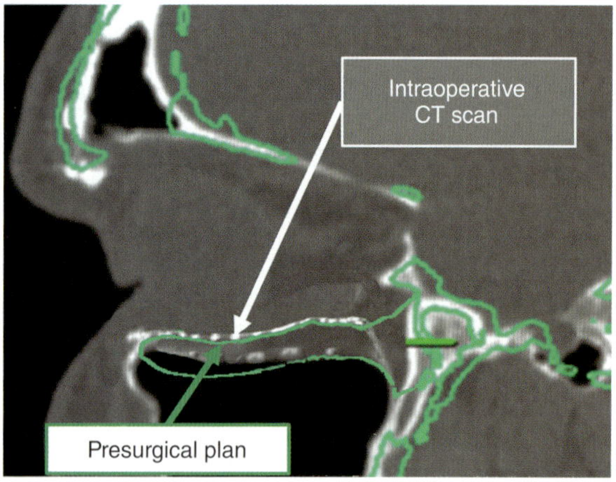


**Fig. 4.8** Data fusion of presurgical plan *(green)* superimposed on intraoperative CT scan to evaluate the accuracy of the orbital floor implant position relative to the presurgical plan.

## Virtual environments

Whereas 3D computer-assisted planning is usually performed on flat panel monitors, the rapid evolution of virtual environments offers both surgeons and patients unprecedented visualization opportunities. There are several types of virtual environments (also called "extended reality"). These can be depicted on a "reality spectrum," with virtual reality on one end, augmented reality on the other, and mixed reality in the middle (Fig. 4.9). Each environment has different goals and applications.

**Virtual reality:** Virtual reality applications use occlusive goggles (and sometimes gloves and earphones) to completely separate the user from their environment. Virtual reality is often used when information needs to be transferred, but interaction with other users (or the environment) are not necessary (e.g., video games, anatomy illustrations, individual educational activities, etc.) (Fig. 4.10).

**Augmented reality:** Augmented reality superimposes outside information onto the external environment. Common examples include the use of google glass (Alphabet Inc., Mountain View, CA) by physicians to access medical information while seeing patients or a heads-up display as used by pilots (Fig. 4.11). This works well when the information to be transferred is in an alphanumeric format.

**Mixed reality:** Mixed reality combines characteristics of virtual and augmented reality, allowing the user to interact with both physical and virtual objects at the same time. This can be ideal for patients and medical education where the user wants to see virtual objects, and real objects, as well as interact with other users (Fig. 4.12).

Multiple studies have validated the use of extended reality in craniomaxillofacial reconstruction, and some intraoperative applications have been examined.[4,9-12] Unfortunately, there are significant hurdles in a surgical environment, including equipment sterility and registration accuracy for virtual objects. Because there are no defined reimbursement pathways, equipment costs can also be prohibitive.[13,14] As with all new technologies, increasing demand and improved manufacturing efficiency will likely drive down production costs.

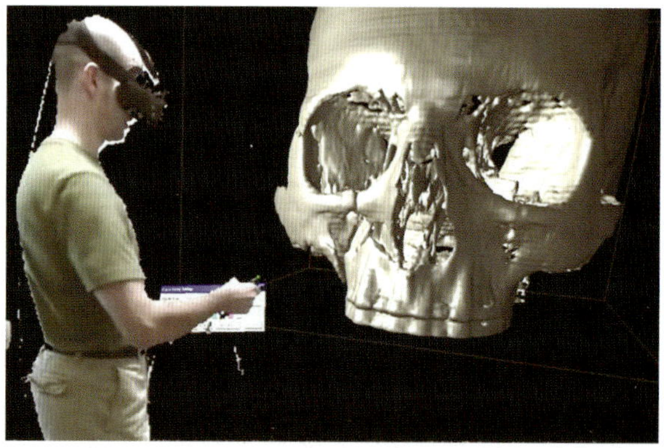

**Fig. 4.10** Demonstration of a virtual reality environment which utilizes occlusive goggles to create a completely virtual experience. (Credit: Oliver Kreylos PhD)

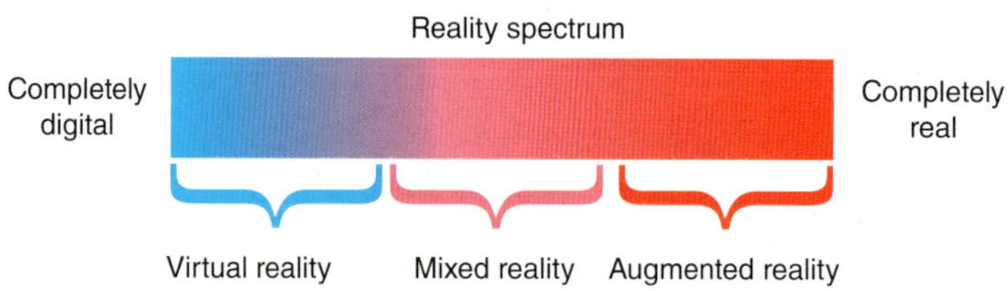


**Fig. 4.9** Illustration of the "reality spectrum", with a completely real environment on the right and completely digital environment on the left. Augmented, mixed, and virtual reality environments are on a spectrum between the two.

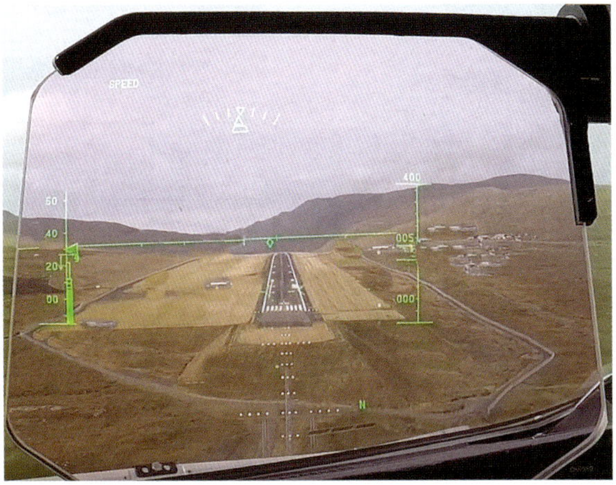


**Fig. 4.11** Example of an augmented reality environment that superimposes alphanumeric digital information onto the external environment.

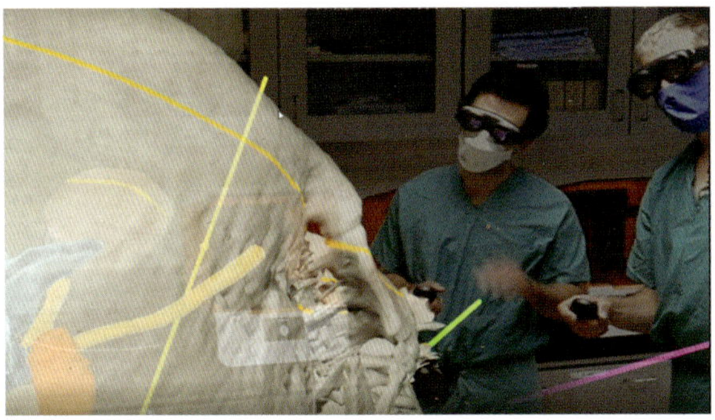

**Fig. 4.12** Example of a mixed reality environment in which the users can see both the virtual objects and the real environment, allowing for interaction with other users.

## Surgical models

Some 3D printed surgical models can be used for presurgical planning. Some examples include:

**Patient-specific implant contouring:** A computer-assisted surgical plan that can be used to fabricate a physical model (see "3D models" later for more detailed description of this process). The surgeon then bends standard surgical implants onto the patient-specific model, generating an ideal shape for reconstruction (Fig. 4.13). The plates are then sterilized and used to guide intraoperative bone reduction and stabilization.[15] This strategy eliminates the need for intraoperative bending, increasing accuracy and reducing operative time. Common applications include mandibular reconstruction (Fig. 4.14) and complex midface reconstruction (Fig. 4.13). Precontoured plates improve the accuracy and symmetry because they have only one "proper fit location" (i.e., the inferior border of the mandible or onto complex 3D midfacial contours). It is more challenging to utilize this technique with flat contours or for areas that lack bony margins to assist with plate placement.

**Osteotomy simulation:** Some surgeons find it helpful to use patient-specific surgical models to practice complex osteotomies prior to the surgical procedure.[16]

**Anatomic simulation:** Physical models can also be beneficial for presurgical planning of complex soft tissue procedures (e.g., neurosurgery, cardiac, abdominal surgery) (Fig. 4.15).

## Surgical execution

Surgical execution tools accurately transfer a surgical plan from the virtual environment to the physical environment. The computer-assisted planning software data is transferred in standard tessellation language (STL) format to a 3D printer or milling device.[17-19] A 3D printer uses a technique called "additive manufacturing" (or "rapid prototyping") for fabrication of these tools. Additive manufacturing devices work by building up sequential layers of a material to create a 3D object.[20] Using a 3D print improves implant design/accuracy and reduces operative time.[21-23] Common additive manufacturing modalities include stereolithography (SLA), selective laser sintering (SLS), inkjet printing, and fused-deposition modeling (FDM). Each technique has advantages and disadvantages related to cost, rigidity, sterilization, and ease of use.[24]

Common surgical execution tools used in maxillofacial reconstruction include 3D models, cutting/drill guides, and patient-specific implants.

**3D models:** Once the computer-assisted surgical plan is transferred to the physical environment in the form of a 3D model, it can be sterilized and taken into the operating room. Sterilization strategies vary depending on the printing material. Two common methods are autoclave and gas plasma sterilization (Sterrad, Johnson & Johnson, New Brunswick, NJ). In the operating room, models are used for the execution of the surgical plan. Standard flat titanium implants (Fig. 4.16) can be molded onto the 3D model to generate patient-specific shapes (Fig. 4.13). The plates are then used as guides for intraoperative bone reduction and stabilization. As mentioned (see Patient-specific implant contouring above), this strategy is most effective for complex midface reconstruction (where the contours improve the accuracy of plate placement by providing only one

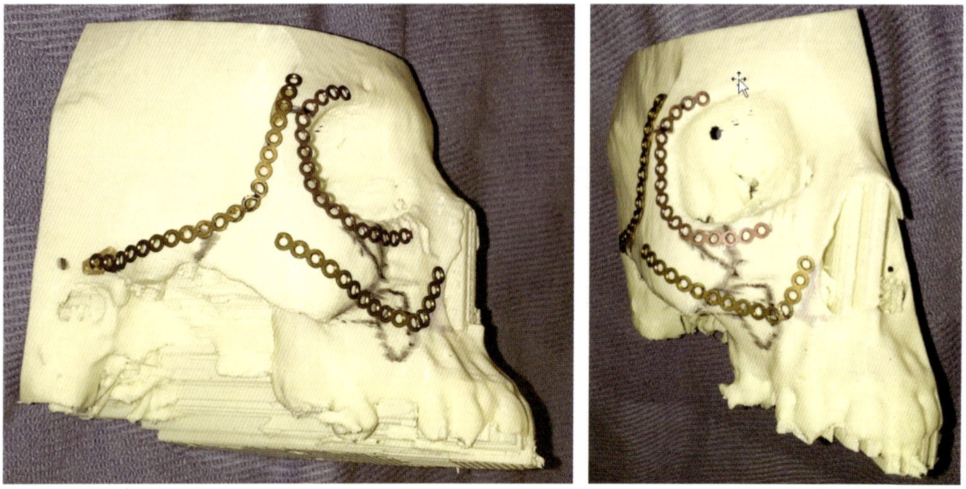

**Fig. 4.13** A 3D printed patient-specific model of a zygomaticomaxillary fracture. Preoperative plate contouring was performed on the patient-specific model to create accurate shapes of implants for intraoperative fixation.

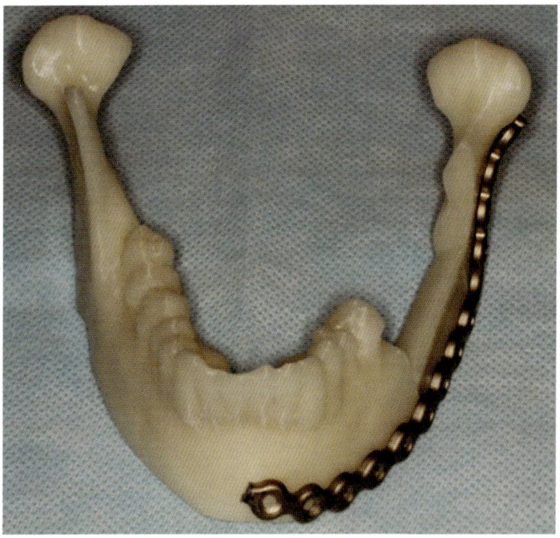

**Fig. 4.14** A 3D printed patient-specific model of a mandibular reconstruction with fibula free flap. Preoperative contouring of the reconstruction plate was performed to create an accurate shape for intraoperative fixation.

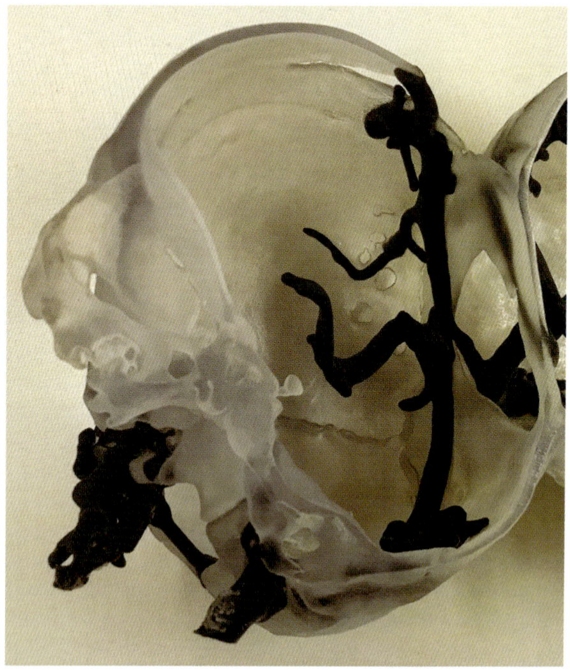

**Fig. 4.15** A 3D print of conjoined twins demonstrating the intracranial vascular architecture.

"proper fit location" on the patient's anatomy) and mandible reconstruction (where the inferior border can assist with an accurate implant placement).

"Generic" (i.e., non—patient-specific) skull models can be sterilized for intraoperative use (Fig. 4.17). There are no studies comparing the efficacy of intraoperative bending utilizing "patient-specific" versus "generic" models. However, the authors believe that generic models significantly improved accuracy over freehand bending and use this method regularly when patient-specific implants (see surgical implants below) and patient-specific bending strategies cannot be used.

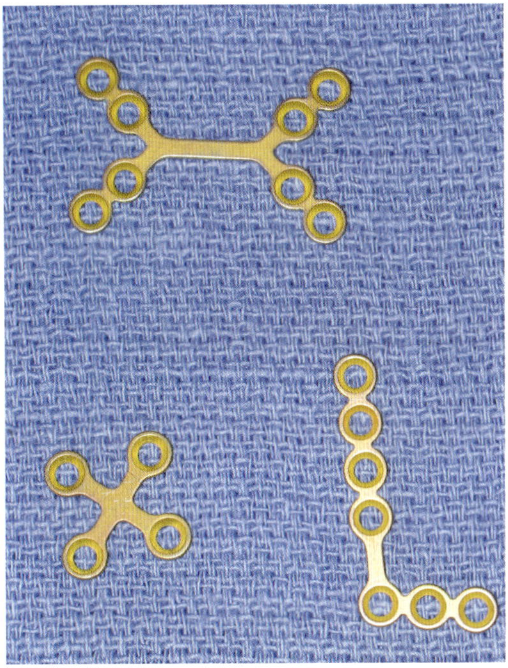

Fig. 4.16 Standard flat titanium implants.

**Cutting/drill guides:** Cutting and drill guides can also be used to transfer information from the virtual to physical environment. Drill guides can be used for precise placement of dental implants (Fig. 4.18). Cutting guides can be used in fibular free flap reconstruction and orthognathic surgery. Fibula free flap cutting guides provide a more accurate and rapid localization of the mandibular and fibular osteotomies (Fig. 4.19).[25-27] Drill guides can be added to the fibula cutting guides, allowing for precise implant placement in a single stage fibular/dental rehabilitation procedure.[28] Cutting and drill guides have also become popular for orthognathic surgery (Fig. 4.20).[29]

**Surgical implants:** Patient-specific surgical implants (PSI) provide an elegant solution to complex reconstructive problems. Applications include orbital, midface, cranial, and mandibular reconstruction. There is no FDA approval for PSI fabrication from individual hospitals or universities, therefore implants are fabricated exclusively through industrial partners. The surgeon initially provides the patient's data and follows up with a 10- to 45-minute video conference with a planning engineer to determine the appropriate shape, size, and functionality of the implant. Implant costs

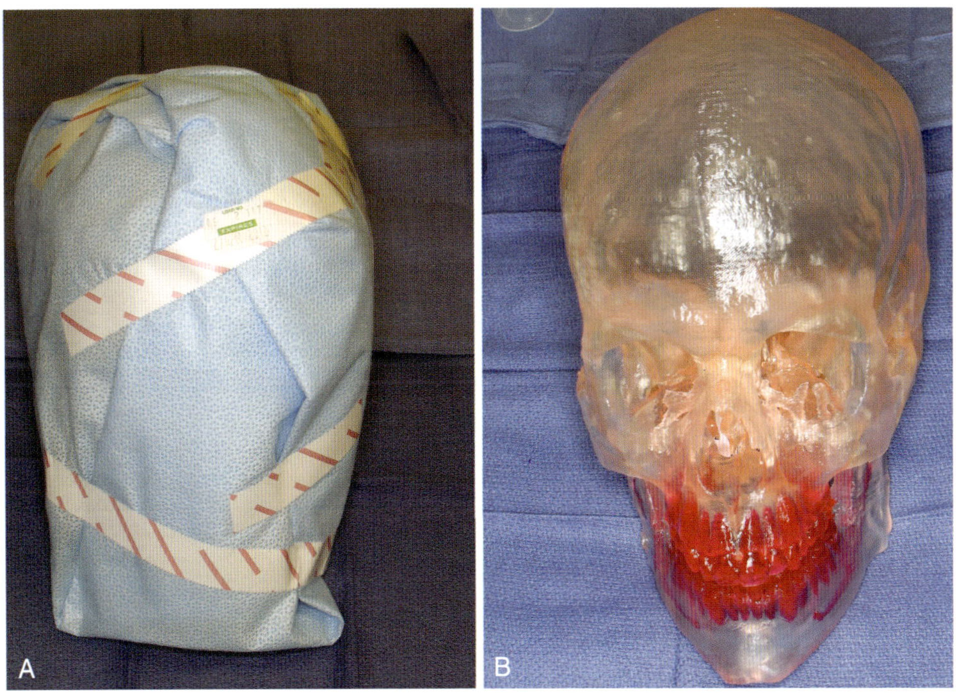


Fig. 4.17 Illustration of a "generic" (non—patient-specific) skull model sterilized and packaged (A) prior to being used in the operating room (B).

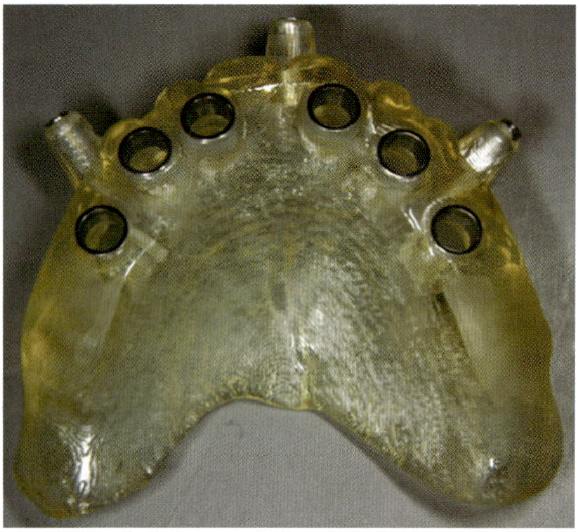

Fig. 4.18 Example of a dental drill guide for precise placement of dental implants. (Credit: Alexander Schramm MD, DDS)

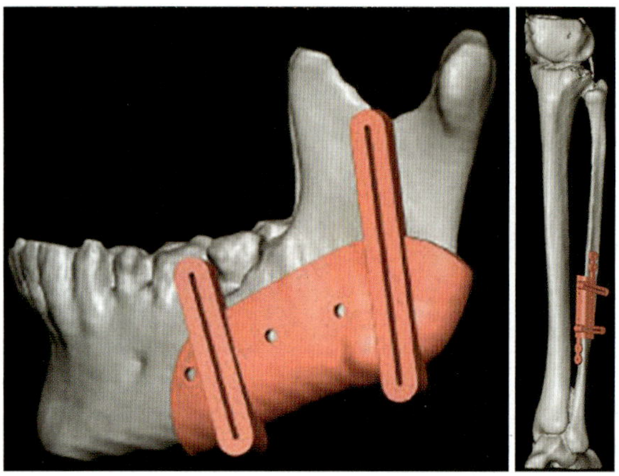

Fig. 4.19 Example of a computer-assisted surgical plan with fibula free flap and mandibular cutting guides.

are high, with orbital implants ranging from $2000 to $6000 USD and large cranioplasty implants ranging from $5000 to $20,000 USD (at the time of writing). Midface and mandibular implants are most commonly printed from titanium, while cranial implants are more commonly printed from polyetheretherketone (PEEK), porous polyethylene, or titanium. Fabrication times vary depending on the implant and company, but 1- to 3-week turnaround times are typical. As demand continues to grow, the authors would anticipate reduced cost and delivery times.

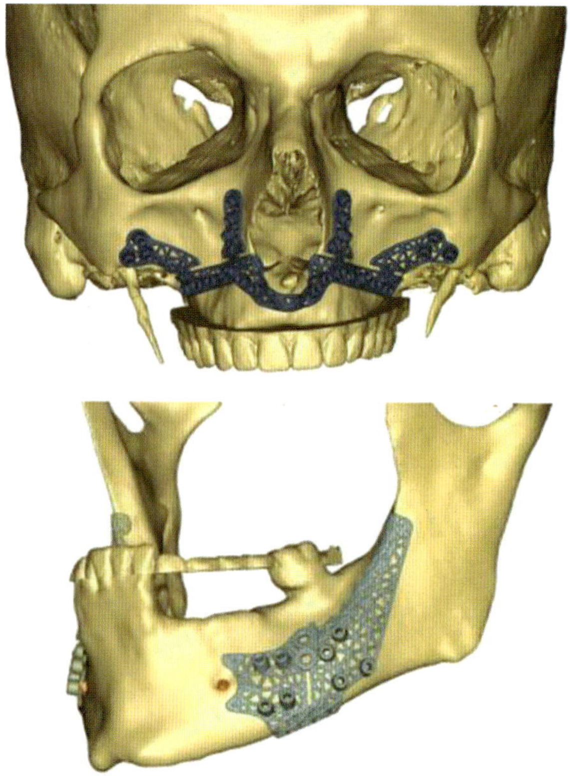

Fig. 4.20 Example of computer-assisted surgical planning for mandibular and maxillary osteotomies.

## Anatomic verification

The third phase of the CAS workflow is anatomic verification. Although this step is not necessary or possible for all procedures, the authors feel strongly that it is indicated for reconstructive procedures where clear visualization of the surgical field is difficult or impossible (i.e., orbital, midface, skull base, and some mandibular reconstructions). Surgical navigation and CT imaging are the most useful modalities.

### Intraoperative navigation

Intraoperative navigation is commonly used in sinus and neurosurgery to assist with anatomic localization. It can also be used in maxillofacial reconstruction. A computer-assisted surgical plan can be incorporated into the navigation data set, uploaded onto the navigational hardware, and used to guide intraoperative localization of bone segments and implant placement. Current navigational tools limit this application to bony reconstructive procedures.

To navigate, a reference array (patient tracker) must be rigidly attached to the patient. A similar reference array must be attached to the instrumentation (instrument tracker). The navigation system utilizes reflected infrared light to track both the patient and instrument in 3D space (Fig. 4.21). The precision of this tool is highly dependent on the accuracy of registration. Registration is the process whereby the navigation system precisely overlies the virtual patient (computer-assisted planning software plan) onto the physical patient. This is accomplished by identification of fiducial markers (i.e., stable, identifiable landmarks) on both the virtual and real patient. Operative time for registration is approximately 5 to 15 minutes. Bony landmarks are most predictable, but skin surface landmarks can be used if a recent CT is utilized and there are minimal soft tissue changes (<24 to 48 hours). Significant changes in facial swelling will change the patient's surface anatomy, and soft tissue registration will be impossible. Clinical studies have found the accuracy of intraoperative navigation to approximately 2 to 5 mm, with significantly higher accuracy in firm bony areas as compared to soft tissue.[18,21,22,24,30]

The major advantage of navigation over intraoperative CT is the lack of radiation exposure. While the data presented on the monitor has the potential for registration inaccuracies, measurements can be taken repeatedly throughout the case without concern for radiation exposure. The authors have found this strategy to be most useful in anatomic regions where visualization is difficult (i.e., internal orbit and skull base reconstruction) as well as procedures that require significant bone mobilization. In these situations, final positioning often requires repeated testing, which would be impractical using intraoperative CT due to excessive radiation exposure.

## Intraoperative imaging

Intraoperative imaging plays an integral role in orthopedic surgery, providing real-time feedback and the ability to perform intraoperative revisions for malreduction and implant repositioning. It has similar benefits in maxillofacial surgery. Intraoperative imaging can be separated into two distinct categories: fan-beam CT and cone-beam CT. Fan-beam scanners use a collimator to generate a fan-shaped radiation beam. This produces "slices" of data that can be combined to generate a 3-dimensional volume. Cone-beam scanners emit a cone-shaped x-ray beam that is recorded as a 3-dimensional volume. This volume can then be sliced into 2-dimensional images at varying slice thicknesses. Fan-beam CT scanners have a higher radiation dose and superior "soft tissue to bone" image resolution.

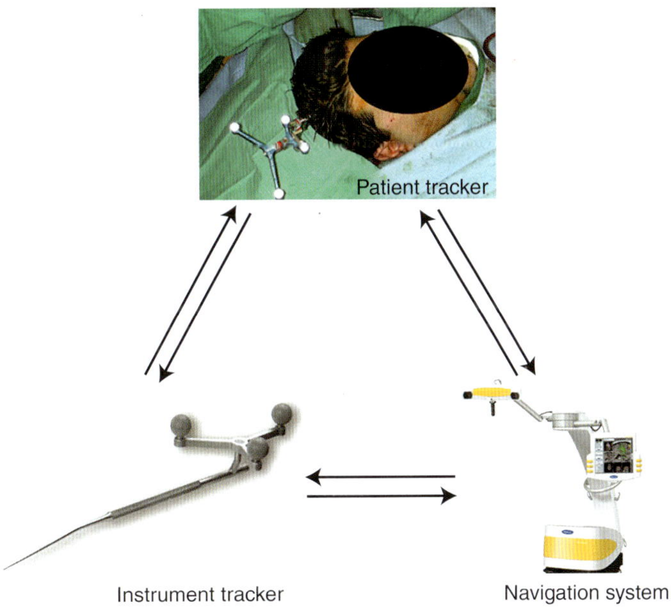


**Fig. 4.21** Illustration of the intraoperative navigation setup. The three components include: (1) navigation system, (2) patient tracker, (3) trackable instrumentation. The navigation system emits infrared light that reflects off the tracking arrays on the patient and instrument and allows for accurate instrument tracking in the operating room.

Cone-beam scanners are often smaller and more maneuverable, with a significantly lower radiation dose. This results in reduced soft tissue resolution, but adequate bone visualization for intraoperative decision-making. For this reason, most maxillofacial reconstructive surgeons currently utilize cone-beam CT technology.

The potential risks associated with intraoperative imaging include added operative time and radiation exposure. Several studies have addressed these questions. Shaye et al. found that intraoperative imaging added 15 minutes per case.[31] The question of radiation exposure is more difficult to answer. Multiple authors have tried to examine the long-term risk of CT imaging.[32-34] Unfortunately, the longitudinal nature of such studies makes them difficult to interpret for any given patient. Radiation dosage for a maxillofacial fan-beam CT scan is approximately 600 to 800 μSv and for a cone-beam CT scan is approximately 40 to 80 μSv. Relative radiation doses from other common sources include mammogram: 400 μSv; 2-view chest radiograph: 100 μSv; and daily background radiation: 8 μSv every 24 hours.[35]

A literature review reveals at least seven different studies looking at the utility of intraoperative imaging in maxillofacial reconstruction.[31,36-41] Each study has shown that intraoperative correction rates are significant (14%–44%; mean 26%). Although this does not mean that every intraoperative correction would result in an improved clinical outcome, it does mean that if we are attempting to optimize our surgical results, intraoperative imaging is a readily available strategy to improve implant placement. If we look at surgeon utilization, it is safe to assume that a surgeon's threshold for revision will be significantly lower if an error is noted intraoperatively as opposed to postoperatively. The current authors utilize intraoperative imaging in most orbital and complex reconstructive procedures.

## Conclusion

Maxillofacial reconstruction involves vital anatomic structures and requires high precision to achieve good quality postoperative outcomes. Advancements in CAS are introducing adjunctive tools to assist surgeons with these complex surgical repairs. The authors have presented their three-phase CAS workflow including presurgical planning, surgical execution, and intraoperative verification. Computer-assisted planning software uses CT or MRI imaging data to generate virtual 3D objects utilized in presurgical planning. Virtual environments, including augmented, virtual, and mixed reality, allow surgeons enhanced visualization of these virtual preoperative plans. Surgical models, guides, and implants can be fabricated through additive manufacturing. They can improve the accuracy of surgical repair and are valuable intraoperative tools in reconstruction. Lastly, intraoperative navigation and imaging provide real-time verification of the surgical repair, potentially reducing surgical revision rates. CAS technology continues to evolve and will play an integral role in the future of maxillofacial reconstructive surgery.

## References


1. Doi K. Computer-aided diagnosis in medical imaging: historical review, current status and future potential. *Comput Med Imaging Graph.* 2007;31(4-5):198-211. doi:10.1016/j.compmedimag.2007.02.002.
2. Efanov JI, Roy AA, Huang KN, Borsuk DE. Virtual surgical planning: the pearls and pitfalls. *Plast Reconstr Surg Glob Open.* 2018;6(1):e1443. doi:10.1097/GOX.0000000000001443.
3. Mischkowski RA, Zinser M, Kübler A, Seifert U, Zöller JE. Clinical and experimental evaluation of an augmented reality system in cranio-maxillofacial surgery. *Int Congr Ser.* 2005;1281:565-570.
4. Badiali G, Ferrari V, Cutolo F, et al. Augmented reality as an aid in maxillofacial surgery: validation of a wearable system allowing maxillary repositioning. *J Craniomaxillofac Surg.* 2014;42(8):1970-1976. doi:10.1016/j.jcms.2014.09.001.
5. Kalavakonda N, Sekhar L, Hannaford B. Augmented reality application for aiding tumor resection in skull-base surgery. *Int Symp Med Robot ISMR.* 2019;1-6. doi:10.1109/ISMR.2019.8710203.
6. Tack P, Victor J, Gemmel P, Annemans L. 3D-printing techniques in a medical setting: a systematic literature review. *Biomed Eng Online.* 2016;15(1):115. doi:10.1186/s12938-016-0236-4.
7. Pham AM, Rafii AA, Metzger MC, Jamali A, Strong EB. Computer modeling and intraoperative navigation in maxillofacial surgery. *Otolaryngol Head Neck Surg.* 2007;137(4):624-631. doi:10.1016/j.otohns.2007.06.719.
8. Yu H, Shen SG, Wang X, Zhang L, Zhang S. The indication and application of computer-assisted navigation in oral and maxillofacial surgery – Shanghai's experience based on 104 cases. *J Craniomaxillofac Surg.* 2013;41(8):770-774. doi:10.1016/j.jcms.2013.01.016.

9. Rose AS, Kim H, Fuchs H, Frahm JM. Development of augmented-reality applications in otolaryngology-head and neck surgery. *Laryngoscope*. 2019;129(suppl 3):S1-S11. doi:10.1002/lary.28098.
10. Chen G, Zeng W, Yin H, Yu Y, Ju R, Tang W. The preliminary application of augmented reality in unilateral orbitozygomatic maxillary complex fractures treatment. *J Craniofac Surg*. 2020;31(2):542-548. doi:10.1097/SCS.0000000000006238.
11. Ferrari V, Megali G, Troia E, Pietrabissa A, Mosca F. A 3-D mixed-reality system for stereoscopic visualization of medical dataset. *IEEE Trans Biomed Eng*. 2009;56(11):2627-2633. doi:10.1109/TBME.2009.2028013.
12. Freschi C, Troia E, Ferrari V, Megali G, Pietrabissa A, Mosca F. Ultrasound guided robotic biopsy using augmented reality and human-robot cooperative control. *Annu Int Conf IEEE Eng Med Biol Soc*. 2009;2009:5110-5113. doi:10.1109/IEMBS.2009.5332720.
13. Hupp JR. Advanced technology—hammers looking for nails. *J Oral Maxillofac Surg*. 2013;71(3):465-466. doi:10.1016/j.joms.2012.12.002.
14. Turchetti G, Spadoni E, Geisler EE. Health technology assessment. Evaluation of biomedical innovative technologies. *IEEE Eng Med Biol Mag*. 2010;29(3):70-76. doi:10.1109/MEMB.2010.936553.
15. Memon AR, Wang E, Hu J, Egger J, Chen X. A review on computer-aided design and manufacturing of patient-specific maxillofacial implants. *Expert Rev Med Devices*. 2020;17(4):345-356. doi:10.1080/17434440.2020.1736040.
16. Ho M, Goldfarb J, Moayer R, et al. Design and printing of a low-cost 3d-printed nasal osteotomy training model: Development and feasibility study. *JMIR Med Educ*. 2020;6(2):e19792. doi:10.2196/19792.
17. Hauser R, Westermann B, Probst R. Noninvasive tracking of patient's head movements during computer-assisted intranasal microscopic surgery [published correction appears in Laryngoscope 1997 Jul;107(7):1000-1001]. *Laryngoscope*. 1997;107(4):491-499. doi:10.1097/00005537-199704000-00012.
18. Hassfeld S, Zöller J, Albert FK, Wirtz CR, Knauth M, Mühling J. Preoperative planning and intraoperative navigation in skull base surgery. *J Craniomaxillofac Surg*. 1998;26(4):220-225. doi:10.1016/s1010-5182(98)80017-6.
19. Hassfeld S, Mühling J. Comparative examination of the accuracy of a mechanical and an optical system in CT and MRT based instrument navigation. *Int J Oral Maxillofac Surg*. 2000;29(6):400-407.
20. Xia J, Ip HH, Samman N, et al. Computer-assisted three-dimensional surgical planning and simulation: 3D virtual osteotomy. *Int J Oral Maxillofac Surg*. 2000;29(1):11-17.
21. Hauser R, Westermann B. Optical tracking of a microscope for image-guided intranasal sinus surgery. *Ann Otol Rhinol Laryngol*. 1999;108(1):54-62. doi:10.1177/000348949910800108.
22. Marmulla R, Hilbert M, Niederdellmann H. Inherent precision of mechanical, infrared and laser-guided navigation systems for computer-assisted surgery. *J Craniomaxillofac Surg*. 1997;25(4):192-197. doi:10.1016/s1010-5182(97)80075-3.
23. Kikinis R, Gleason PL, Moriarty TM, et al. Computer-assisted interactive three-dimensional planning for neurosurgical procedures. *Neurosurgery*. 1996;38(4):640-651.
24. Zamorano L, Jiang Z, Kadi AM. Computer-assisted neurosurgery system: Wayne State University hardware and software configuration. *Comput Med Imaging Graph*. 1994;18(4):257-271. doi:10.1016/0895-6111(94)90050-7.
25. Roser SM, Ramachandra S, Blair H, et al. The accuracy of virtual surgical planning in free fibula mandibular reconstruction: comparison of planned and final results. *J Oral Maxillofac Surg*. 2010;68(11):2824-2832. doi:10.1016/j.joms.2010.06.177.
26. Metzler P, Geiger EJ, Alcon A, Ma X, Steinbacher DM. Three-dimensional virtual surgery accuracy for free fibula mandibular reconstruction: planned versus actual results. *J Oral Maxillofac Surg*. 2014;72(12):2601-2612. doi:10.1016/j.joms.2014.07.024.
27. Weitz J, Bauer FJ, Hapfelmeier A, Rohleder NH, Wolff KD, Kesting MR. Accuracy of mandibular reconstruction by three-dimensional guided vascularised fibular free flap after segmental mandibulectomy. *Br J Oral Maxillofac Surg*. 2016;54(5):506-510. doi:10.1016/j.bjoms.2016.01.029.
28. Patel A, Harrison P, Cheng A, Bray B, Bell RB. Fibular reconstruction of the maxilla and mandible with immediate implant-supported prosthetic rehabilitation: Jaw in a day. *Oral Maxillofac Surg Clin North Am*. 2019;31(3):369-386. doi:10.1016/j.coms.2019.03.002.
29. Farrell BB, Franco PB, Tucker MR. Virtual surgical planning in orthognathic surgery. *Oral Maxillofac Surg Clin North Am*. 2014;26(4):459-473. doi:10.1016/j.coms.2014.08.011.
30. Birkfellner W, Watzinger F, Wanschitz F, et al. Systematic distortions in magnetic position digitizers. *Med Phys*. 1998;25(11):2242-2248. doi:10.1118/1.598425.
31. Shaye DA, Tollefson TT, Strong EB. Use of intraoperative computed tomography for maxillofacial reconstructive surgery. *JAMA Facial Plast Surg*.

2015;17(2):113-119. doi:10.1001/jamafacial.2014.1343. Erratum in: JAMA Facial Plast Surg. 2015;17(3):227.
32. Berrington de González A, Darby S. Risk of cancer from diagnostic X-rays: estimates for the UK and 14 other countries. *Lancet*. 2004;363(9406):345-351. doi:10.1016/S0140-6736(04)15433-0.
33. Lee CI, Haims AH, Monico EP, Brink JA, Forman HP. Diagnostic CT scans: assessment of patient, physician, and radiologist awareness of radiation dose and possible risks. *Radiology*. 2004;231(2):393-398. doi:10.1148/radiol.2312030767.
34. Brody AS, Frush DP, Huda W, Brent RL, American Academy of Pediatrics Section on Radiology. Radiation risk to children from computed tomography. *Pediatrics*. 2007;120(3):677-682. doi:10.1542/peds.2007-1910.
35. National Council on Radiation Protection and Measurements. *Ionizing Radiation Exposure of the Population of the United States* (NCRP Report No 160). Bethesda, MD: National Council on Radiation Protection and Measurements; 2009.
36. Stanley RB Jr. Use of intraoperative computed tomography during repair of orbitozygomatic fractures. *Arch Facial Plast Surg*. 1999;1(1):19-24. doi:10.1001/archfaci.1.1.19.
37. Hoelzle F, Klein M, Schwerdtner O, et al. Intraoperative computed tomography with the mobile CT Tomoscan M during surgical treatment of orbital fractures. *Int J Oral Maxillofac Surg*. 2001;30(1):26-31. doi:10.1054/ijom.2000.0014.
38. Stuck BA, Hülse R, Barth TJ. Intraoperative cone beam computed tomography in the management of facial fractures. *Int J Oral Maxillofac Surg*. 2012;41(10):1171-1175. doi:10.1016/j.ijom.2012.06.006.
39. Wilde F, Lorenz K, Ebner AK, Krauss O, Mascha F, Schramm A. Intraoperative imaging with a 3D C-arm system after zygomatico-orbital complex fracture reduction. *J Oral Maxillofac Surg*. 2013;71(5):894-910. doi:10.1016/j.joms.2012.10.031.
40. Borad V, Lacey MS, Hamlar DD, Dresner HS, Yadava GK, Schubert W. Intraoperative imaging changes management in orbital fracture repair. *J Oral Maxillofac Surg*. 2017;75(9):1932-1940. doi:10.1016/j.joms.2017.05.002.
41. Cuddy K, Khatib B, Bell RB, et al. Use of intraoperative computed tomography in craniomaxillofacial trauma surgery. *J Oral Maxillofac Surg*. 2018;76(5):1016-1025. doi:10.1016/j.joms.2017.12.004.

Chapter | 5 |

# Computer-assisted surgical planning in orthognathic surgery: a practical workflow

*Dmitriy Kravchenko, Joseph Lopez, Derek M. Steinbacher*

CHAPTER OUTLINE



## Introduction

Orthognathic surgery outcomes depend not only on surgical technique, but also on appropriate diagnosis and treatment planning. The adoption of computer-assisted design/ computed-assisted manufacturing (CAD/CAM) technology, computer-assisted surgical planning (CaSP), and three-dimensional (3D) printing has created a paradigm shift for patients with maxillofacial deformities and for the surgeons treating them.[1] The advent of noninvasive 3D visualization of the maxillofacial skeleton has allowed for the conversion of a preoperative plan to the manufacture of patient-specific guides and implants. These applications of CAD/CAM technology often share a common workflow, which entails the following: (1) performing a clinical exam, paying particular attention to patient anthropometrics in the frontal and profile views (in addition to obtaining a global appraisal to determine areas of imbalance, weakness, and asymmetry); (2) obtaining patient photographs, both facial and intraoral (preoperatively, photographs can be used with 3D imaging software to simulate treatment outcomes while intraoperatively, photographs can serve as a point of reference); (3) obtaining dental records, either in the form of stone models or digitally fabricated dental models; (4) obtaining conventional or cone-beam computed tomographic data (these images will be used for cephalometric analysis and for 3D planning); (5) conversion of CT data to digital imaging and communications in medicine (DICOM) format for digital image manipulation and 3D reconstruction by a bioengineering company; (6) setting idealized occlusion, either virtually or by hand articulation of dental models; (7) video teleconference between surgeons and biomedical engineers to virtually perform surgery and create planned osteotomies; and lastly, (8) fabrication of patient-specific implants and cutting guides.[2,3]

There are many advantages to utilizing 3D CaSP. Several treatment options can be considered simultaneously, allowing the ability to determine the best approach. Planned bony movements may alter soft tissue position, which may be more easily evaluated preoperatively with the CaSP software. Location and extent of dysmorphology and asymmetry can be better appreciated. The degree to which occlusal changes affect bony relationships can be evaluated, and the need for adjunctive procedures can be determined. 3D surgical planning allows assessment of actual patient anatomy, correction of deformities in all three planes of space, evaluation of soft tissue, as well as comparison of actual results with planned movements. Being able to perform all these analyses and visualize surgical skeletal movements has provided surgeons with a wealth of information that conventional orthognathic surgery preoperative planning could not provide.[4]

There are no known absolute contraindications to CaSP, and the disadvantages are usually related to cost and logistics. The ability of an office or institution to purchase the necessary software and hardware may preclude CaSP. A recent and accurate CT data set is required by the bioengineering team in order to fabricate precise surgical guides or patient-specific implants. Collaborative planning with the orthodontist to ensure the appropriate orthodontic brackets, surgical wires, and hooks prior to obtaining final dental models requires advanced preparation and can present logistic setbacks if not anticipated. With the advent of onsite 3D printing capability, current challenges will likely be less relevant in the future.[5]

In this chapter, the authors presents their preferred CAD/CAM workflow to perform orthognathic surgery. This approach has been validated by numerous studies performed at our institution by the senior author (D.S.).[6-10] This chapter will focus on this approach and provide information to surgeons who hope to utilize CAD/CAM-based orthognathic surgery.

## Clinical considerations

Dentofacial deformities present a challenge for reconstructive surgeons, who must approach the repair of bony architecture and overlying soft tissue with the goal of restoring function while optimizing aesthetics. Of paramount importance is the proper means of comprehensively assessing the orthognathic patient. A problem list must be generated and diagnoses itemized in order for the surgical plan to meet all functional and aesthetic objectives. The clinical exam must be methodical and organized, looking at static and dynamic relationships. A series of measurements is then taken—both cephalometric and anthropometric—and compared to "standards" to help guide diagnosis and treatment planning.

The clinical examination should begin with a global assessment to determine areas of asymmetry, lack of support, and disharmony. Certain reproducible hard and soft tissue landmarks must be evaluated to determine what is normal and what is abnormal. It is essential that the surgeon identify soft tissue discrepancies that, by virtue of the planned movements, will correct after surgery and those that will not. From the frontal view, the face should be divided into vertical fifths and horizontal thirds. With the patient in normal head position, the profile view is used to assess the anteroposterior dimension for skeletal relationship and its effect on other facial features. Various aesthetic subunits deserve specific consideration. The external nose, ears, eyes, cheeks, and lips display a wide range of variation, and correction of the presenting incongruity may improve or worsen harmony between various facial subunits. A complete examination of the oral cavity and occlusion must not be overlooked, as facial disharmony may be caused by subpar dentoalveolar relationships. Whether performing mandible- or maxilla-first surgery, the planned position of the maxilla should be based on maxillary incisal show at rest, which is generally accepted to be 2 to 4 mm. Orthognathic surgery occasionally affects the temporomandibular joint, and those with temporomandibular joint dysfunction (TMD) should be identified and evaluated. While there is disagreement among clinicians as to when to treat TMD, there is a consensus that orthognathic surgery may improve or aggravate symptoms of TMD.[11]

Patient facial and intraoral photographs are an integral piece of treatment planning for orthognathic surgery. Photographs aid with documentation and authorization for insurance purposes, may be combined with 3D surgical planning systems to simulate potential results, and can be used to evaluate the degree to which various objectives were met. Dental models are obtained to evaluate tooth structure, positioning of teeth, and interocclusal relationships in order to determine the need and/or duration of presurgical orthodontics. Radiographic data is essential to 3D planning for orthognathic surgery. Conventionally, a panorex, lateral, and PA cephalograms were obtained to assess the teeth and facial skeleton. Today, cone-beam computed tomography (CBCT) is utilized to capture, with minimal radiation, skeletal anatomy of the maxillomandibular complex in the sagittal, vertical, and transverse dimensions. Of note, when treating individuals with dentofacial deformity, it is imperative that the surgeon develop a systematic approach for collecting and interpreting data based on patient history and physical examination. This will aid in arriving at the proper diagnosis and formulating an appropriate treatment plan that addresses both form and function.

## Workflow for computer-assisted design/computer-assisted manufacturing

The workflow for CAD/CAM-based orthognathic surgery is presented in Fig. 5.1.

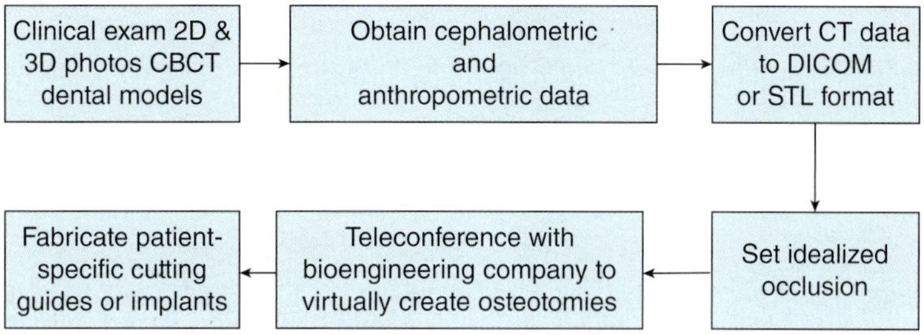


**Fig. 5.1** Workflow for computer-assisted design/computer-assisted manufacturing.

## Computer-assisted design

The senior author has utilized CAD planning for all orthognathic procedures for over a decade. Although the use of CAD for orthognathic planning can vary by surgeon, there are several benefits to its use. First, it offers the unique opportunity to integrate clinical data, patient photos, and three-dimensional skeletal data concurrently. Moreover, it offers the opportunity to ensure centric occlusion/centric relation virtually without the use of a facebow. Third, using CAD facilitates three-dimensional visualization of the planned skeletal movements highlighting any potential flaws in the operative plan such as skeletal or dental interferences. Lastly, CAD facilitates the ability to customize hardware. In the senior author's practice, custom-designed genioplasty cutting guides and custom titanium plates are used to ensure high fidelity and accuracy in the genio movements. The following figures 5.2-5.9 provide a broad overview of the senior authors preferred CaSP work-flow (see Figs. 5.2–5.9).

## Computer-assisted manufacturing

The use of CAD provides many benefits as described above. Although CAD can also be used to computer-assisted manufacture custom titanium plates for fixation, the senior author prefers to only routinely use CAM for 3D-printed occlusal-based intermediate and final splints (in addition to Hawley-type palatal splints for maxillary segmentation cases) and custom genioplasty titanium plates/cutting guides. Using only CAM

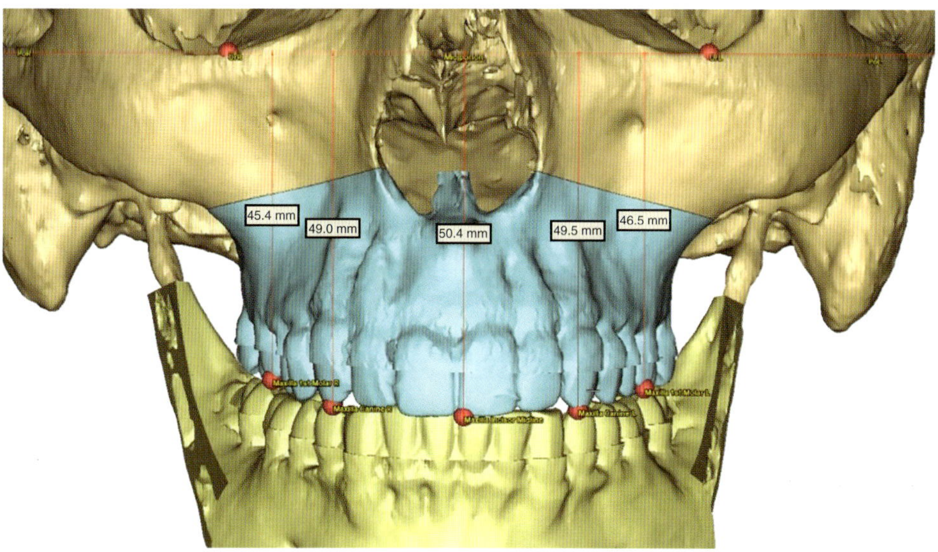


**Fig. 5.2** Level the cant. Begin leveling the cant by measuring the distance from the inferior orbital rim to the occlusal surface of the canine and first molar bilaterally.

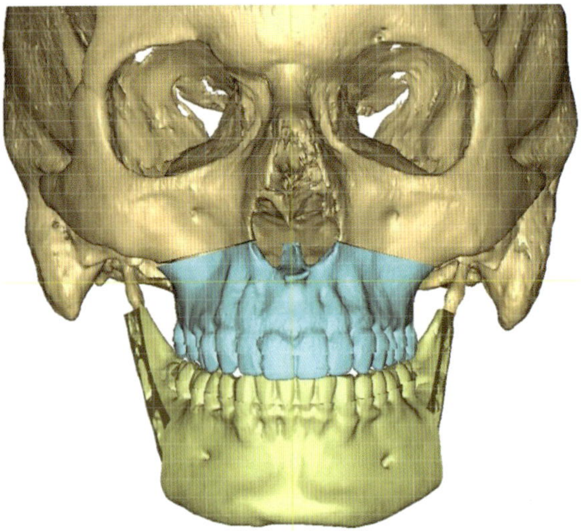

Fig. 5.3 Make skeletal and dental midline coincident. Next, bring the maxillary dental midline toward the midline so that it coincides with the skeletal midline.

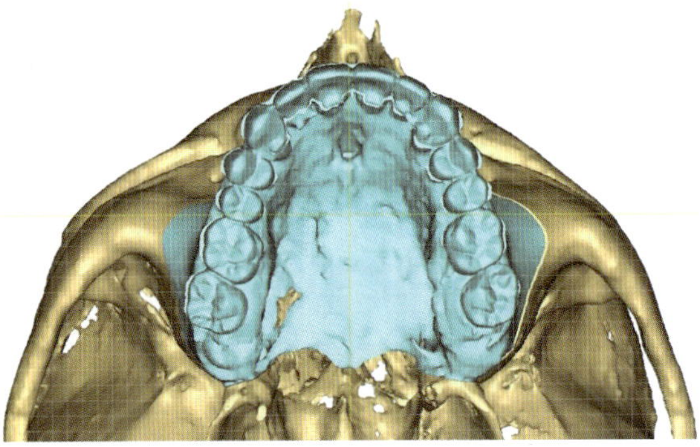

Fig. 5.4 Adjust the yaw. Next, adjust the yaw by visualizing the position of the first molar and canine.

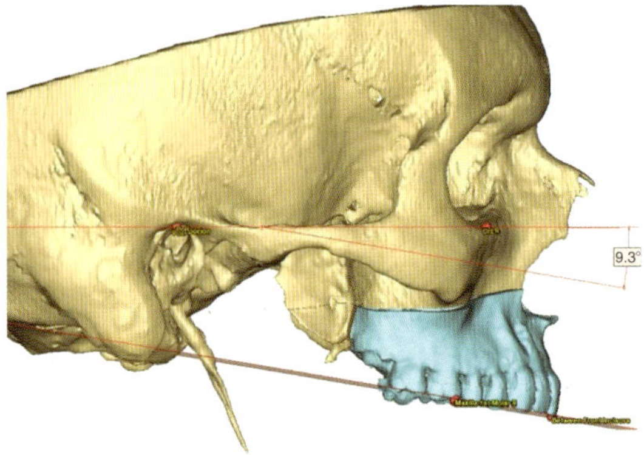


Fig. 5.5 Adjust the pitch. Next, adjust the occlusal plane as necessary.

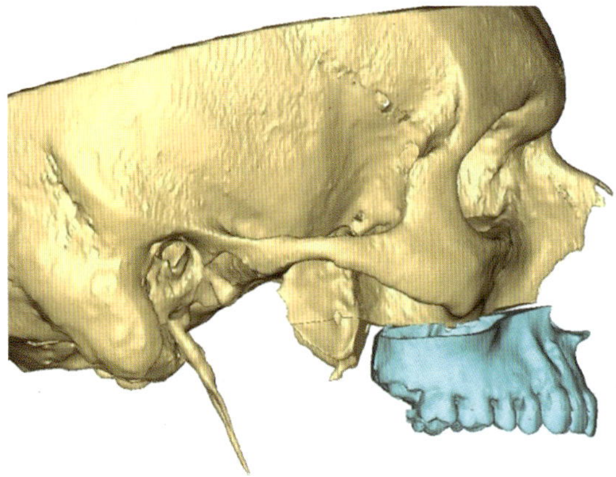

Fig. 5.6 Adjust the A–P movement of Le Fort. Next, adjust bodily the position of the maxilla in the anterior-posterior dimension per plan.

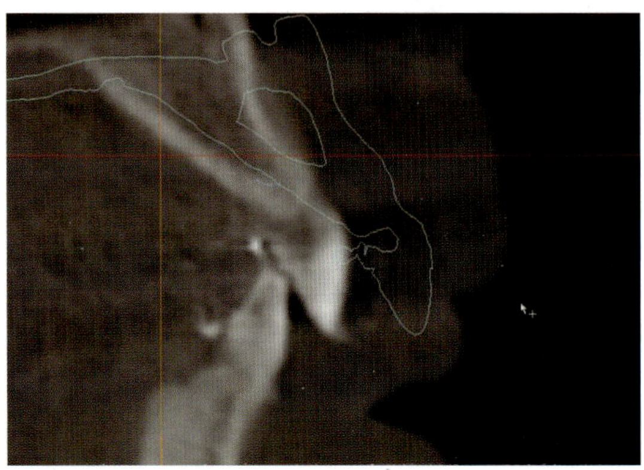

Fig. 5.7 Evaluate incisor show with movement. Next, evaluate incisal show using soft-tissue sagittal computed tomography data to confirm position of maxilla.

3D-printed occlusal-based intermediate and final splints and custom genio-plates/guides not only saves costs, but more importantly gives the surgeon the ability to make any artistic adjustments that could otherwise not be performed with CAM, custom maxillary or mandibular plates. The following figures (Figs. 5.10–5.14) provide an overview of the various orthognathic surgery-related items that could be 3D printed via CAM.

## Operative technique

The operative steps to perform orthognathic surgery can vary, especially in the setting of mandible- or maxillary-first

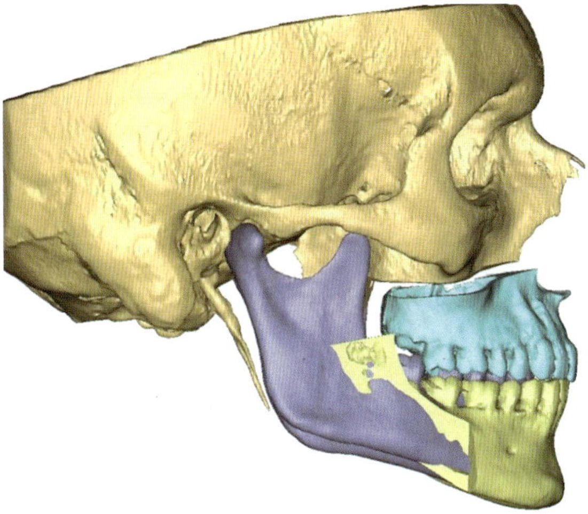

Fig. 5.8 Bring mandible to occlusion. Once maxilla is in final position, bring mandible to occlusion.

approaches. The preferred sequence for the senior author for the majority of cases is mandible first.

Steps:

- Bilateral Sagittal Split Osteotomy
  - A mandible-first orthognathic sequence is often elected.
  - Bilateral sagittal split osteotomy with pitch and yaw correction is performed in a standard fashion.
  - Local anesthesia is injected followed by a hockey-stick-like incision to expose the external oblique ridge.
  - The inferior alveolar nerve is exposed and the first corticotomy is made using a reciprocating saw, extending from just behind the lingula coursing down and anterior.[12]
  - The anterior, mid-body, dissection and corticotomy is then performed. The same approach is taken on the opposite side, followed by splitting the mandible, ensuring the nerve is laid on the distal segment.[13]
  - An intermediate splint is used and mandibular internal fixation applied bilaterally.
- Le Fort 1
  - A standard Le Fort I segmental maxillary osteotomy is performed.
  - Local anesthesia with vasoconstrictor is injected into the labio-buccal sulcus extending from the midline to the pterygomaxillary areas. We often utilize a V–Y incision at the upper lip frenulum to lengthen the upper sulcus if necessary.
  - A subperiosteal dissection is extended posteriorly to the level of the pterygomaxillary fissure, allowing complete exposure of the anterior surface of the maxilla.

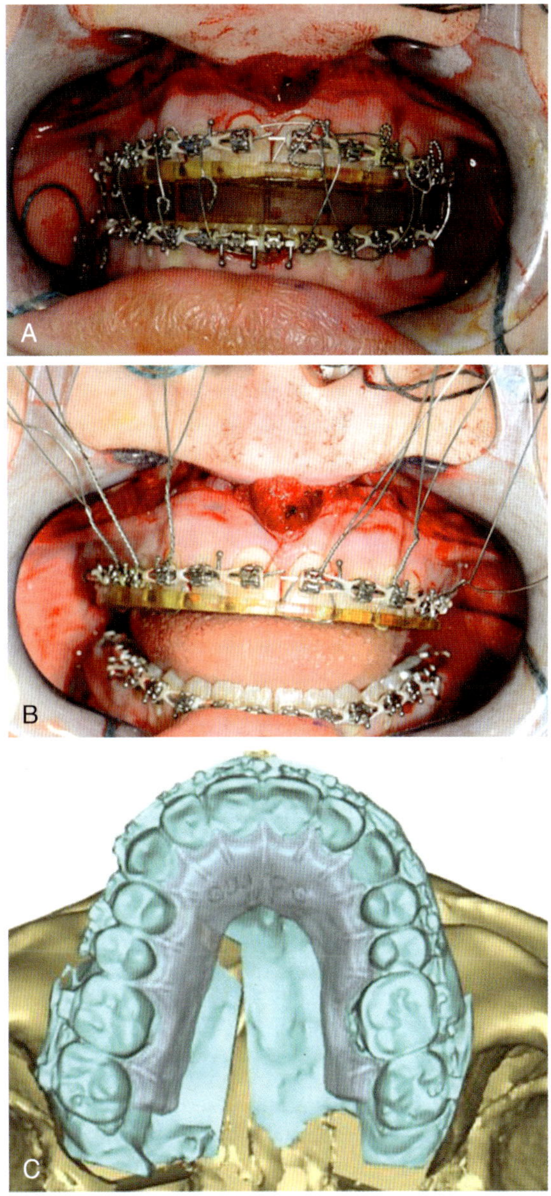


Fig. 5.9 Splints. Based on final occlusion, intermediate and final occlusal splints are designed and 3D printed. If maxillary segmentation is planned, Hawley-type palatal splints are designed and printed as well. (A) Intermediate splint. (B) Final splint. (C) Hawley-type splint.

  - The nasal mucosa is dissected anteriorly, exposing the septum, nasal floor, and walls.
  - A reciprocating saw is then used to create the osteotomy extending anteriorly toward the piriform recess. Lateral nasal wall and septal

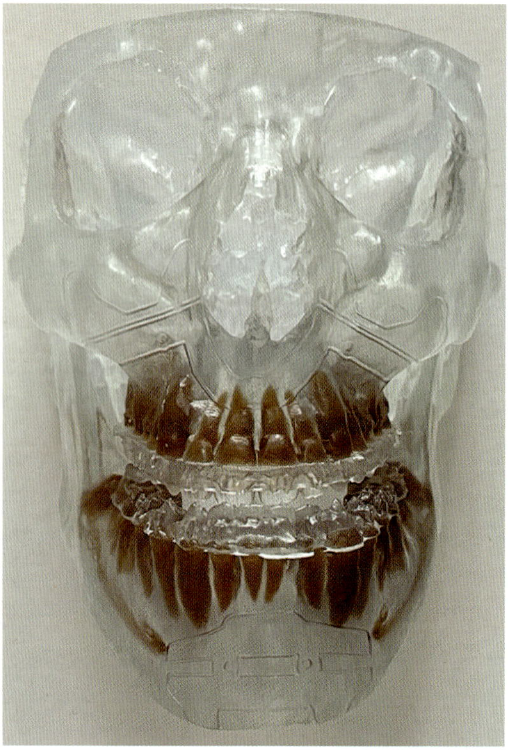

**Fig. 5.10** Models.

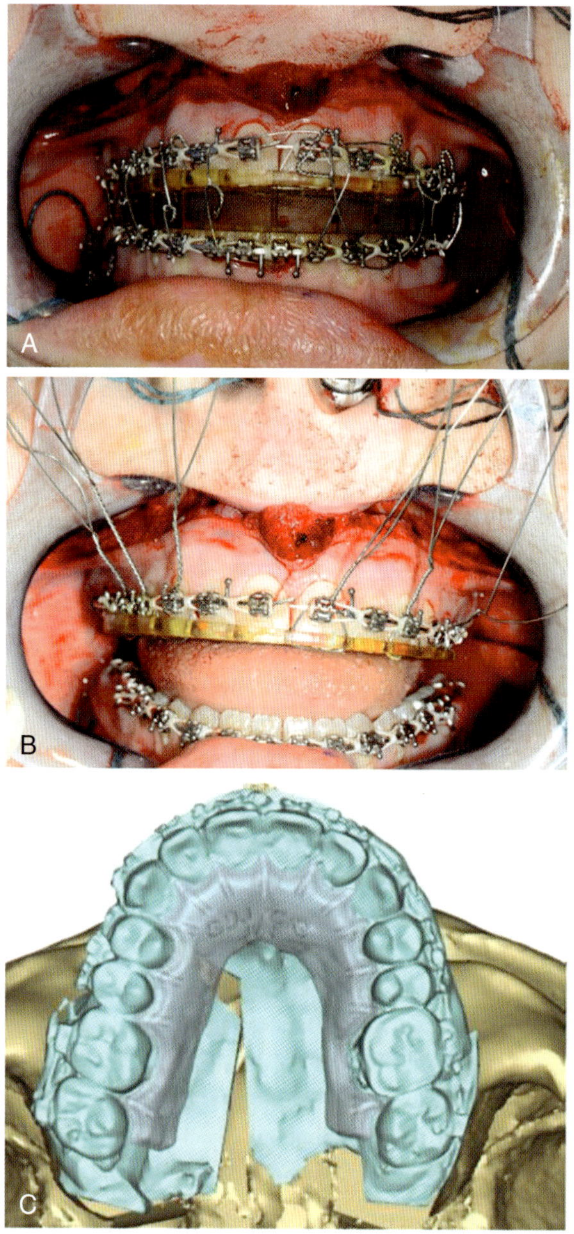


**Fig. 5.11** Splints. (A) Intermediate splint. (B) Final splint. (C) Hawley-type palatal splint.

osteotomies are performed. A series of osteotomes are used to allow for maxillary down-fracture and mobilization.

- If segmentation is to be performed, the maxilla is divided into segments with piezo saw and fine osteotomes. The maxillary segments are repositioned using a Hawley-type palatal splint.
- Internal fixation ensures correct maxillary positioning at the lateral and medial buttresses. A septal reset and repositioning, alar cinching, and V–Y mucosal closure is performed

- Genioplasty
    - A single-piece sliding genioplasty with advancement for asymmetry correction and lengthening is often also performed if needed.

## Clinical Case

A 33-year-old male presented with a history of left, unilateral cleft lip and palate (CLP) with maxillary hypoplasia, alveolar cleft, cleft-dental gap with missing lateral incisor, and an impacted, buccally-erupting canine (see Video 5.1). Significant nasal deformity with asymmetry, lack of tip support and projection, rim deficiency and scarring were also evident. The patient underwent presurgical orthodontic alignment, maintaining the fistula and impacted canine to be addressed at the time of orthognathic surgery. A mandible-first orthognathic sequence was elected.

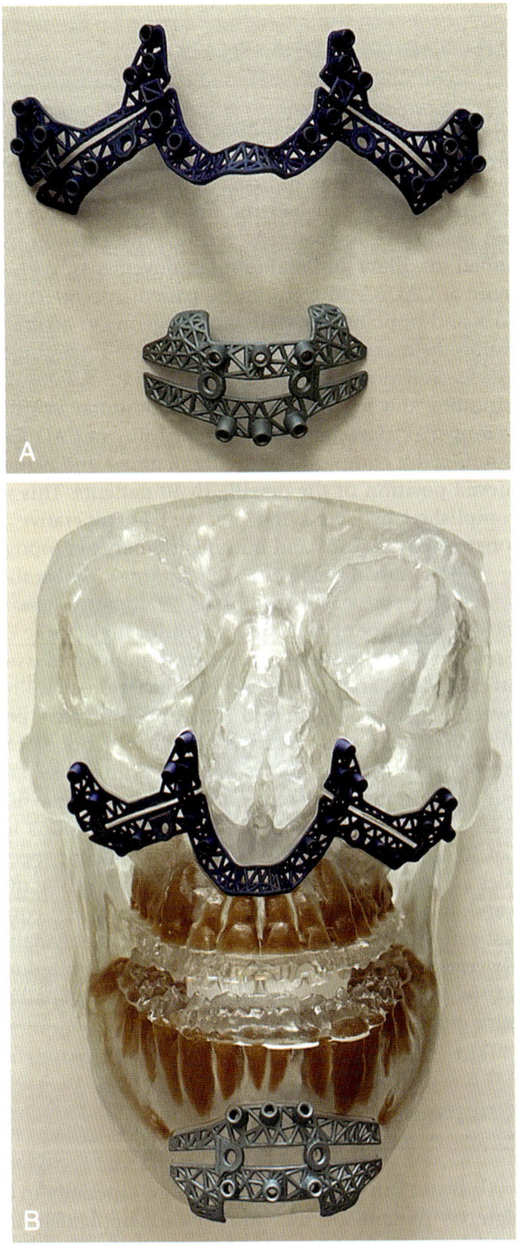


Fig. 5.12 Cutting guides.

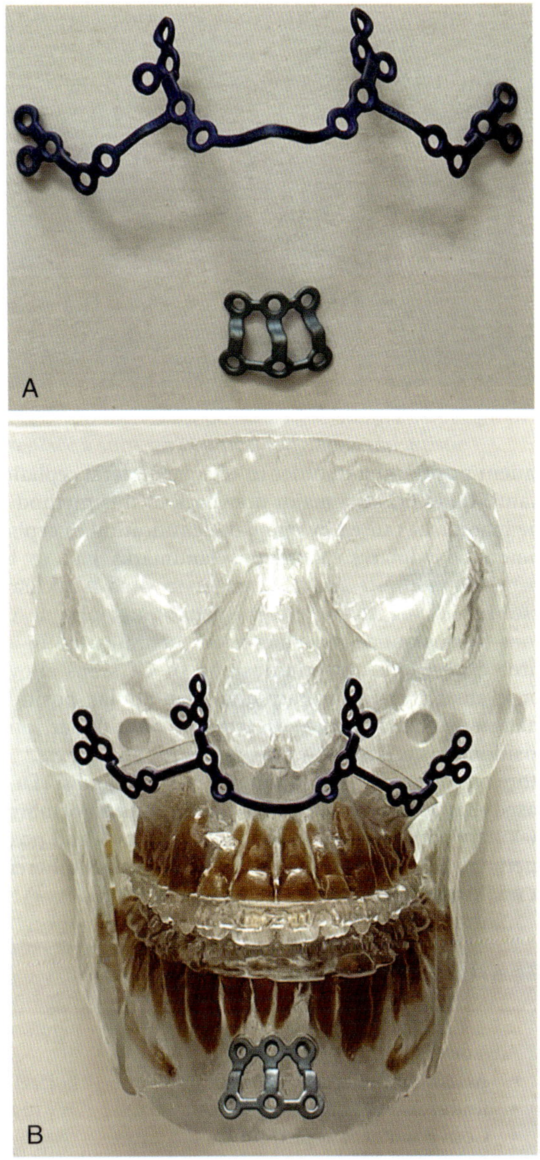


Fig. 5.13 Custom three-dimensional printed plates.

## Fidelity/verification

Objective and accurate evaluation of CAD/CAM technology and 3D CaSP is imperative in a time when operator experience, patient values, and use of best available scientific knowledge to guide decision-making are integrated. CaSP can increase proficiency and accuracy, but cannot replace a surgeon's clinical judgment and ability. One of the core components of virtually-assisted orthognathic surgery is the comparison of planned results with those that were actually obtained. Historically, comparison of cephalometric landmarks from preoperative and postoperative lateral cephalograms were evaluated to determine precision of outcome. This required exact

craniofacial cone-beam computed tomographies for facial soft tissue assessment: reproducibility and segmentation effects. *Am J Orthod Dentofacial Orthop*. 2021;59(3):343-351.e1.

19. Mazzoni S, Bianchi A, Schiariti G, et al. Computer-aided design and computer-aided manufacturing cutting guides and customized titanium plates are useful in upper maxilla waferless repositioning. *J Oral Maxillofac Surg*. 2015;73(4):701-707.
20. Kraeima J, Jansma J, Schepers RH. Splintless surgery: does patient-specific CAD-CAM osteosynthesis improve accuracy of Le Fort I osteotomy? *Br J Oral Maxillofac Surg*. 2016;54(10):1085-1089.
21. Greenberg S, Buchbinder D, Turner MD, et al. Three-dimensional repositioning of the maxilla in orthognathic surgery using patient-specific titanium plates: a case series. *J Oral Maxillofac Surg*. 2021;79(4):902-913.

# Chapter 6

# Computer-assisted surgical planning in head and neck reconstruction: cranium

*Leila Musavi, Amir H. Dorafshar*

**CHAPTER OUTLINE**



## Introduction

The goal of cranioplasty is to restore structure and function of missing cranial bone while providing support to soft tissues.[1] Choice of surgical approach and reconstructive material depends on the nature and size of the defect, the patient's history, and surgeon preference. Cranioplasty techniques are broadly divided into two categories: alloplastic and autologous. Alloplastic material is useful for very large defects or when the underlying defect is of a complex contour, but it is more prone to foreign body reaction, infection, extrusion, and plate breakdown.[2] Autologous bone graft can reduce the risk of infectious complications and technical failures associated with synthetic material but presents its own challenges. These include difficulty in shaping the bone and donor site morbidity when harvesting grafts for large cranial defects.[3]

Computer-assisted design, computer-assisted manufacturing (CAD/CAM) technology can mitigate the challenges associated with both alloplastic and autologous cranioplasty techniques. In recent years, CAD/CAM has become increasingly popular for the prefabrication of patient-specific implants (PSIs). The ability to construct a well-fitting implant preoperatively may reduce procedure time and infection risk and is particularly important in cases where a large defect spans an area of intricate contour, such as the fronto-orbital region. CAD/CAM technology has been described in the fabrication of custom titanium,[4-7] hydroxyapatite,[8,9] polyetheretherketone (PEEK),[7,10-13] porous polyethylene (Medpor),[14,15] and polymethyl methacrylate (PMMA)[16-18] implants, as well as for production of intraoperative molds to be used with acrylic prostheses.[19] Based on the computed tomography (CT) scan of the patient, an implant or mold is virtually designed using CAD software and then manufactured either through subtraction (high-speed milling) or additive manufacturing methods.[10] Additive manufacturing has grown in popularity as it allows for the rapid production of complex 3D shapes from a CAD file in a layer-by-layer fashion, thus reducing the waste and cost associated with traditional subtractive techniques.[20]

PSIs have been applied in a broad range of cases, including very large calvarial defects,[12] repeatedly reconstructed cases,[10] and pediatric craniectomy defects.[7] However, the fabrication of these implants are associated with significant cost, based on size and complexity. The average cost for custom-made PEEK or titanium implants has been cited anywhere between an estimated \$7000 to \$15,000 USD,[10,12] limiting its availability in low-resource settings.

CAD/CAM is also a powerful tool in the realm of autologous cranioplasty, particularly in split calvarial bone grafting. Many of the commonly cited disadvantages of autologous cranioplasty, such as longer operative times, contour unpredictability, and donor-site morbidity, can be addressed by this technology.[21] Through calculated measurements of the calvarium and estimation of three-dimensional constructs, the surgeon can determine the optimal site to harvest a graft in one piece to provide the most natural contour while avoiding critical structures such as dural venous sinuses.[3,22] Thus, CAD/CAM may improve efficiency and safety in split-calvarial bone grafting while helping the surgeon to avoid an irregular final construct.

## Clinical considerations

The surgeon must consider several anatomic and clinical factors to achieve a successful cranial reconstruction with CAD/CAM technology. Defect size and location are primary concerns. The complexity of implant design increases with defect size, crossing of the sagittal midline, and involvement of the orbital rim, as it is difficult to model accurate contour symmetry in these cases.[23] Prior reconstructive history is also important. In repeatedly reconstructed cases where residual material is often present at the defect site, the irregular wound bed surface can be modeled with CAD software to facilitate accurate implant placement intraoperatively. Koper et al. presented a series of 20 patients undergoing repeated reconstruction with PSIs and demonstrated no difference in operative time among those patients with residual reconstruction material still present compared to those without.[10] Additionally, there was no need for intraoperative manipulation of the implants in either patient group.

A number of implant modifications using CAD/CAM technology have been reported to enhance surgical efficiency and safety.[24] Holes may be designed in the implant for fluid drainage, dural suspension sutures, and temporalis muscle resuspension. Fixation points along the perimeter of the implant, including screw holes or indentations for plate placement, may be specified. These points can be angled precisely to facilitate screwdriver or drill access and avoid injury to the superior sagittal sinus for defects near the midline. The edges of the implant can be tapered to overlap the surrounding skull in to decrease strain forces on the implant and limit palpability of the edges. When there is concern about the ability to achieve tension-free closure, such as repeat reconstructions or irradiated fields, the contour of the implant may be slightly decreased to allow easier soft tissue coverage. Implant manipulation via CAD/CAM technology has also been used to correct temporal hollowing caused by bone resorption, temporalis muscle malposition, and/or temporal fat pad atrophy.[25]

Additionally, CAD/CAM facilitates the use of split calvarial bone grafting for the reconstruction of complex defects traditionally considered not amenable to autologous techniques. Preoperative planning can help the surgeon identify the optimal donor site for large or previously reconstructed defects and avoid the need to harvest separate calvarial segments in a "piecemeal" approach. Measurements of the cranial diploe allow for identification of areas with sufficient width for splitting. Dural venous sinuses can be mapped to avoid craniotomy-associated damage during graft harvest.[22] The final result can be visualized and further refinements to shape can be decided in the planning stage. The utility of CAD/CAM was demonstrated in a series of five patients with large cranial defects (mean defect size of 69 $cm^2$) undergoing secondary cranioplasty. In this series, there were no dural tears, sagittal sinus bleeds, or other intraoperative complications, and no immediate postoperative complications requiring extended hospital stay or reoperation. All patients achieved successful reconstruction with satisfactory cranial contour on follow-up.[3]

## Workflow for computer-assisted design, computer-assisted manufacturing

A 3D CT scan is obtained to characterize the cranial defect. The surgical team and bioengineer meet to plan the operative approach. Depending on the chosen approach and complexity of the case, the design phase may span several days. Once the operative plan is finalized, manufacturing begins. In the case of alloplastic cranioplasty, custom implants and molds are usually produced within 7 to 14 days. They are then shipped to the medical facility and sterilized. In total, alloplastic implants are typically ready for surgery in fewer than 3 weeks. In the case of autologous cranioplasty, osteotomy guides are usually manufactured within 10 days and ready for surgical use within 2 weeks (Fig. 6.1).

## Computer-assisted design

Preoperative 1-mm spiral CT scan of the calvarium is obtained in axial, coronal, and sagittal planes. The data is converted to a 3D reconstruction. The area for cranioplasty is then mapped by the operator.

In the case of alloplastic reconstruction, a mirror image of the contralateral calvarium is transposed onto the affected side (if the defect does not cross midline), or an

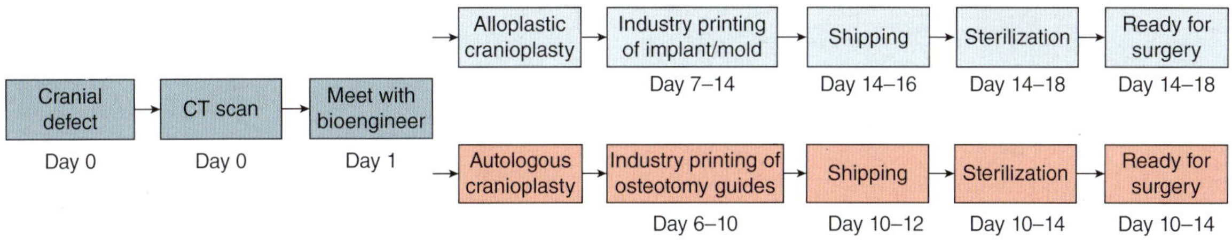


**Fig. 6.1** The computer-assisted design/computer-assisted manufacturing workflow, from implant design to surgical implementation, is shown for both alloplastic and autologous cranioplasty.

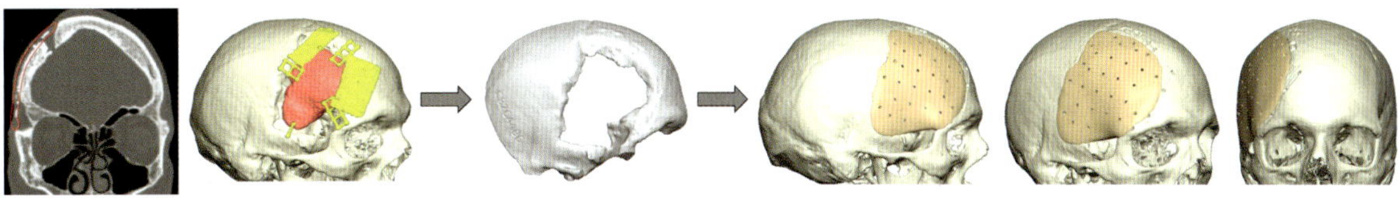

**Fig. 6.2** The computer-assisted design, computer-assisted manufacturing planning process is shown for Patient A, a 63-year-old male undergoing secondary cranioplasty with a polyetheretherketone (PEEK) implant. He had a history of right frontal craniotomy for recurrent meningioma, with replacement of the bone flap and titanium mesh. He subsequently developed a prominent frontotemporal contour deformity. A 1-mm spiral computed tomography scan was obtained and three-dimensional reconstruction performed showing areas of bony deficiency. The bone flap is presented in *pink* and the titanium plates in *yellow*. The full defect was then recreated. A PEEK implant was modeled to restore cranial symmetry of the right frontotemporal defect based on the contralateral normal cranial contour.

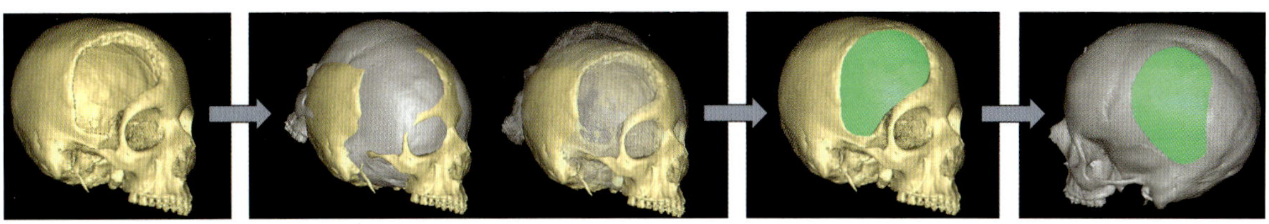

**Fig. 6.3** The computer-assisted design planning process is demonstrated for Patient B, a 59-year-old female patient undergoing secondary cranioplasty with split calvarial bone. She had a history of titanium mesh cranioplasty after meningioma resection and subsequently developed an infection requiring hardware removal. She presented with a 70-$cm^2$ right frontotemporal defect. A 1-mm spiral computed tomography scan was obtained and a three-dimensional reconstruction of the calvarium performed. A duplicate calvarium was created and transposed on the original to find a new region that optimally fit the defect. A region of the left parietal calvarium was selected for its size and contour match.

average skull image is superimposed on the patient's calvarium (if the defect is midline). To model the implant, the defect-filling portion of the template is sequentially "cookie-cut" and thickness is added to create a tapered edge that abuts or overlaps the surrounding calvarium. The surgeon can determine fixation points at this time. In addition to confirming proper fit of the implant, this process ensures that there is no intersection with the adjacent dural sac. Consideration should also be given as to whether there is sufficient scalp to cover the implant or if additional measures (e.g., galeal scoring, tissue expansion) may be needed.[26]

In autologous split calvarial bone cranioplasty, special attention is given to the contour of the remaining skull, diploe thickness, and location of the sagittal sinus to find an appropriate donor site. Using CAD software, a duplicate calvarium is transposed on the original skull and carefully repositioned to find a new region that best replicates the anatomical contour of the defect. Care is taken to select an area of calvarium with adequate diploe thickness for splitting. A template of the defect is generated and positioned over the determined donor site. From this transposition, an osteotomy guide can be manufactured for intraoperative use.

The CAD planning process is demonstrated for a patient undergoing alloplastic reconstruction (patient A; Fig. 6.2) and a patient undergoing autologous cranioplasty (patient B; Fig. 6.3 and Video 6.1).

## Computer-assisted manufacturing

Additive manufacturing has become the preferred method for fabrication of custom cranial implants and intraoperative guides.[20] An implant is built layer by layer from a CAD file, allowing the manufacture of complex contours with predefined porosity. Various techniques, including photopolymerization, laser sintering, and extrusion-based printing, have been used successfully.[20,26]

Implant modifications can be made to improve surgical accuracy and efficiency, shown for Patient A (Fig. 6.4) and Patient B (Fig. 6.5).

## Operative technique

### 1. Design

**a.** Alloplastic cranioplasty: using the 3D CT reconstruction, a mirror image of the contralateral calvarium is transposed on the defect to create an implant of optimal contour and fit.

**b.** Autologous split calvarial bone grafting: a duplicate skull is transposed on the original to find a donor site with ideal contour, and an osteotomy guide is modeled.

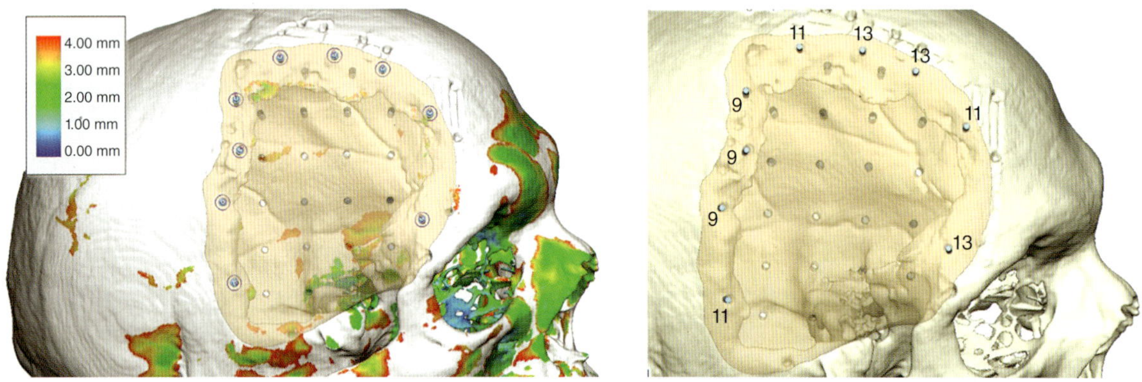


**Fig. 6.4** The polyetheretherketone implant for Patient A was further customized to facilitate accurate inset. The surrounding cranial bone contour and thickness were carefully mapped. Fixation points and screw lengths for the implant *(shown in blue)* were determined using this information.

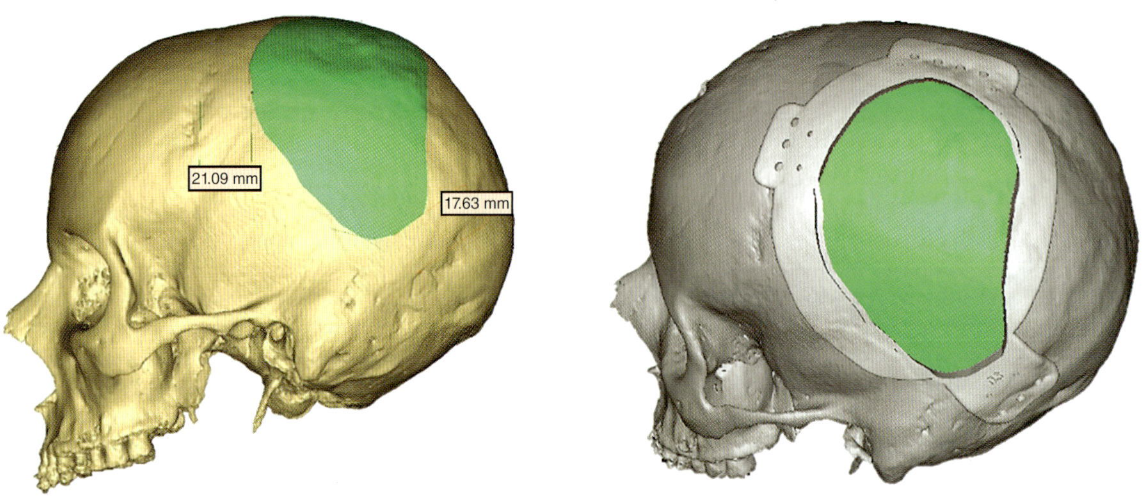


**Fig. 6.5** The osteotomy guide for Patient B is presented. A 60-cm$^2$ donor site of the left parietal region was marked for graft harvest. Distances from bony landmarks, including the left coronal and lambdoid sutures, were measured to facilitate intraoperative positioning. An osteotomy guide with burr hole sites was created.

## 2. Manufacturing

a. Using the CAD file, the custom cranial implant, mold, or osteotomy guide is created via subtractive or additive manufacturing.

## 3. Surgery

a. Alloplastic cranioplasty.
   i. The custom implant is checked for fit over the defect and secured with titanium miniplates. If necessary, contouring is performed using a burr drill.
b. Autologous split calvarial bone grafting.
   i. A full-thickness craniectomy is performed of the donor site. The osteotomy guide is placed over the donor site, burr holes are created as indicated by the guide, and the underlying dura is freed. A craniotome is used to complete the craniectomy.
   ii. The harvested calvarium is split into inner and outer tables using a sagittal saw with splitting osteotomy.
   iii. The outer table is placed onto the calvarial defect and secured in place with titanium plates. The inner table is placed on the donor site and secured.

## 4. Confirmation

a. Restoration of cranial contour is confirmed via clinical assessment before the patient leaves the operating room.
b. Postoperative CT scan is obtained to evaluate contour at recipient and donor sites, skull symmetry, and fidelity to the model.

Figs. 6.6 and 6.7 demonstrate the clinical course for Patient A and Patient B, respectively.

Postoperative CT scans for Patients A and B are shown demonstrating fidelity with the preoperative models (Figs. 6.8 and 6.9, respectively).

## Fidelity/verification

Intraoperatively, a satisfactory cranial reconstruction is verified by complete defect coverage without large gaps or overlap, symmetry with the contralateral side, and a smooth transition between the implant/graft and native bone. In addition to clinical evaluation, early postoperative CT scans should be taken to assess the fidelity of the reconstruction to the operative plan. Congruency of the implant or graft can be assessed by transposition of the CAD model or a mirror image of the nonaffected side onto the reconstructed side. The cranial index of symmetry or volumetric calculations can be used as quantitative measures.[27] In the case of split calvarial bone grafting, the surface areas of the CAD-modeled graft and harvested graft can be compared to ensure accuracy. The patient is followed in clinic to ensure satisfactory contour and durability of the reconstruction.

## Pearls/pitfalls

- An experienced team of bioengineers and surgeons is necessary for the accurate virtual design of custom cranial implants and osteotomy guides.
- The complexity of implant or graft design increases with defect size, crossing of the sagittal midline, and involvement of the orbital rim.
- Implant design should provide precise defect coverage, congruency with the native calvarium, and overall skull symmetry. Consideration should also be given to adequate soft tissue coverage and correction of temporal hollowing during the planning phase.
- Implant modifications, such as perforations for fluid drainage and dural suspension sutures, angled fixation points, and tapered implant edges, will facilitate safe and efficient implant placement.
- In autologous split calvarial bone cranioplasty, care should be taken during computer-assisted planning to select an area of calvarium with adequate diploe thickness for splitting and a safe distance from the sagittal sinus.

## Outcomes/complications

CAD/CAM has been applied successfully in a wide range of cranioplasty procedures with low complication rates, efficient operative times, and satisfactory skull-shape symmetry. In a series of 33 patients undergoing cranioplasty of defects of more than 100 $cm^2$ with PSI (titanium or PEEK) versus bone flap reimplantation, Lethaus demonstrated significantly lower complication rate, reoperation rate, and hospital length of stay in the PSI group.[12] In another large series of 131 patients undergoing bone flap reimplantation, PMMA intraoperative molding, or custom fabricated PMMA implant, Lee et al. found significantly less operative time and blood loss in the custom implant group compared to the intraoperative molding group.[16] Several other studies have demonstrated successful CAD/CAM implant reconstruction with low rates of infection, seroma, implant exposure, or contour irregularity on long-term follow-up.[6,28,29] Rating of patient satisfaction after PSI reconstruction has generally been very high, with patients reporting improved quality of life, decreased pain and headache, and good aesthetic results.[4,11] CAD/CAM technology has been used safely in pediatric cranioplasty as well. In one of the largest

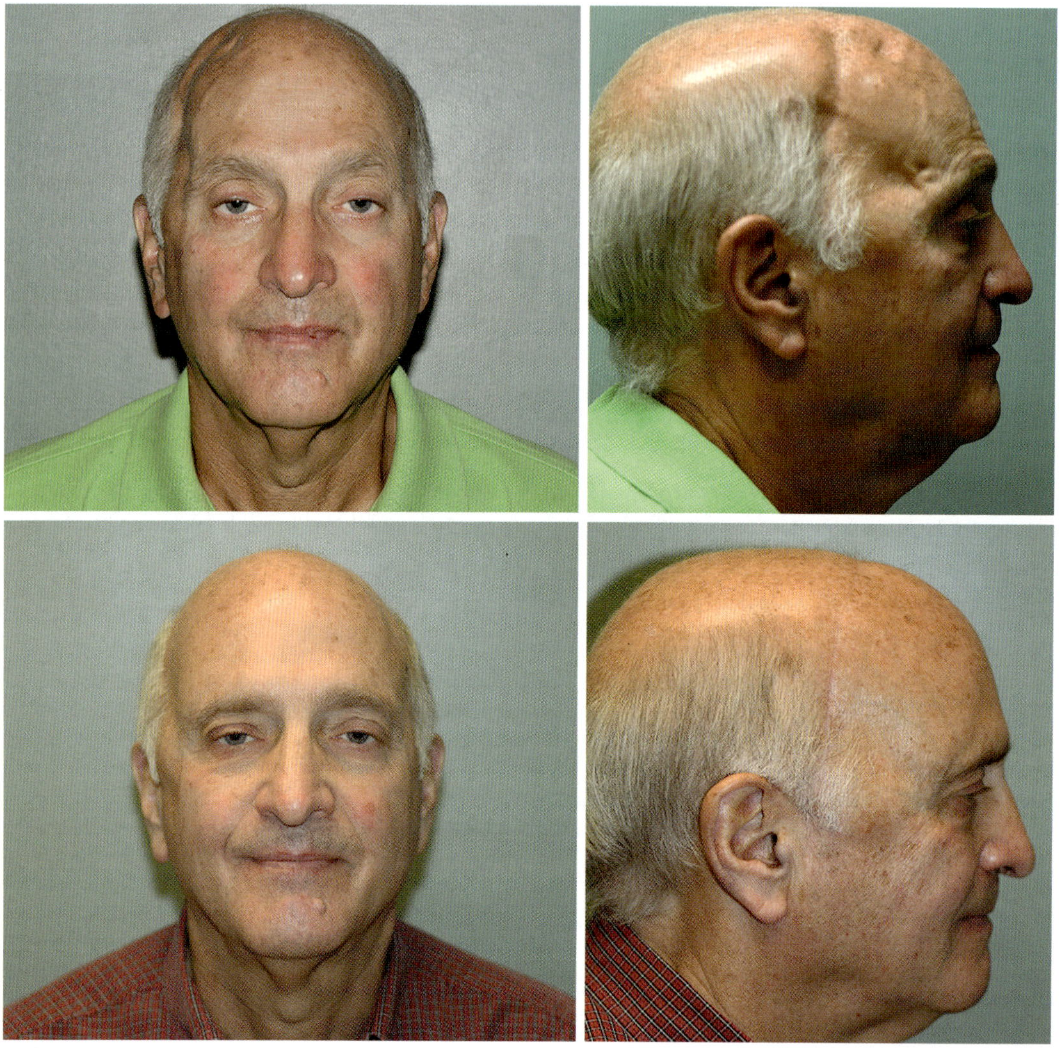

**Fig. 6.6** Patient A presented to clinic with concavity and contour irregularity of the frontotemporal region after right frontal craniotomy. The previously placed bone flap and hardware were removed and a custom-made polyetheretherketone implant was placed. Postoperative photos demonstrate restoration of frontotemporal contour and smooth transition from implant to native calvarium.

pediatric series to date, including a subset of 93 patients undergoing full-thickness cranioplasty, Nguyen reported the successful use of custom PEEK, PMMA, and titanium implants with low infection rate (4.4%) and implant failure (3.7%).[7]

The use of CAD/CAM in autologous split calvarial bone grafting has not been as widely published, but the proof of concept is promising. In a case series of five patients with prior failed reconstruction undergoing split calvarial cranioplasty, CAD/CAM technology was used to enhance graft selection and improve contour accuracy, with postoperative graft surface areas on average within 2% of the planned graft.[3]

As with other craniofacial applications, the main drawback of CAD/CAM technology in cranioplasty is production expense. Custom-made implant costs have been reported anywhere between an estimated $7000 to $15,000 USD, and titanium implants are generally associated with higher production cost than PEEK or PMMA.[7,10,12] More recently, the use of low-cost commercial 3D printers with stereolithography models has been reported to increase application of this technology in low resource settings.[5,30,31]

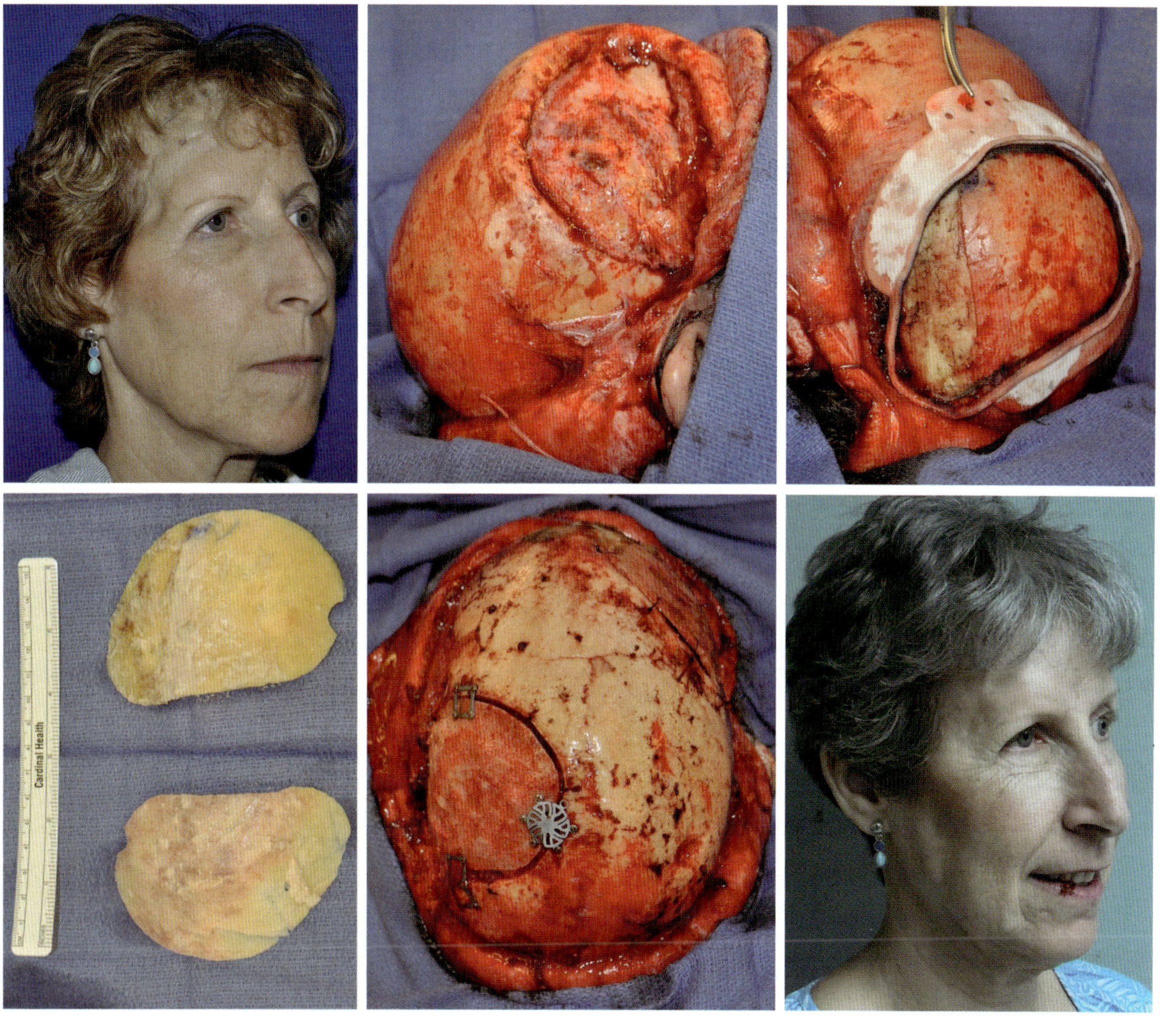


**Fig. 6.7** Patient B presented with exposed hardware and contour deficiencies after failed titanium mesh cranioplasty. The hardware was removed, and the osteotomy guide generated from computer-assisted design/computer-assisted manufacturing was used to harvest the graft. The calvarium was split into inner and outer tables and used to reconstruct the frontal bone and donor site. Postoperative photo demonstrates satisfactory restoration of frontal contour.

## Conclusion

The ideal cranial reconstruction provides precise defect closure with a material of good durability and biocompatibility. Whether the surgeon pursues alloplastic or autologous reconstruction, CAD/CAM is a useful tool to enhance surgical accuracy, efficiency, and safety. Operative time, surgical complications, and blood loss can be reduced, while achieving excellent contour symmetry and patient satisfaction. Importantly, CAD/CAM has allowed for the more streamlined reconstruction of traditionally complex cases, including very large defects, midline or fronto-orbital defects, repeat reconstructions, and prior irradiated or infected fields. The main drawback of this technique, the production cost, may be mitigated by inexpensive commercially available 3D printers that allow for in-house implant manufacture.

Future directions include the integration of CAD/CAM technology with tissue engineering. Manufacture of new resorbable ceramic scaffolds, application of growth factors, and antibiotic coating of implants are areas of ongoing investigation.[1,26,32] Addition of stem cells to potentiate the

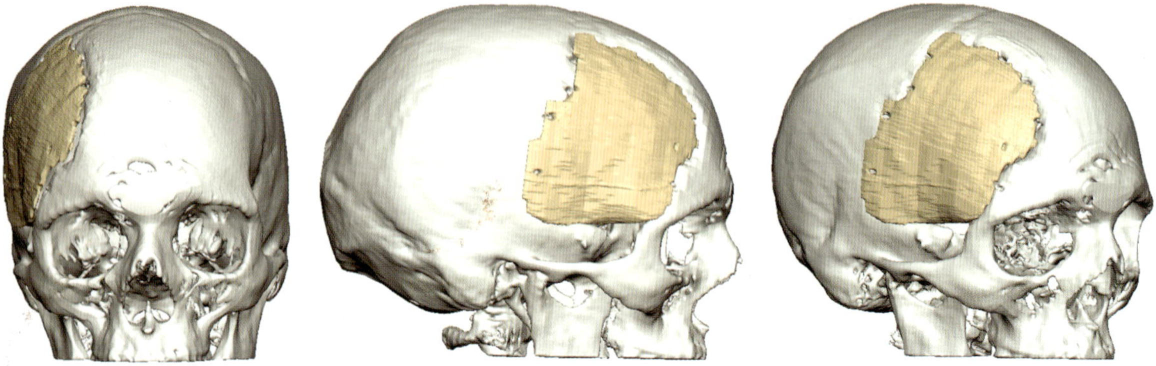

Fig. 6.8 Postoperative three-dimensional computed tomography reconstruction of Patient A demonstrated a well-positioned implant without gaps or overlap. Symmetry with the contralateral side was restored.

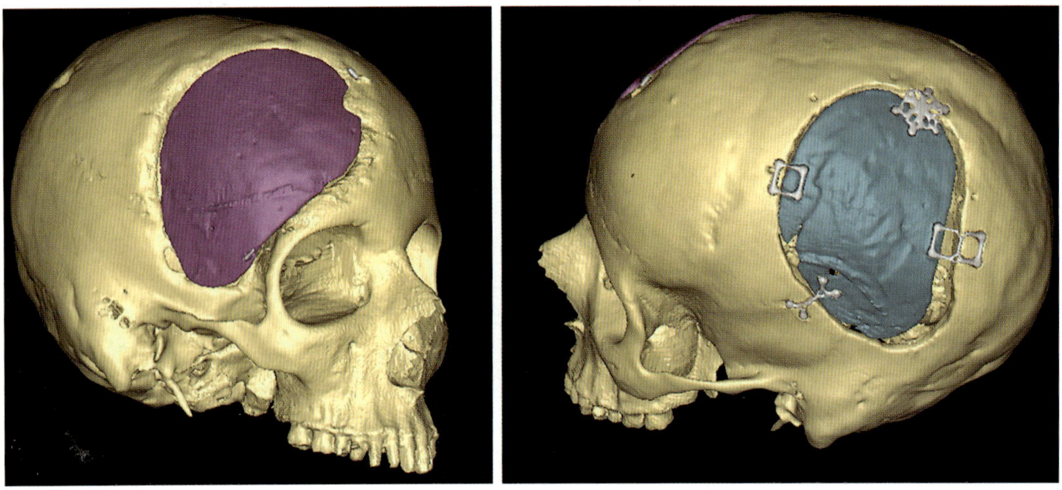

Fig. 6.9 Postoperative three-dimensional computed tomography reconstruction of Patient B demonstrated restoration of contour of the right frontoparietal defect and left parietal donor site. The predicted graft surface area based on computer-assisted design measurements and the actual harvested graft area were within 3.2% of each other (64.2 vs 62.2 $cm^2$, respectively).

osteoconductive and osteoinductive properties of scaffolds is also under exploration.[1] These advances in tissue engineering, combined with the accuracy and versatility of CAD/CAM technology, hold promise for the manufacture of more ideal native bone replacements.

## Take-home points

- CAD/CAM technology allows the surgeon to design congruous and symmetric cranial reconstructions using normal contralateral contours or average skull models.
- The ability to construct a well-fitting implant preoperatively may contribute to reductions in operative time, blood loss, and infection risk. Careful measurements ensure no intersection of the implant with the underlying dural sac or structures like the superior sagittal sinus.
- CAD/CAM facilitates split calvarial bone grafting of complex defects through the transposition of a duplicate calvarium to find a donor site of optimal contour and fit.

- Additive manufacturing of cranial implants/guides has grown in popularity as it allows for the rapid production of complex shapes in a layer-by-layer fashion, thus reducing the waste and cost associated with traditional subtractive techniques.
- Advancements in this field include the integration of CAD/CAM technology with new biologic scaffolds and tissue factors to improve the durability and biocompatibility of cranial reconstruction.

## References


1. Goldstein JA, Paliga JT, Bartlett SP. Cranioplasty: indications and advances. *Curr Opin Otolaryngol Head Neck Surg*. 2013;21(4):400-409. doi:10.1097/MOO.0B013E328363003E.
2. Piazza M, Grady MS. Cranioplasty. *Neurosurg Clin N Am*. 2017;28(2):257-265. doi:10.1016/J.NEC.2016.11.008.
3. Musavi L, Macmillan A, Lopez J, Dorafshar AH. Using computer-aided design/computer-aided manufacturing for autogenous, split calvarial bone graft-based cranioplasty: Optimizing reconstruction of large, complex skull defects. *J Craniofac Surg*. 2019;30(2):347-351. doi:10.1097/SCS.0000000000005010.
4. Cabraja M, Klein M, Lehmann TN. Long-term results following titanium cranioplasty of large skull defects. *Neurosurg Focus*. 2009;26(6):E10. doi:10.3171/2009.3.FOCUS091.
5. Dash C, Dasukil S, Boyina KK, Panda R, Ahmad SR. A novel prefabricated patient-specific titanium cranioplasty: reconsideration from a traditional approach. *Oral Maxillofac Surg*. 2021;1:1-6. doi:10.1007/S10006-021-00977-5.
6. Park EK, Lim JY, Yun IS, et al. Cranioplasty enhanced by three-dimensional printing: custom-made three-dimensional-printed titanium implants for skull defects. *J Craniofac Surg*. 2016;27(4):943-949. doi:10.1097/SCS.0000000000002656.
7. Nguyen PD, Khechoyan DY, Phillips JH, Forrest CR. Custom CAD/CAM implants for complex craniofacial reconstruction in children: our experience based on 136 cases. *J Plast Reconstr Aesthet Surg*. 2018;71(11):1609-1617. doi:10.1016/J.BJPS.2018.07.016.
8. Rossini Z, Franzini A, Zaed I, Zinagretti N, Nicolosi F, Zanotti B. Custom-made porous hydroxyapatite cranioplasty in patients with tumor versus traumatic brain injury: a single-center case series. *World Neurosurg*. 2020;138:e922-e929. doi:10.1016/J.WNEU.2020.03.144.
9. Moles A, Heudes PM, Amelat A, et al. Long-term follow-up comparative study of hydroxyapatite and autologous cranioplasties: complications, cosmetic results, osseointegration. *World Neurosurg*. 2018;111:e395-e402. doi:10.1016/J.WNEU.2017.12.082.
10. Koper D, ter Laak-Poort M, Lethaus B, et al. Cranioplasty with patient-specific implants in repeatedly reconstructed cases. *J Craniomaxillofac Surg*. 2019;47(5):709-714. doi:10.1016/J.JCMS.2019.01.034.
11. Zegers T, ter Laak-Poort M, Koper D, Lethaus B, Kessler P. The therapeutic effect of patient-specific implants in cranioplasty. *J Craniomaxillofac Surg*. 2017;45(1):82-86. doi:10.1016/J.JCMS.2016.10.016.
12. Lethaus B, Bloebaum M, Koper D, ter Laak-Poort M, Kessler P. Interval cranioplasty with patient-specific implants and autogenous bone grafts: success and cost analysis. *J Craniomaxillofac Surg*. 2014;42(8):1948-1951. doi:10.1016/J.JCMS.2014.08.006.
13. Hanasono MM, Goel N, DeMonte F. Calvarial reconstruction with polyetheretherketone implants. *Ann Plast Surg*. 2009;62(6):653-655. doi:10.1097/SAP.0B013E318184ABC7.
14. Wolff A, Santiago GF, Belzberg M, et al. Adult cranioplasty reconstruction with customized cranial implants: preferred technique, timing, and biomaterials. *J Craniofac Surg*. 2018;29(4):887-894. doi:10.1097/SCS.0000000000004385.
15. Lin AY, Kinsella CR, Rottgers SA, et al. Custom porous polyethylene implants for large-scale pediatric skull reconstruction: early outcomes. *J Craniofac Surg*. 2012;23(1):67-70. doi:10.1097/SCS.0B013E318240C876.
16. Lee SC, Wu CT, Lee ST, Chen PJ. Cranioplasty using polymethyl methacrylate prostheses. *J Clin Neurosci*. 2009;16(1):56-63. doi:10.1016/J.JOCN.2008.04.001.
17. Ridwan-Pramana A, Idema S, Te Slaa S, et al. Polymethyl methacrylate in patient-specific implants: description of a new three-dimension technique. *J Craniofac Surg*. 2019;30(2):408-411. doi:10.1097/SCS.0000000000005148.
18. Cheng CH, Chuang HY, Lin HL, Liu CL, Yao CH. Surgical results of cranioplasty using three-dimensional printing technology. *Clin Neurol Neurosurg*. 2018;168:118-123. doi:10.1016/J.CLINEURO.2018.03.004.
19. Schön SN, Skalicky N, Sharma N, Zumofen DW, Thieringer FM. 3D-printer-assisted patient-specific polymethyl methacrylate cranioplasty: a case series of 16 consecutive patients. *World*

*Neurosurg*. 2021;148:e356-e362. doi:10.1016/J.WNEU.2020.12.138.
20. Jindal S, Manzoor F, Haslam N, Mancuso E. 3D printed composite materials for craniofacial implants: current concepts, challenges and future directions. *Int J Adv Manuf Technol*. 2020;112(3):635-653. doi:10.1007/S00170-020-06397-1.
21. Fearon JA, Griner D, Ditthakasem K, Herbert M. Autogenous bone reconstruction of large secondary skull defects. *Plast Reconstr Surg*. 2017;139(2):427-438. doi:10.1097/PRS.0000000000002941.
22. Iyer RR, Wu A, Macmillan A, et al. Use of computer-assisted design and manufacturing to localize dural venous sinuses during reconstructive surgery for craniosynostosis. *Childs Nerv Syst*. 2018;34(1):137-142. doi:10.1007/s00381-017-3601-0.
23. Poukens J, Laeven P, Beerens M, et al. A classification of cranial implants based on the degree of difficulty in computer design and manufacture. *Int J Med Robot*. 2008;4(1):46-50. doi:10.1002/RCS.171.
24. Nout E, Mommaerts MY. Considerations in computer-aided design for inlay cranioplasty: technical note. *Oral Maxillofac Surg*. 2018;22(1):65. doi:10.1007/S10006-017-0668-4.
25. Zhong S, Huang GJ, Susarla SM, Swanson EW, Huang J, Gordon CR. Quantitative analysis of dual-purpose, patient-specific craniofacial implants for correction of temporal deformity. *Neurosurgery*. 2015;11(suppl 2):220-229. doi:10.1227/NEU.0000000000000679.
26. Bonda DJ, Manjila S, Selman WR, Dean D. The recent revolution in the design and manufacture of cranial implants: modern advancements and future directions. *Neurosurgery*. 2015;77(5):814-824. doi:10.1227/NEU.0000000000000899.
27. Basu B, Bhaskar N, Barui S, et al. Evaluation of implant properties, safety profile and clinical efficacy of patient-specific acrylic prosthesis in cranioplasty using 3D binderjet printed cranium model: a pilot study. *J Clin Neurosci*. 2021;85:132-142. doi:10.1016/J.JOCN.2020.12.020.
28. Turgut G, Özkaya Ö, Kayali MU. Computer-aided design and manufacture and rapid prototyped polymethylmethacrylate reconstruction. *J Craniofac Surg*. 2012;23(3):770-773. doi:10.1097/SCS.0B013E31824DBCAF.
29. Goh RCW, Chang CN, Lin CL, Lo LJ. Customised fabricated implants after previous failed cranioplasty. *J Plast Reconstr Aesthet Surg*. 2010;63(9):1479-1484. doi:10.1016/J.BJPS.2009.08.010.
30. Metwali H, Hassanin M, Ibrahim T. A customized technique of cranioplasty for patients with large skull defects: a technical note. *World Neurosurg*. 2021;148:110-114. doi:10.1016/J.WNEU.2020.12.157.
31. Tan ETW, Ling JM, Dinesh SK. The feasibility of producing patient-specific acrylic cranioplasty implants with a low-cost 3D printer. *J Neurosurg*. 2016;124(5):1531-1537. doi:10.3171/2015.5.JNS15119.
32. Nyberg EL, Farris AL, Hung BP, et al. 3D-printing technologies for craniofacial rehabilitation, reconstruction, and regeneration. *Ann Biomed Eng*. 2016;45(1):45-57. doi:10.1007/S10439-016-1668-5.

Chapter | 7 |

# Computer-assisted design/computer-assisted modeling in maxillary reconstruction

*Farooq Shahzad, Evan Matros*

**CHAPTER OUTLINE**



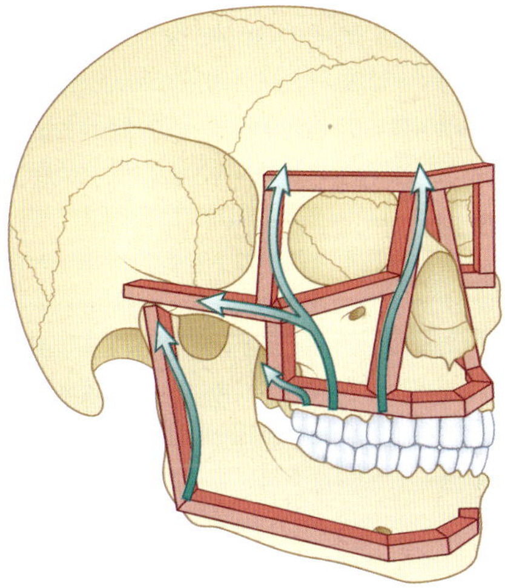

**Fig. 7.1** Horizontal and vertical pillars of the midface.

## Introduction

The midface is a complex skeletal framework that is composed principally of the maxilla and zygoma. Structural support is provided by a set of horizontal and vertical pillars (Fig. 7.1).[1] The main horizontal buttresses are the maxillary alveolus and the infraorbital rim, while the vertical buttresses are the nasomaxillary and the zygomaticomaxillary buttress. Defects of the midface are reconstructed by bony restoration of these buttresses which provide a base for dental implant placement, orbital floor reconstruction, and nasal airway preservation.[2] Furthermore, aesthetics of the midface are maintained by reestablishing facial width, height, and projection.

The midface can be conceptualized as a hexahedron with six walls (Fig. 7.2).[3] The roof is the orbital floor (infraorbital rim buttress), the floor is the alveolus and palate (maxillary buttress), the medial wall is the outer border of the nasal cavity (nasomaxillary buttress), and the lateral wall is the zygomaticomaxillary buttress. One of the earliest classifications of oncologic maxillary resections is based on an imaginary line from the medial canthus to the angle of the mandible (Ohngren's line).[4] Resections below this line are called infrastructure maxillectomies and those above this line are called suprastructure maxillectomies. More comprehensive classification schemes have since been described, the most commonly used of which are the Cordeiro and Brown systems (Figs. 7.3 and 7.4).[3,5]

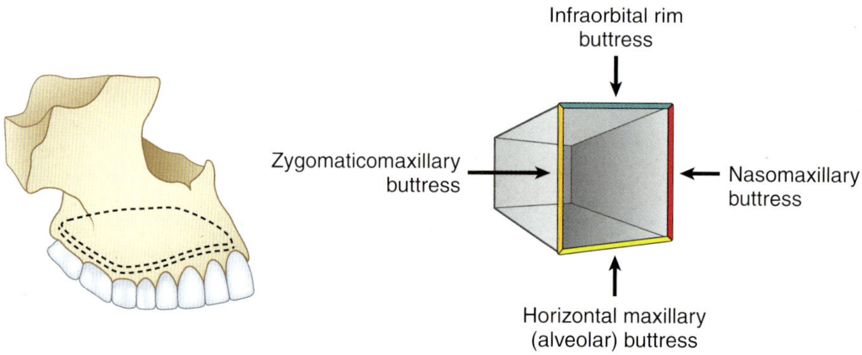


**Fig. 7.2** Hexahedral structure of the midface.

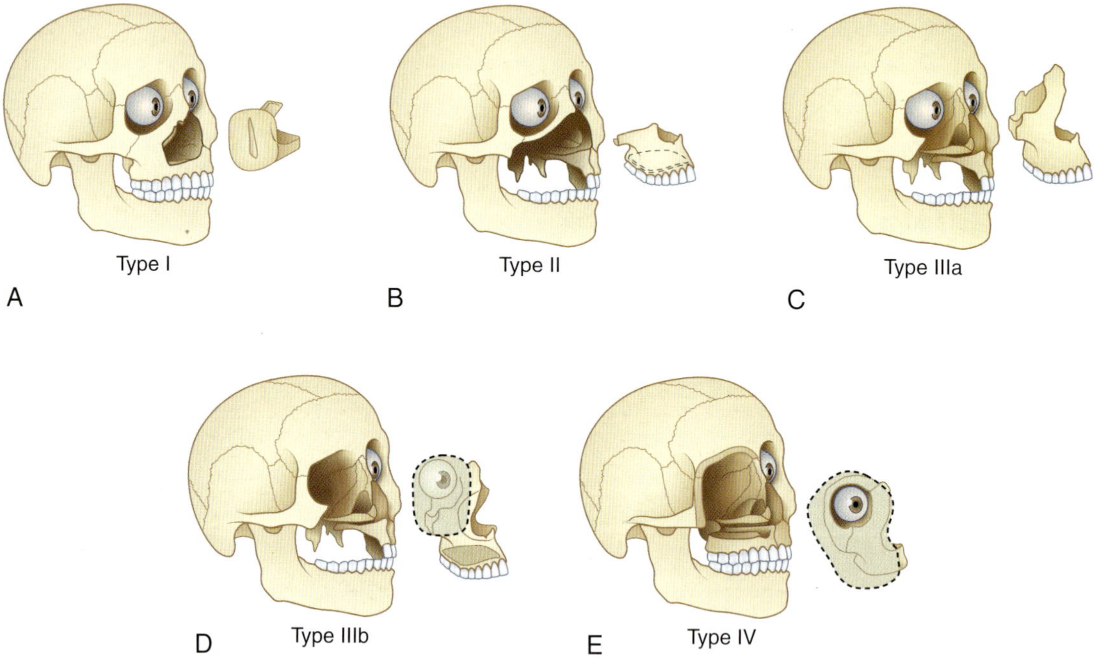


**Fig. 7.3** Cordeiro classification of midface defects. (A) Type I: one or two walls of the maxilla excluding the palate. (B) Type II: lower five walls i.e., maxillary arch, palate, anterior and lateral walls. (C) Type IIIa: all six walls of the maxilla with orbital preservation. (D) Type IIIb: all six walls of the maxilla with orbital exenteration. (E) Type IV: upper five walls of the maxilla along with orbital contents, but with preservation of the palate.

Maxillary reconstruction is a challenging undertaking. There is very limited working area and reduced exposure in the midface. Small bone segments have to fit in a tight space. Depending on defect type, complex geometric plate configurations may be needed.[6] If multiple bone segments are needed (e.g., total maxillectomy), it is imperative that cuts be accurate; even a small change in the angulation of the osteotomies will affect the shape of the entire construct.[6] Bone position needs to be in proper relation to the mandible for dental implants to be usable for prosthetic dental restoration. Accurate infraorbital rim reconstruction is essential to prevent lower lid malposition and create a platform for orbital floor reconstruction to prevent enophthalmos and hypoglobus.[7] The midfacial bony framework also allows for optimal draping of soft tissue for prevention of orocutaneous and nasocutaneous fistulae.

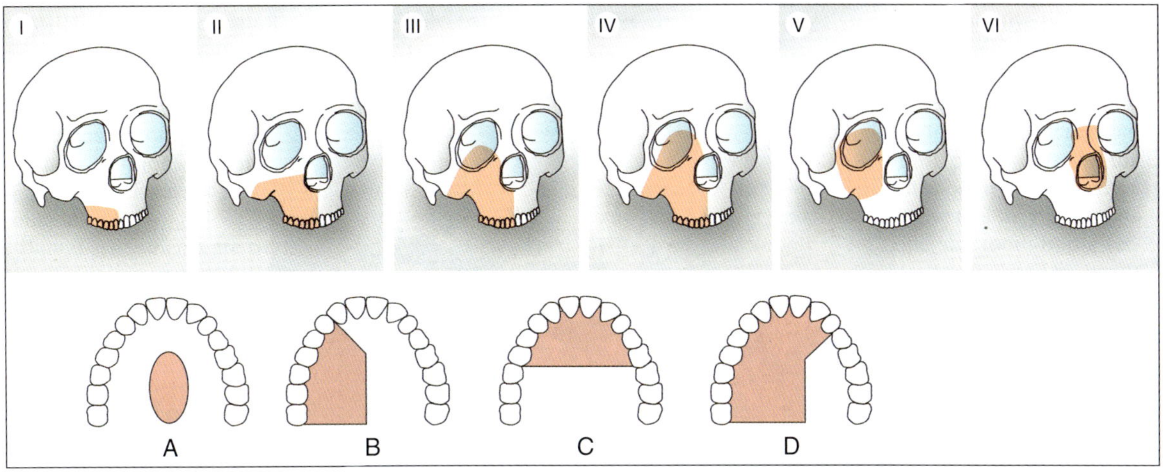


**Fig. 7.4** Brown classification. Vertical classification: I—maxillectomy not causing an oronasal fistula; II—not involving the orbit; III—involving the orbital adnexae with orbital retention; IV—with orbital enucleation or exenteration; V—orbitomaxillary defect; VI—nasomaxillary defect. Horizontal classification: A—palatal defect only, not involving the dental alveolus; B—less than or equal to 1/2 unilateral; C—less than or equal to 1/2 bilateral or transverse anterior; D—greater than 1/2 maxillectomy. Letters refer to the increasing complexity of the dentoalveolar and palatal defect and qualify the vertical dimension.

Computer-assisted design/computer-assisted modeling (CAD/CAM) and three-dimensional (3D) printing technology allows creation of customized flap and plate designs that are specific to the defect and patient's anatomy. It provides unlimited possibilities for designing complex osteotomies and plate configurations. This has decreased the traditionally steep learning curve for midface reconstruction resulting in accurate reconstructions that are reproducible across surgeons and centers. Computer-assisted surgery (CAS) is especially useful for delayed reconstruction in which there is no specimen to base the bone lengths and osteotomy angles on. Furthermore, there may be significant soft tissue contraction, making assessment of the original defect very difficult.[6] One CAS technique to assist in delayed reconstruction is mirroring of the contralateral uninvolved maxilla onto the defect.[8] For total maxillectomy defects there is no contralateral normal for mirroring; therefore, vendors can provide stock normative data of the midface during the CAS process. An alternative is to obtain a computed tomography (CT) scan of the patient with an obturator in place to provide information about the occlusal height and angulation.

A major advantage of CAS is the ability to place osseointegrated dental implants at the time of reconstruction. Implants can be positioned in a functionally favorable location and trajectory and optimal areas of fibula bone thickness. It also allows implants to be placed in nonradiated bone, thus reducing risk of wound healing complications and osteoradionecrosis.[9] Placement of dental implants prior to radiation has higher rates of osseointegration than when implants are placed into irradiated bone.[10] Primary implant placement has resulted in higher rates of dental rehabilitation, as traditionally a very small percentage of patients underwent delayed dental implant placement.[11] Furthermore, it saves an extra operation for the patient.

CAD/CAM also allows fabrication of patient-specific hardware. Novel shaped plates can be designed, including extension arms in multiple planes, to capture buttresses for more stable fixation (Fig. 7.5). A 3D printed plate also eliminates inaccuracies in contouring plates freehand and avoids screw hole distortion from trial-and-error bending. For delayed reconstructions where normal anatomy is distorted the printed plate serves as a useful reference to guide the construct position. Stereolithographic models can also be generated, and plates can be adapted to these models. Orbital floor reconstruction can be performed more accurately by fabricating custom orbital implants or bending titanium meshes on stereolithographic models.[12] Obturators can also be fabricated using CAD/CAM technology.[13] This simplifies the process for clinicians by decreasing the tedious hands-on work traditionally required with getting impressions. It thus increases patient comfort, especially for individuals with restricted mouth opening.

CAS can also help with tumor resection through the creation of osteotomy guides on the maxilla. In the compact and complex structure of the midface, it may be difficult to determine appropriate margins in the operating room. Computer imaging allows visualization of tumor in 3D, we fabricate both bone- and occlusal-based guides, since sometimes the inability to clear soft tissue off adjacent normal maxilla due to space constraints makes placement of a cutting guide on the bone very difficult. Stereolithographic models are used for bending fixation plates and orbital floor plates. They are useful to have as a reference for the bone flap construct. 3D-printed patient-specific fixation plates are extremely useful as they allow accurate bone fixation even with limited visualization.

**Stereolithographic model**

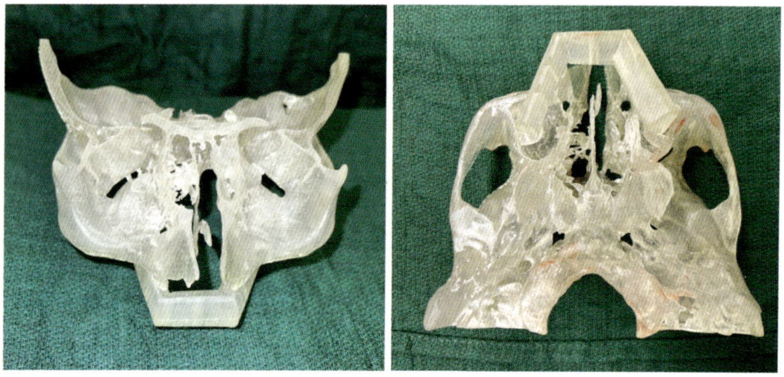

**Maxillary cutting guides**

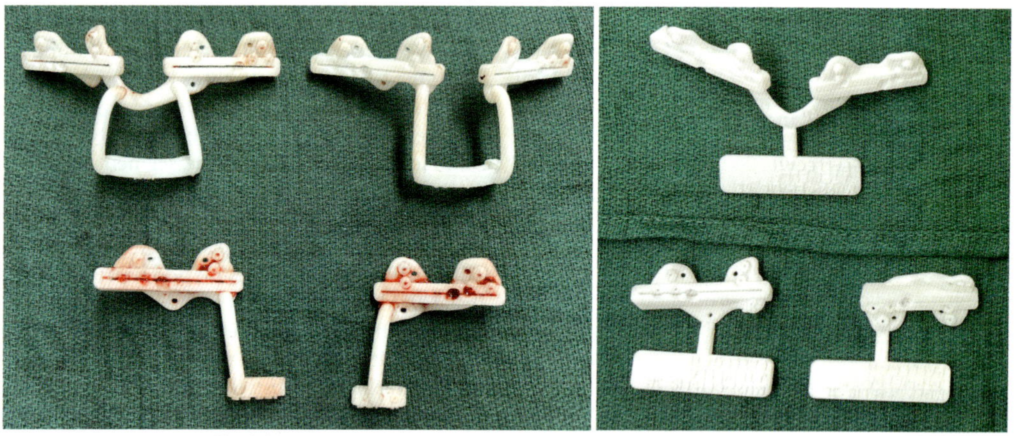

Tooth-borne guides

Bone-borne guides

**Dental implant alignment guide**

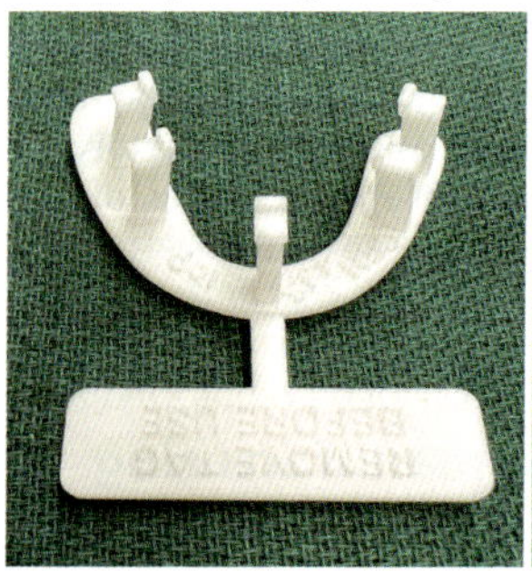

**Fibula cutting guide**

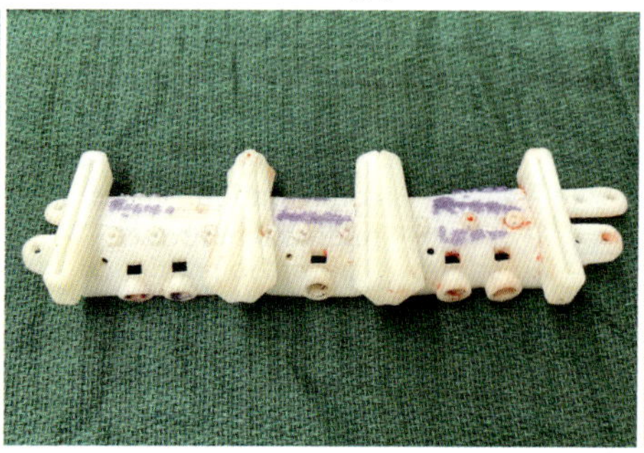

**3D printed plate**

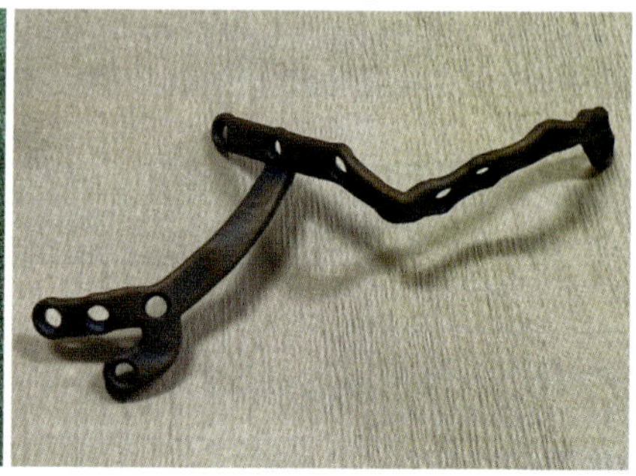

## Operative technique

The operative steps for midface reconstruction using computer-assisted technology are demonstrated in Video 7.2. A brief description is as follows:

- Tumor extirpation is performed by the ablative team. Access is typically via an intraoral gingivobuccal sulcus or a Weber-Ferguson incision.
- Cutting guides, either bone or tooth borne, are placed. Proper guide placement is indicated by press fit of guide on the bone or teeth and by confirming the position of the cutting segment in relation to the teeth as planned by CAD.
- Predictive holes for the plate are drilled into the non-affected bone using the slots in the guide. A drill guide is used as the trajectory of the predictive holes needs to be correct.
- Osteotomies are made with a sagittal saw. Cutting guide is removed.
- A fibula flap is harvested in the standard fashion.[18] Cutting guides are placed on the fibula. They should be placed on the exact location of the fibula as planned by CAM; the septal perforator can serve as a reference. The fibula shape is not uniform throughout its length.[17] Any deviation in location of guide placement on the fibula from the preoperative plan will result in the patient-specific plates not adapting properly to the bone. Predictive holes for the plate are drilled with the aid of drill guides.
- Dental implants are placed by the dental service. The guides for dental implants ensure proper implant location and trajectory.
- The periosteum is cleared behind the fibula at osteotomy sites and an instrument is placed immediately behind the bone to protect the pedicle. Osteotomies are made with a sagittal saw. The cutting guide is removed.
- The patient-specific plate is fixated to the bone segments by placing screws into the predictive holes. There should be good bone to bone contact between the segments.
- Perfusion of the skin paddle is assessed. We use indocyanine green (ICG) angiography. Areas with suboptimal perfusion are removed.
- The anterior surface of the pedicle is marked with methylene blue. The pedicle is ligated. The flap is brought to the defect. The pedicle is passed through the retromandibular tunnel into the neck with the aid of a Penrose drain. The methylene blue markings are checked to confirm that pedicle has not twisted.
- The construct is fixated to the native maxilla by placing screws into the previously drilled predictive holes. Good bone to bone contact should be obtained. The skin paddle is then inset.
- Microvascular anastomosis is performed. The most commonly used arteries in our practice are the facial and superior thyroid arteries. The most commonly used veins are the common facial vein or the internal jugular vein end to side.
- Lip and cheek closure is performed. Neck is washed out. An implantable Doppler is placed around the artery for postoperative monitoring. Drains are placed in the neck and skin closure is performed.

### CLINICAL CASE 1

A 51-year-old female was diagnosed with squamous cell carcinoma of the right posterior maxilla (Fig. 7.6A). A right-sided infrastructure maxillectomy was planned. Computer-assisted design/computer-assisted modeling was used to plan reconstruction with a right-sided fibula osteocutaneous flap, along with immediate dental implant placement and a 3D printed plate (Figs. 7.6B–E). Resection was performed via a Weber-Ferguson approach. The fibular construct fit like a puzzle piece into the defect (Fig. 7.6F). The fibular bone was used for alveolar reconstruction and the skin paddle was used to resurface the palate (Fig. 7.6G). The patient did well postoperatively and resumed a regular diet.

### CLINICAL CASE 2

A 65-year-old male developed a recurrent adenoid cystic carcinoma of the maxilla, after previous resection and radiation (Fig. 7.7A). A total maxillectomy was planned. Computer-assisted design/computer-assisted modeling (CAD/CAM) was used to plan reconstruction with a left-sided fibula osteocutaneous flap, along with immediate dental implant placement and three-dimensional printed plate (Figs. 7.7B–G). CAD/CAM is especially useful in these cases with multiple osteotomies, as even a small error in each osteotomy angle is magnified, cumulatively altering the shape of the construct (Fig. 7.7F). The fibula bone was used for alveolar reconstruction and the skin paddle was used to resurface the palate (Figs. 7.7H–J).

## Fidelity/verification

The biggest advantage of CAD/CAM technology is that it allows for highly accurate reconstruction based on the patient's unique anatomy. Intraoperatively, indicators of concordance with the preoperative plan are good bone to bone contact and apposition of plate to the bone. Moreover,

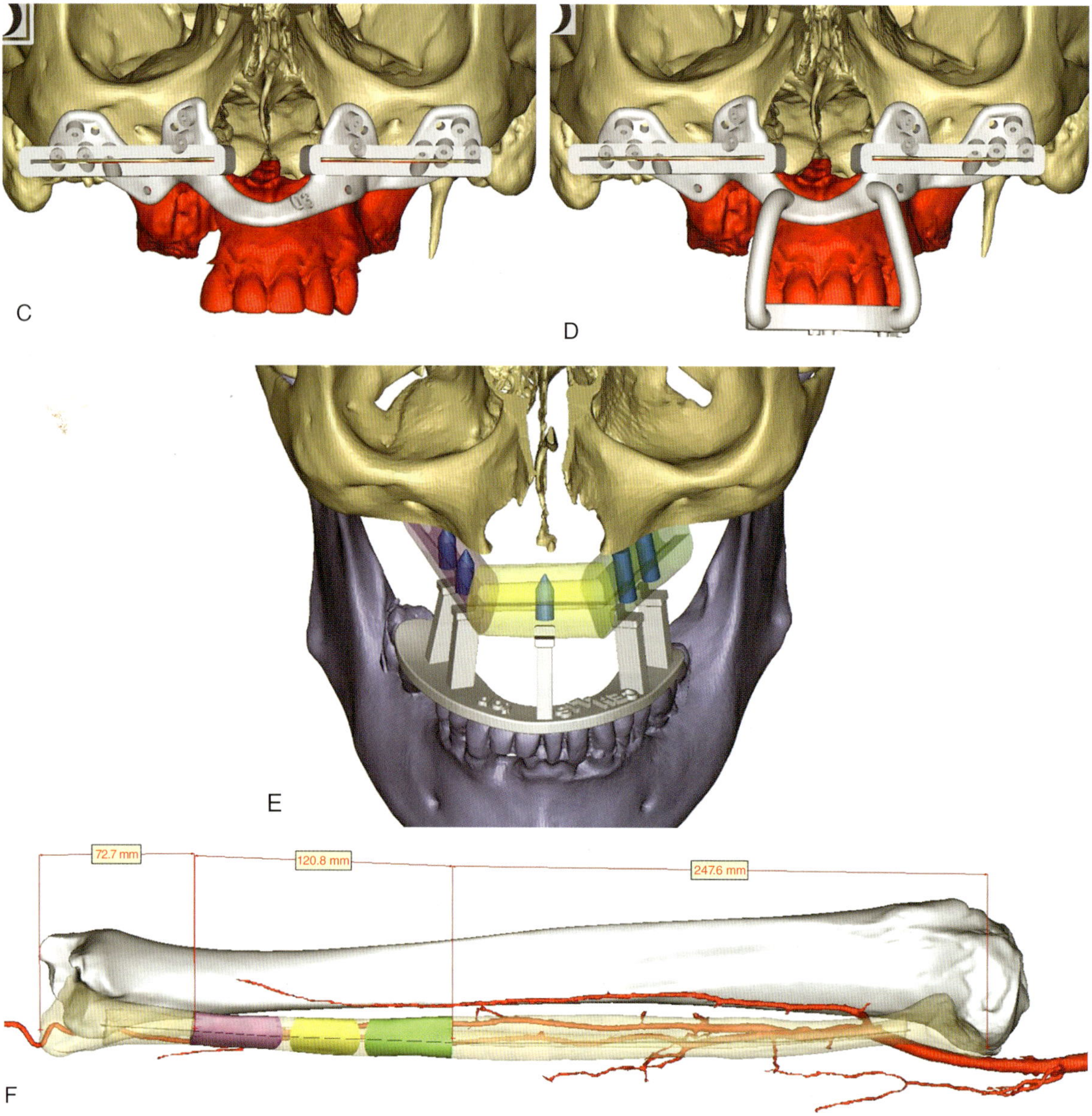


**Fig. 7.7, cont'd** (C) Bone-based cutting guides. (D) Tooth-borne cutting guides. (E) Dental implant alignment guide, used to confirm proper positioning of dental implants before rigid fixation. (F) Fibula osteotomies.

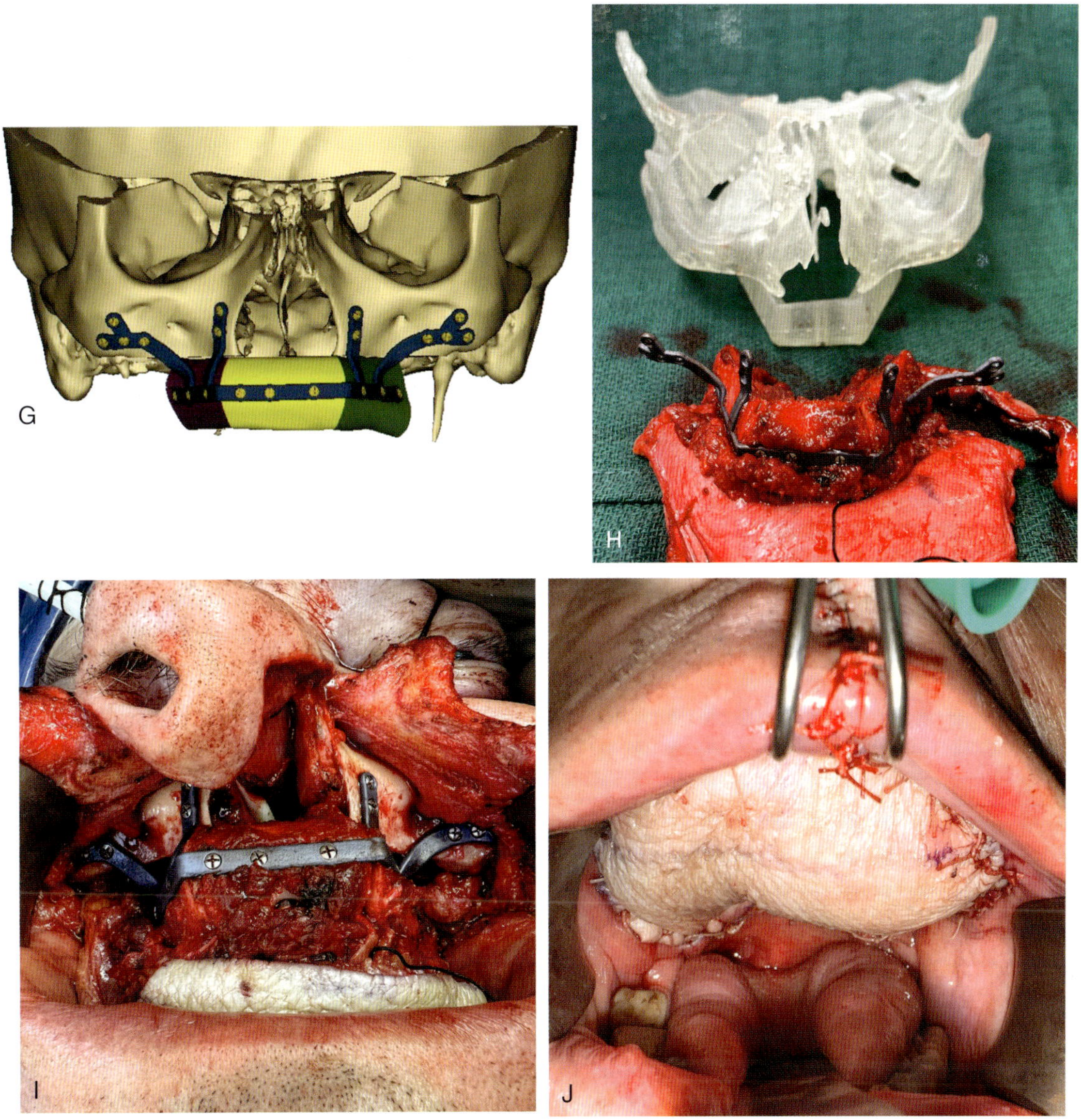


**Fig. 7.7, cont'd** (G) Three-dimensional printed plate. (H) Fibula flap construct matches the stereolithographic model. (I) Flap inset. (J) Skin paddle used to resurface the palate.

the fibula reconstruction with the adapted plate is highly accurate so serves as a reference to guide insetting. The surgeon should consider modifying the midface defect if there are problems during insetting. After inset, the occlusal relationship of the upper and lower jaw is observed. Anatomic bone positioning is critical for dental rehabilitation as the implants need to be in proper position for prosthesis fabrication. Postoperative assessment can be performed via imaging with computed tomography and orthopantomogram. Zhu et al. used open-source software to create 3D digital models to assess accuracy of reconstruction.[7] They assessed pre- and postoperative differences on infraorbital rim height, globe height, lower lid height, and orbital volume.

## Pearls/pitfalls

- The fibula has an alpha helical twist and therefore the shape of the bone is not uniform throughout.[17] When making fibular osteotomies, cutting guides should be placed on the exact location planned via CAD/CAM, otherwise the guides will not sit flush with the fibula and therefore bone cuts may not be completely accurate.
- Accurate bone cuts are especially important if a computer-generated plate is used. Otherwise, as the plate is fixated on to the bone segments, there will be maladaptation and/or bone gaps.
- Ensure that all hardware is covered with vascularized tissue. Otherwise, hardware infections may occur due to communication with sinuses and oronasal cavities. These infections can occur long term.
- In scapular flaps, soft tissue attachments on the bone may be bulky. Maintenance of these attachments is paramount for bone perfusion. Guides may thus not oppose well to bone. This problem can be tackled in a few ways. The guides can be offset by 3 to 5 mm to account for the soft tissue over the bone.[16] Alternatively, "negative cutting guides" can be manufactured that fixate on the part of the bone that is staying in situ; soft tissue can be removed off this bone and then repaired after bone is harvested.[16]
- In the operating room, it may be discovered that the planned resection margins are not sufficient (e.g., due to tumor growth or unappreciated extent of radionecrotic bone). We routinely create a second set of cutting guides with a wider margin, just in case this situation arises.[19]

## Outcomes/complications

CAS ensures that the ablative, reconstructive, and dental surgeons communicate and formulate a definitive surgical strategy prior to the operation. Most critical decisions are made beforehand, facilitating a smooth conduct of the operation. CAD/CAM has been shown to decrease ischemia and operative times.[20,21] Chang et al. compared 92 mandible reconstructions performed with CAS to 43 reconstructions with stereolithic models.[22] The CAS group required less intraoperative revisions and saved an average of 2 hours.[22] Similarly, Navarro Cuellar et al.[20] found ischemia time was shorter by 25 minutes and the total operative time by 1.5 hours in patients who had CAS compared to those who did not.

CAS has also been shown to result in more accurate reconstruction compared with standard bone shaping techniques.[20,23] Zhang et al. compared the accuracy of maxillectomy reconstruction with and without computer-assisted techniques and found that computer-assisted reconstruction was significantly more accurate than conventional freehand techniques.[24] The difference in position of fibula segments and the computer-assisted plan was <5 mm. Swendseid et al. compared 9 patients who had midface defects reconstructed with CAS with 14 cases.[16] CAS was associated with a higher number of successfully reconstructed subunits, higher number of successful bony contact between segments, and a higher percentage of segments in anatomic position. Postoperative bone position was within less than 1 cm of ideal bone position in 82% of CAS reconstructed cases. Navarro Cuellar et al. compared reconstructive outcomes between patients with and without CAS and found that the fibula bones were in anatomic position in 100% of CAS patients compared to 66% in the conventional group.[20] Bone apposition was 100% vs 83.3% in the CAS and conventional groups, respectively. Aesthetic results were significantly better in the CAS group. Similarly, Tarsitano et al. reported good reproducibility between the CAS plan and the reconstruction with less than 1 mm of deviation between the plan and the final outcomes.[25] A recent systematic review of computer-assisted surgery in maxillary reconstruction showed that the accuracy of bone segment positioning was 0.44 to 7.8 mm and 2.90 degrees to 6.96 degrees.[23] The postoperative dental implant position compared to preoperative computer-assisted planning, showed a mean center point deviation of 4.95 mm and a mean angulation deviation of 6.26 degrees. Bone to bone contact was achieved in 88% cases.

Pang et al. used CAD/CAM to perform staged reconstruction of oncologic maxillary defects.[26] The first operation consisted of maxillary tumor resection. After final pathology confirmed margins, neck dissection and reconstruction were performed at a second stage using CAD/CAM technology. This strategy allowed definitive margin confirmation prior to undertaking a challenging reconstruction.

The biggest barrier to adaptation of CAD/CAM is cost. CAS saves time in the operating room, which may arguably offset the expense of this technology. Some institutions are setting up in-house CAS, using open-source software for computer-assisted modeling.[7,27] Manufacturing of models and guides is then done by 3D printers.

## Conclusion

Computer-assisted surgery allows highly accurate reconstruction of complex and delayed maxillary defects, which is reproducible across centers and surgeons of varying expertise. Custom plates can be manufactured that conform to specific bony design and capture facial buttresses more accurately for secure fixation. CAD/CAM allows for placement of immediate dental implants, resulting in higher rates of dental rehabilitation and potentially lower complication rates by avoiding placement of implants in radiated bone. Patient-specific obturators and orbital floor implants can be designed, resulting in more accurate functional restoration. CAS also helps the ablative surgeon plan resection margins as it may be difficult to visualize tumor extent in the small working space of the midface.

## Take-home points

- CAD/CAM allows precise design of osteotomies and plates for accurate bony reconstruction.
- The most important utility of this technology may be for delayed or secondary defects, where there is soft tissue distortion and a specimen is not present for reference.
- Primary dental implant placement is a major benefit of CAD/CAM, allowing osseointegrated implants to be placed in optimal location and trajectory.
- Flap ischemia time and total operative time are reduced, potentially resulting in improved outcomes and decreased total costs.

## References


1. Manson PN, Hoopes JE, Su CT. Structural pillars of the facial skeleton: an approach to the management of Le Fort fractures. *Plast Reconstr Surg*. 1980;66(1): 54-62.
2. Rodriguez ED, Bluebond-Langner R, Park JE, Manson PN. Preservation of contour in periorbital and midfacial craniofacial microsurgery: reconstruction of the soft-tissue elements and skeletal buttresses. *Plast Reconstr Surg*. 2008;121(5):1738-1747.
3. Cordeiro PG, Santamaria E. A classification system and algorithm for reconstruction of maxillectomy and midfacial defects. *Plast Reconstr Surg*. 2000;105(7):2331-2346; discussion 2347-2348.
4. Dooley L, Shah J. Management of the neck in maxillary sinus carcinomas. *Curr Opin Otolaryngol Head Neck Surg*. 2015;23(2): 107-114.
5. Brown JS, Shaw RJ. Reconstruction of the maxilla and midface: introducing a new classification. *Lancet Oncol*. 2010;11(10): 1001-1008.
6. Myers PL, Nelson JA, Rosen EB, Allen Jr RJ, Disa JJ, Matros E. Virtual surgical planning for oncologic mandibular and maxillary reconstruction. *Plast Reconstr Surg Glob Open*. 2021;9(9):e3672.
7. Zhu B, Han M, Heaton C, Park AM, Seth R, Knott PD. Assessing free flap reconstruction accuracy of the midface and orbit using computer-aided modeling software. *Facial Plast Surg Aesthet Med*. 2020;22(2):93-99.
8. Nwagu U, Swendseid B, Ross H, Ganti R, Kane A, Curry JM. Maxillectomy reconstruction revision using virtual surgical planning and intraoperative navigation. *Laryngoscope*. 2021;131(10): E2655-E2659.
9. Allen Jr RJ, Shenaq DS, Rosen EB, et al. Immediate dental implantation in oncologic jaw reconstruction: workflow optimization to decrease time to full dental rehabilitation. *Plast Reconstr Surg Glob Open*. 2019;7(1):e2100.
10. Panchal H, Shamsunder MG, Petrovic I, et al. Dental implant survival in vascularized bone flaps: a systematic review and meta-analysis. *Plast Reconstr Surg*. 2020;146(3):637-648.
11. Anne-Gaelle B, Samuel S, Julie B, Renaud L, Pierre B. Dental implant placement after mandibular reconstruction by microvascular free fibula flap: current knowledge and remaining questions. *Oral Oncol*. 2011;47(12):1099-1104.
12. Le Clerc N, Baudouin R, Carlevan M, Khoueir N, Verillaud B, Herman P. 3D titanium implant for orbital reconstruction after maxillectomy. *J Plast Reconstr Aesthet Surg*. 2020;73(4): 732-739.
13. Jiao T, Zhu C, Dong X, Gu X. Rehabilitation of maxillectomy defects with obturator prostheses fabricated using computer-aided design and rapid prototyping: a pilot study. *Int J Prosthodont*. 2014;27(5):480-486.

14. Witjes MJH, Schepers RH, Kraeima J. Impact of 3D virtual planning on reconstruction of mandibular and maxillary surgical defects in head and neck oncology. *Curr Opin Otolaryngol Head Neck Surg*. 2018;26(2):108-114.
15. Breik O, Idle M, Martin T, Praveen P, Parmar S. Three-dimensional computer-assisted surgical planning and manufacturing in complex maxillary reconstruction. *Atlas Oral Maxillofac Surg Clin North Am*. 2020;28(2):151-164.
16. Swendseid BP, Roden DF, Vimawala S, et al. Virtual surgical planning in subscapular system free flap reconstruction of midface defects. *Oral Oncol*. 2020;101:104508.
17. Rosen EB, Kyle Gazdeck R, Goldman DA, et al. An anatomic analysis of fibula flap mandible reconstructions: implications for endosseous implant placement. *Plast Reconstr Surg*. 2022;149(6):1419-1428.
18. Hidalgo DA. Fibula free flap: a new method of mandible reconstruction. *Plast Reconstr Surg*. 1989;84(1):71-79.
19. Shenaq DS, Matros E. Virtual planning and navigational technology in reconstructive surgery. *J Surg Oncol*. 2018;118(5):845-852.
20. Navarro Cuellar C, Martinez EB, Navarro Cuellar I, et al. Primary maxillary reconstruction with fibula flap and dental implants: a comparative study between virtual surgical planning and standard surgery in class IIC defects. *J Oral Maxillofac Surg*. 2021;79(1): 237-248.
21. Avraham T, Franco P, Brecht LE, et al. Functional outcomes of virtually planned free fibula flap reconstruction of the mandible. *Plast Reconstr Surg*. 2014;134(4):628e-634e.
22. Chang EI, Jenkins MP, Patel SA, Topham NS. Long-term operative outcomes of preoperative computed tomography-guided virtual surgical planning for osteocutaneous free flap mandible reconstruction. *Plast Reconstr Surg*. 2016;137(2):619-623.
23. van Baar GJC, Schipper K, Forouzanfar T, et al. Accuracy of computer-assisted surgery in maxillary reconstruction: a systematic review. *J Clin Med*. 2021;10(6):1226.
24. Zhang WB, Wang Y, Liu XJ, et al. Reconstruction of maxillary defects with free fibula flap assisted by computer techniques. *J Craniomaxillofac Surg*. 2015; 43(5):630-636.
25. Tarsitano A, Battaglia S, Ciocca L, Scotti R, Cipriani R, Marchetti C. Surgical reconstruction of maxillary defects using a computer-assisted design/ computer-assisted manufacturing-produced titanium mesh supporting a free flap. *J Craniomaxillofac Surg*. 2016; 44(9):1320-1326.
26. Pang JH, Brooke S, Kubik MW, et al. Staged reconstruction (delayed-immediate) of the maxillectomy defect using CAD/ CAM technology. *J Reconstr Microsurg*. 2018;34(3):193-199.
27. Smithers FAE, Cheng K, Jayaram R, Mukherjee P, Clark JR. Maxillofacial reconstruction using in-house virtual surgical planning. *ANZ J Surg*. 2018;88(9): 907-912.

Chapter | 8 |

# Computer-assisted surgical planning in head and neck reconstruction: mandible and dental restoration

Amanda Silva, Adam S. Jacobson, David Hirsch, Jamie P. Levine

**CHAPTER OUTLINE**



## Introduction

The free fibula flap has become the workhorse for mandible reconstruction. It was popularized by Hidalgo in 1989[1] and in its early iterations, involved creating intraoperative templates to guide osteotomies and hand-bend plates. Although this involved great artistry and skill, this method also carried a greater margin for error and could be time consuming.

In the decades following, advancements have improved the planning, accuracy, and efficiency of osseous free flap mandible reconstruction. In the 1990s, surgeons translated technology utilized in craniofacial surgery, and printed three-dimensional (3D) models of recipient defects and reconstructive templates to aid flap shaping.[2] This also allowed the ability to bend plates preoperatively. In the early 2000s, cutting jigs to create more precise osteotomies were used.[3] Soon after, surgeons started performing preoperative "virtual surgery" to fabricate more precise cutting guides.[4-6] Next, custom milled plates, which are thinner, stronger, and configured to specifically fit the defect were utilized.[7]

Dental restoration has evolved in parallel. Placement of immediate dental implants was introduced at the same time the free fibula was popularized for mandible reconstruction.[8] However, patients still underwent a period of osseointegration before the implants were loaded with a prosthesis, and the initial reconstructive plan was often not centered around occlusion. This led to greater challenges providing ultimate dental restoration. Over time, the use of computer-assisted surgical planning (CaSP) to refine dental implant placement[9,10] and earlier functional loading[11] has expedited the process and allowed the possibility of "jaw in a day" surgery.[12,13]

## Clinical considerations

It is important for the ablative, dental, and reconstructive surgeons to plan the surgery together. Because the fibula is the most often used flap for mandible reconstruction, we will focus on details related to this option. However, there are situations where other flaps may be better suited and CaSP can be utilized to assist reconstruction.

One of the first aspects to consider is the anticipated bony and soft tissue defect location and size. Unless this is a benign case with adequate gingiva, there will likely be a need for a skin paddle. One can plan to place the bony segments centered around the perforators depending on where the needed soft tissue is located. One needs to also determine if a second skin paddle or free flap will be necessary. Situations that may require this additional soft tissue are when there is an external skin defect or other oral cavity structures, such as the floor of mouth or tongue, that are involved.[14]

Another key determination is whether the vascular pedicle will run anterior or posterior. This may be determined by recipient vessel quality and availability, and whether the condyle needs to be reconstructed. This orientation will affect the soft tissue inset and planned laterality of the donor site. There are different schools of thought on how to orient and drape the skin paddle. Traditional thinking is to have the skin paddle septum drape over the posterior fibula in the lingual direction.[15] However, tighter inset may be better suited for dental implants, leading some to advocate having the septum drape over the lateral fibula and reconstruction plate in the buccal direction. This helps avoid skin paddle bulk and creates a buccal sulcus from the pull of the septum.[16]

Once the fibula laterality and orientation are decided, the next step is to determine how many osteotomies to perform for reconstruction. The native mandible can be ghosted or mirrored to help with optimal configuration. If the defect is anterior, a double-barrel configuration to help with lip support, and chin height and projection may be considered. However, the planning needs to maintain enough restorative space for dental rehabilitation.

When planning for dental rehabilitation, it is important to ensure the reconstructed mandible will align with the opposing maxillary dentition, and that the implants are aligned through the occlusal or lingual surface of the teeth. Another consideration is the positioning of the fibula in the superior/inferior direction and its effects on dental rehabilitation versus optimizing lower mandible contour. There may be advantages to aligning the fibula along the mandible alveolus rather than the inferior border, which allows better prosthetic abutment-to-implant ratio.[6] Regardless, one needs to allow at least 15 mm of restorative space for dental rehabilitation.[13] When planning the location of the dental implants along the bone, there may be certain areas of the fibula that are better shaped and suited for placement of implants which will affect where the fibula is harvested in the proximal/distal direction.[10]

## Workflow for computer-assisted design/computer-assisted manufacturing

Please see Fig. 8.1.

## Computer-assisted design

Please see Figs. 8.2 to 8.4.

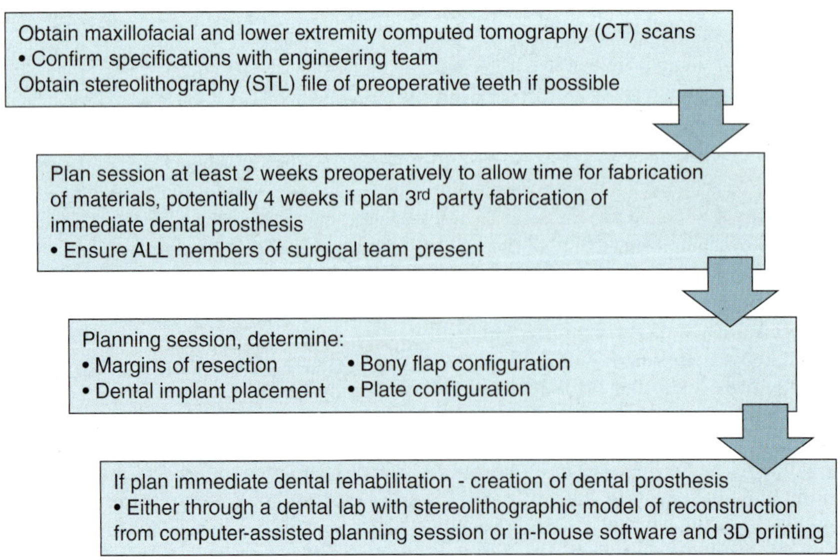


**Fig. 8.1** Workflow for computer-assisted design/computer-assisted manufacturing.

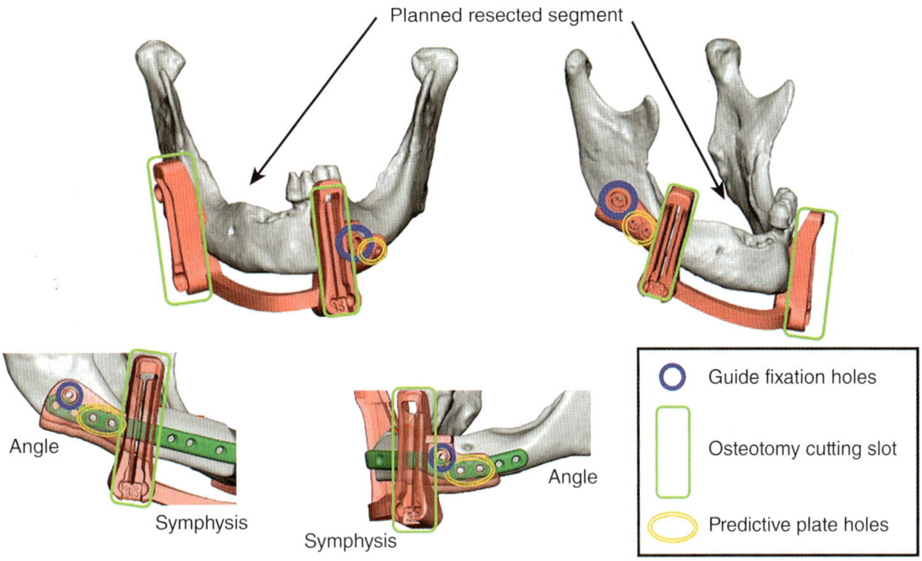


**Fig. 8.2** Mandible cutting guide. The mandible cutting guide affixes to the native mandible and contains osteotomy cutting slots that cut the mandible at the exact angle to fit to the fibula cut. It also contains guide fixation holes to secure it to the mandible and predictive plate holes that allow for predrilling of plate screw holes for accurate reconstruction plate placement.

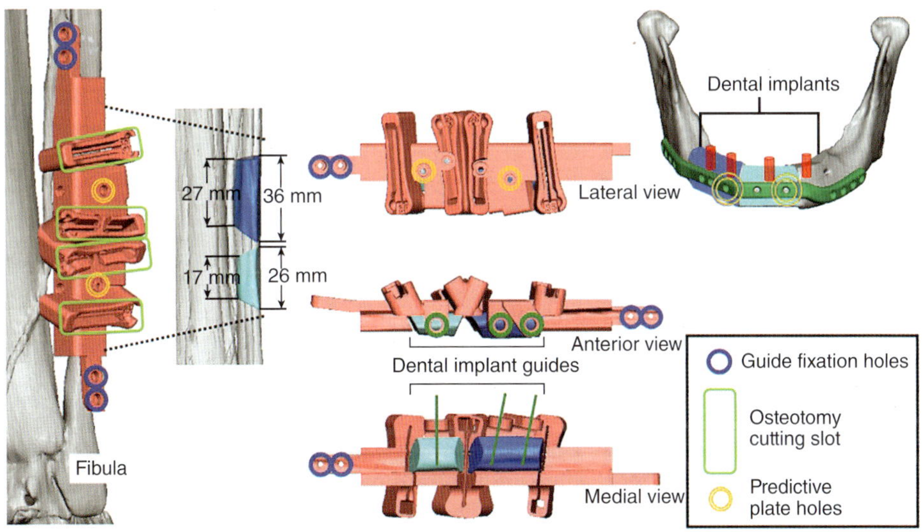


**Fig. 8.3** Fibula cutting guide. The fibula cutting guide affixes to the fibula bone to guide osteotomy cuts between the fibula segments and for inset to the mandible. It contains guide fixation holes to secure it to the mandible and can contain predictive plate holes that allow for predrilling of plate screw holes for accurate reconstruction plate placement. This can only be utilized when a patient-specific plate is planned and made. The precise nature of these predictive holes both in the jaw and the fibula make the reconstruction outcome match exactly to the preoperative plan. The guide can also contain holes to guide dental implant placement. It can be designed to be placed on the fibula in a very precise or less precise fashion. The less precise design may be beneficial to allow sliding of the guide along the fibula to better center the skin paddle over bony segments once the perforator anatomy is more clear or if there are deviations in the ablative plan. However, the more precise fit may be preferred for more accuracy and free hand or plan B options opted for if the ablative plan deviates. If planning for osseointegrated dental implant placement then a more precise fit will likely be necessary since the computer-assisted design/computer-assisted manufacturing plan usually takes into account the three-dimensional variability found in each fibula. If the positioning guide needs to be moved then the preciseness of implant placement cannot be guaranteed.

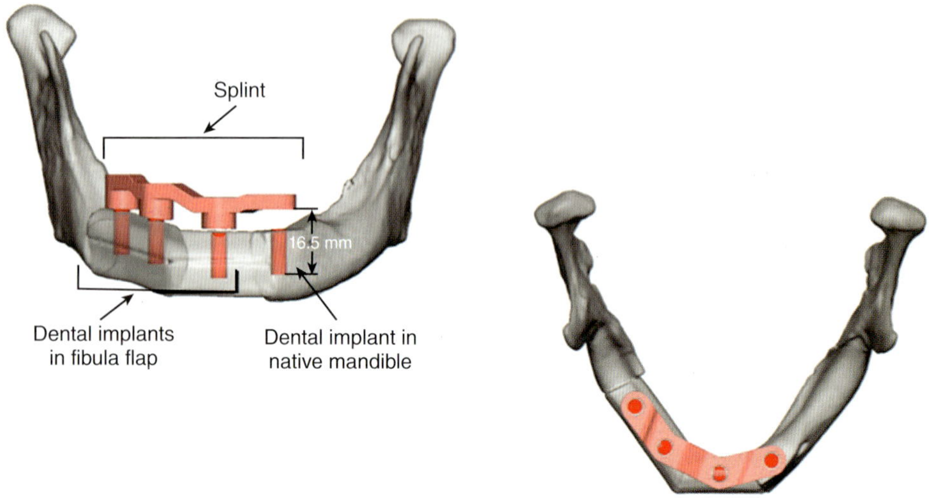


**Fig. 8.4** Dental splint. If planning dental rehabilitation, a dental splint may be fabricated to guide flap inset. The figure shows a splint utilized in a patient with an edentulous mandible. This splint fits on the dental implants to help guide proper flap inset. If a patient has residual dentition, splints may be fabricated to fit on to the occlusive plane and the dental implants.

## Computer-assisted manufacturing

Please see Fig. 8.5.

## Operative technique

Steps of the procedure. Please see Figs. 8.6 to 8.8 (see Video 8.1).

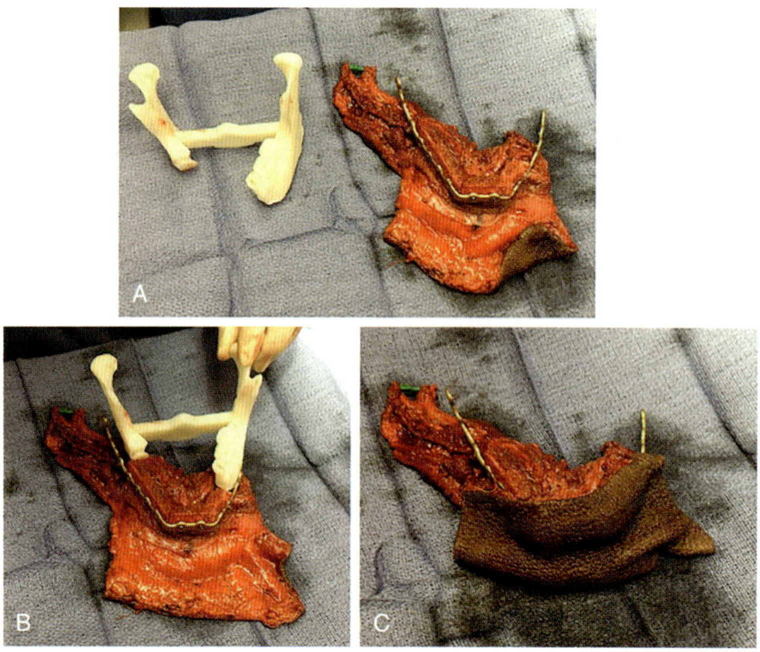


**Fig. 8.5** Stereolithographic model demonstrating defect after resection, allowing test-run of actual flap inset. (A) A stereolithographic model of the planned defect after resection and the harvested osteocutaneous free fibula flap secured to the custom reconstruction plate. (B) Demonstration of the stereolithographic model inset to the osteocutaneous free fibula flap to test inset fit. (C) Osteocutaneous free fibula flap with skin paddle draped as planned to reconstruct external skin defect.

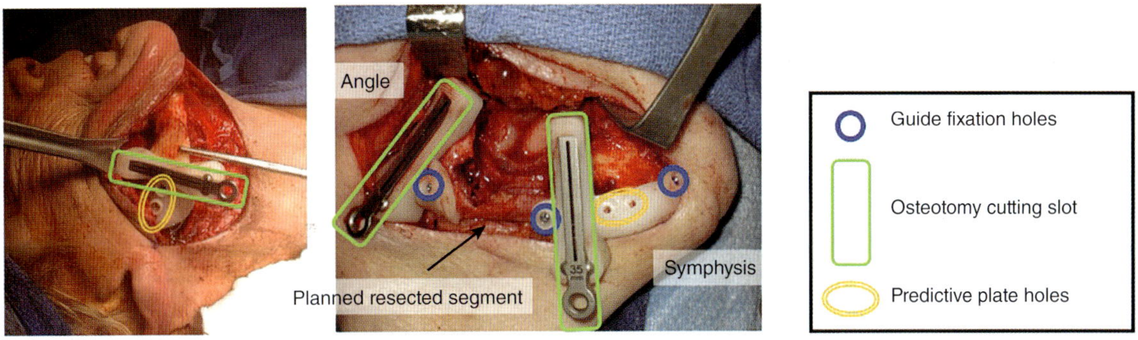


Resection steps:
1. Exposure and fitting of cutting guides. Cutting guides secured in place through guide fixation holes.
2. Predictive holes for reconstruction plate drilled into native mandible.
3. Metal guides snap into osteotomy cutting guide and cuts made with an oscillating saw blade to resect bony specimen.

**Fig. 8.6** Resection.

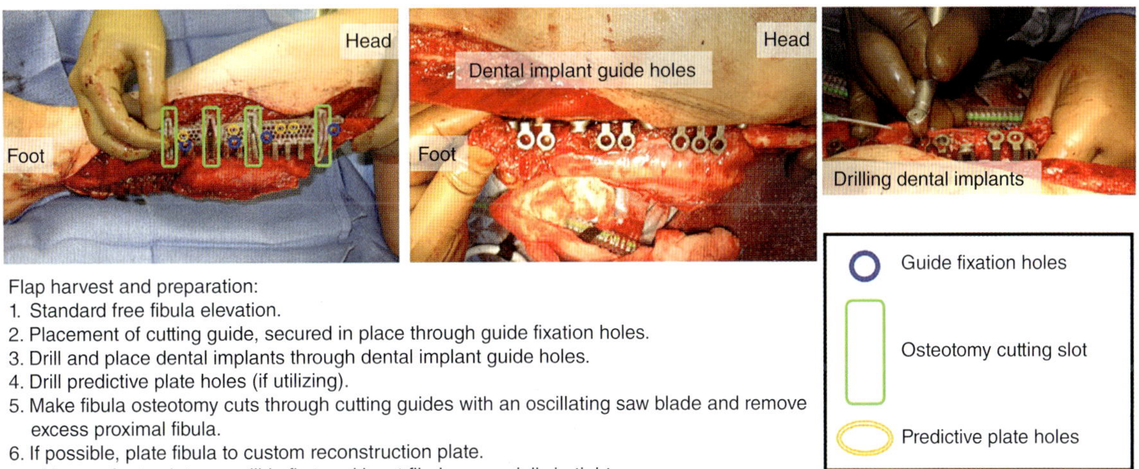


Flap harvest and preparation:
1. Standard free fibula elevation.
2. Placement of cutting guide, secured in place through guide fixation holes.
3. Drill and place dental implants through dental implant guide holes.
4. Drill predictive plate holes (if utilizing).
5. Make fibula osteotomy cuts through cutting guides with an oscillating saw blade and remove excess proximal fibula.
6. If possible, plate fibula to custom reconstruction plate.
   - May prefer to plate mandible first and inset fibula, especially in tighter spaces.
7. Harvest flap.

**Fig. 8.7** Flap harvest and preparation.

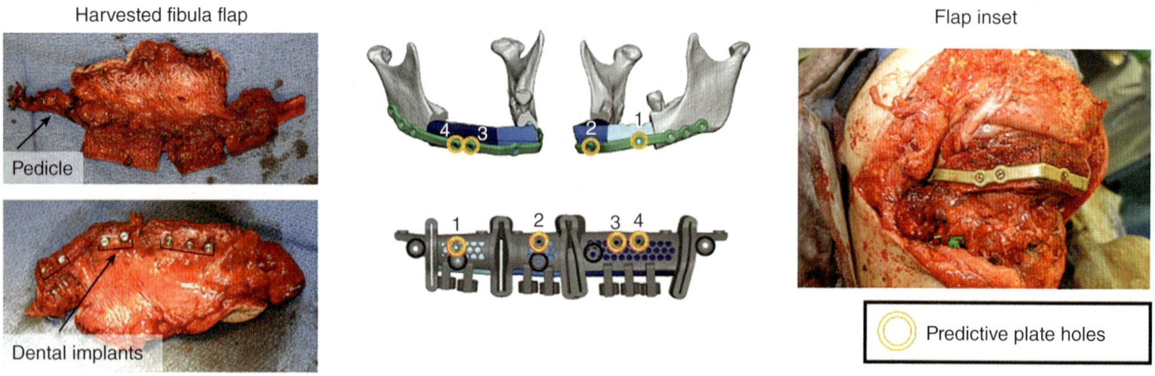


Flap inset:

1. Inset bone and screw reconstruction plate in place via prior drilled predictive holes on mandible. If planning dental rehabilitation, utilize a dental splint to properly guide orientation of fibula for prior dental implant orientation.
2. Inset of soft tissue. If planning immediate dental rehabilitation may need to cut slits in the skin paddle to inset around dental implants. If a benign case it's ideal to use native gingiva or the fibula fascia to avoid skin paddle bulk.
3. Microsurgical anastomosis.
4. If performing immediate dental rehabilitation, place dental prosthesis.

**Fig. 8.8** Flap inset.

## CLINICAL CASE

This is a patient who underwent resection of the anterior mandible and reconstruction with a 3-segment free fibula flap with immediate dental implant placement. Fig. 8.9 shows the patient's preoperative three-dimensional (3D) CT scan. Fig. 8.10 shows her planned resection and mandible osteotomy cutting guides in place. Fig. 8.11 shows her planned 3-segment free fibula reconstruction with immediate dental implant placement. Figs. 8.12 and 8.13 show her postoperative 3D CT scan and panorex. Figs. 8.14 and 8.15 show her healed dental implants and dental prothesis in place. Fig. 8.16 shows her preoperative and postoperative appearance.

### Fidelity/verification

Historically, we evaluated the computer-assisted design/computer-assisted manufacturing plan compared to the postoperative scan and found very good accuracy, usually within 2 mm (unpublished data). However, over time this has proven to be unnecessary as the plates and splints themselves offer verification of fit. Any past inaccuracy could likely be attributed to hand-bending the plates to match the models, but with custom-milled plates, the fit of the plate provides the plan verification. Other inaccuracies were likely due to flexibility in the earlier generation cutting guides. The cutting guides have become stronger, and if using the titanium insert, it doesn't allow for wiggle. Additionally, if the patient is undergoing immediate dental rehabilitation, the intraoperative splint guides the perfect inset. Therefore, with use of current planning, patient-specific guides and plates, there is little need to check for accuracy unless the guides or plate did not appear to fit precisely enough.

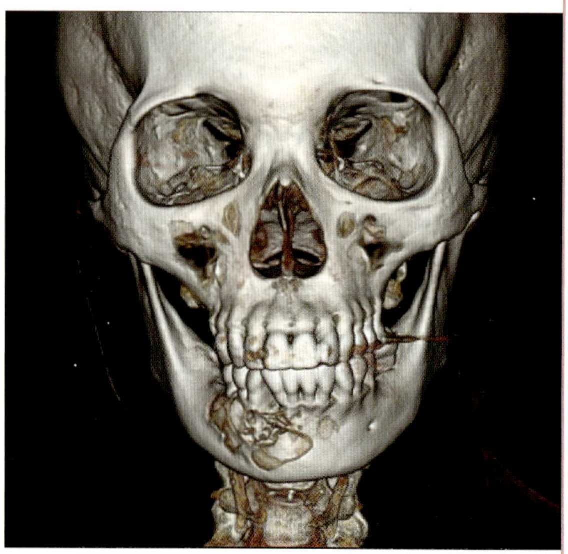

**Fig. 8.9**

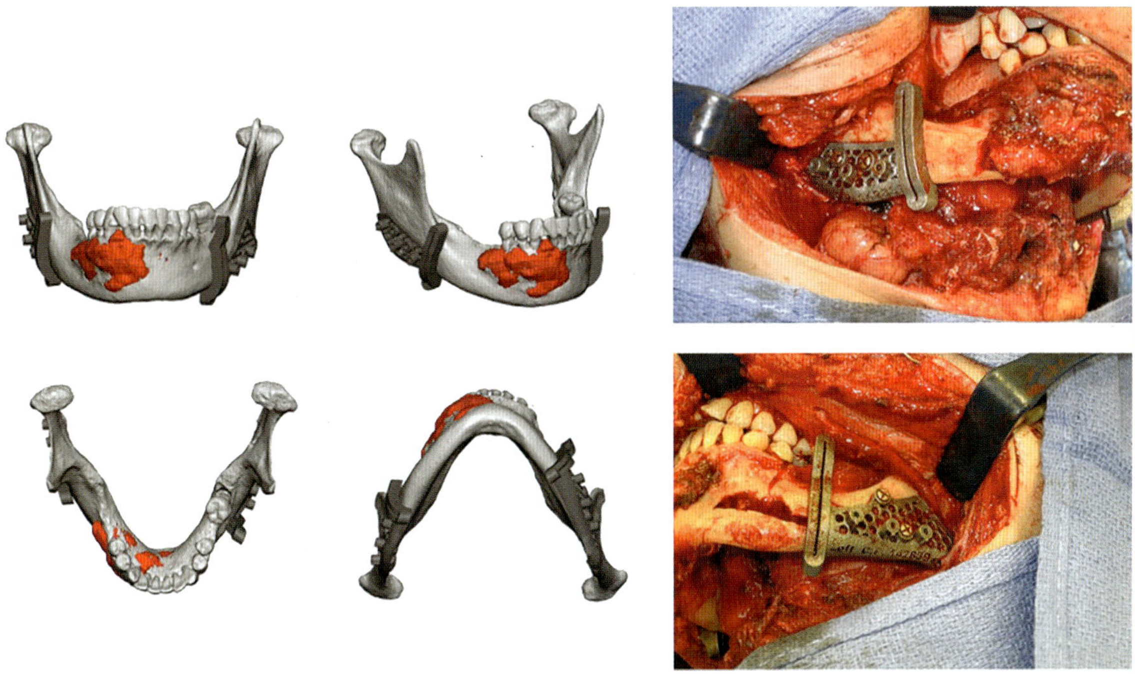

Fig. 8.10

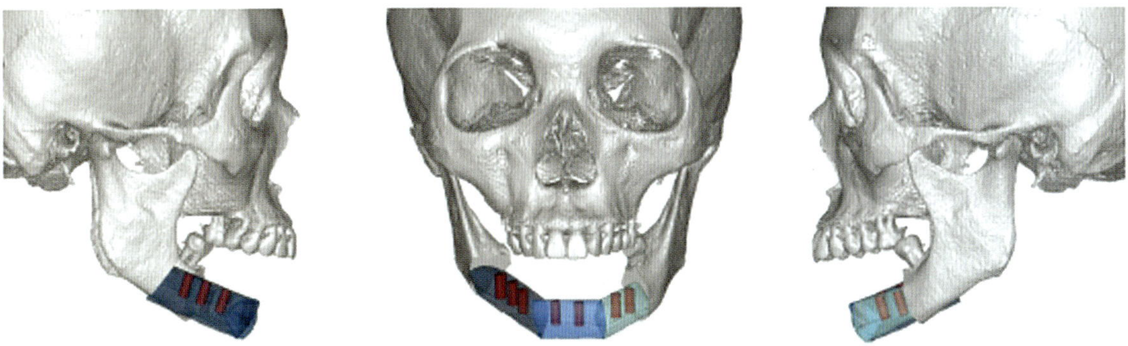

Fig. 8.11

*Continued*

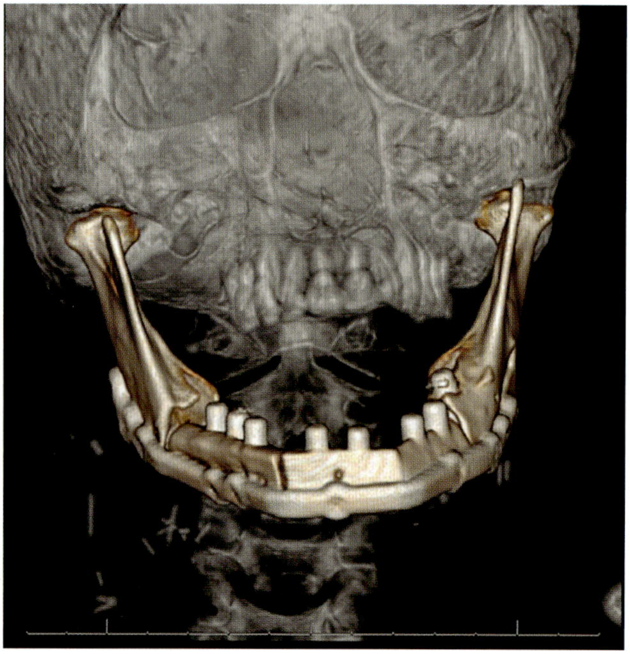

Fig. 8.12

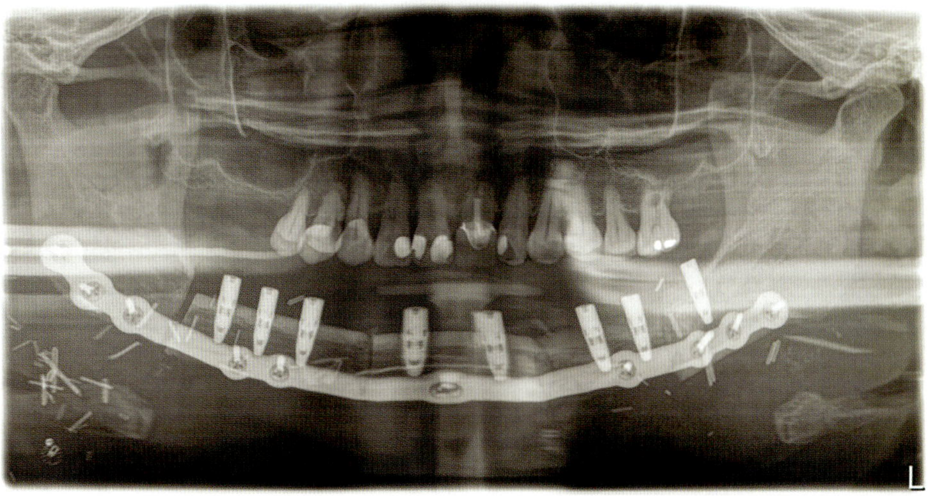


Fig. 8.13

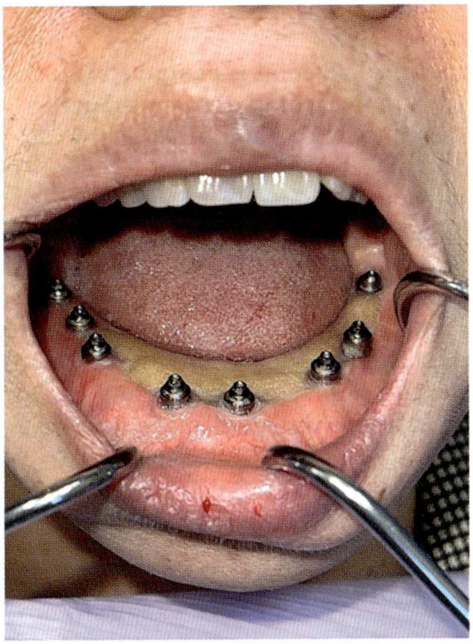

Fig. 8.14

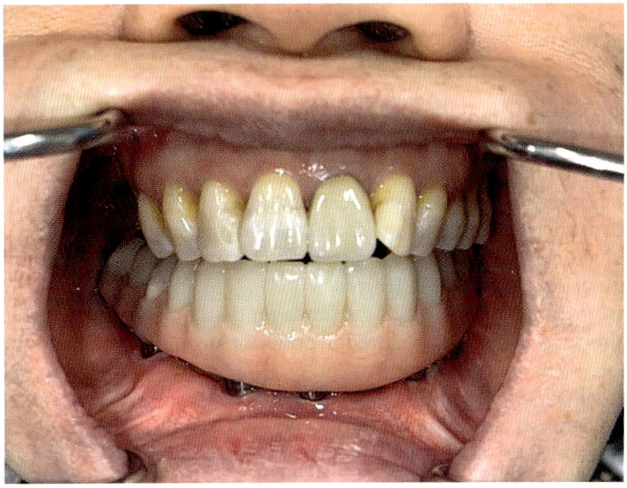

Fig. 8.15

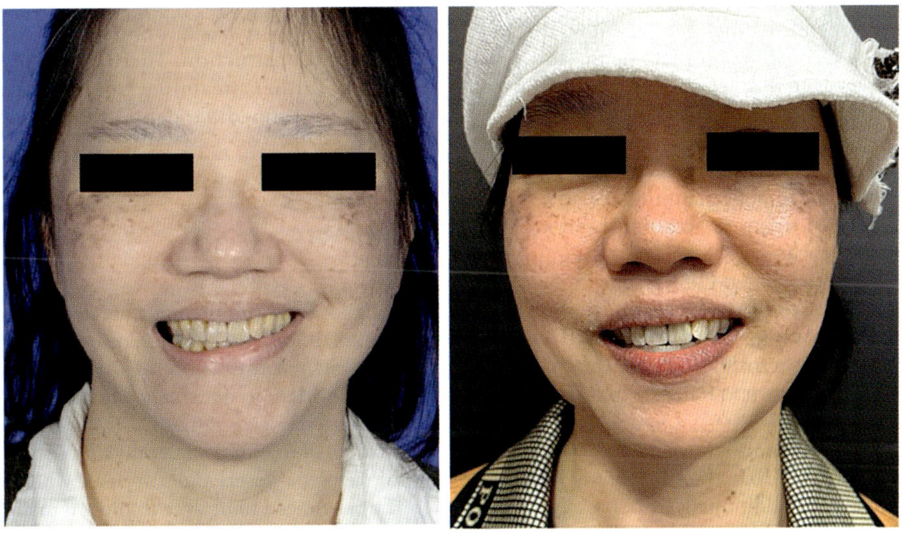

Preoperative Postoperative

Fig. 8.16

immediate dental implant placement in free fibula flaps for oncologic mandibular reconstruction. *Plast Reconstr Surg*. 2020;146:768e-776e.
23. Sandoval ML, Rosen EB, Allen Jr R, Nelson JA, Matros E, Gelblum DY. Immediate dental implants in fibula free flaps to reconstruct the mandible: A pilot study of the short-term effects on radiotherapy for patients with head and neck cancer. *Clin Implant Dent Relat Res*. 2020;22:91-95.
24. Smolka K, Kraehenbuehl M, Eggensperger N, et al. Fibula free flap reconstruction of the mandible in cancer patients: evaluation of a combined surgical and prosthodontic treatment concept. *Oral Oncol*. 2008;44: 571-581.
25. Schepers RH, Slagter AP, Kaanders JHAM, van den Hoogen FJA, Merkx MAW. Effect of postoperative radiotherapy on the functional results of implants placed during ablative surgery for oral cancer. *Int J Oral Maxillofac Surg*. 2006;35:803-808.

Chapter | 9 |

# Computer-assisted surgical planning in head and neck reconstruction: temporomandibular joint replacement

*Sydney H. Arnold, Michelle Seu, Amir Aminzada, Kelly A. Harmon, Christina Tragos*

**CHAPTER OUTLINE**



## Introduction

Total temporomandibular joint replacement (TMJR) is indicated for the treatment of inflammatory arthritis not responsive to other modalities of treatment, recurrent fibrous and/or bony ankylosis, failed tissue grafts, failed alloplastic temporomandibular joint (TMJ) reconstruction, or loss of vertical mandibular height and/or occlusal relationship (secondary to bone resorption, trauma, developmental abnormality, or pathologic lesion).[1] Early joint replacements using autologous tissue had a high rate of complication, particularly ankylosis (32.7%) and overgrowth (16.4%).[2] Alloplastic TMJR more readily conforms to the given anatomy, is less susceptible to systemic disease, does not require a donor site, and allows for early physical therapy. Initial prostheses were derived of proplast-teflon, silicone, or metal, all of which led to high rates of failure. Metal-on-metal stock prostheses were subsequently developed but faced similar challenges. These stock implants had difficulty with large orthognathic movements, issues with posterior TMJ dislocation, and problems treating patients with anomalous anatomy. Large orthognathic movements place significant angulation on the TMJ prosthesis, and previous implants were not designed to handle such strain. Additionally, stock joints may not fit the glenoid fossa or mandibular ramus and body in patients with anatomic variation.

Computer-assisted design/computer-assisted manufacture (CAD/CAM) technology has addressed many of the challenges faced by these traditional implants and is quickly gaining popularity as the custom TMJR components interface well with the host anatomy.[3,4] In 2015, Wolford proposed his protocol for concomitant TMJR and orthognathic surgery using CAD/CAM surgical simulation, which is widely used by surgeons. CAD/CAM allows for the development of custom TMJR prostheses made of titanium alloy and polyethylene. This metal-on-polyethylene design is better suited to handle the angulation that large orthognathic movement places on the implant, and results in less torque on the contralateral TMJ during jaw movement and implant placement. Greater customization also allows for the design of a larger posterior stop on the temporal component of the implant, minimizing the risk of posterior TMJR dislocation.[5] Computer-assisted planning and CAD/CAM design allows the surgeon to view the proposed prosthesis on the models from multiple vantage points to ensure the validity of the design.

Anatomic models are produced from a computed tomography (CT) scan or from the images of the computer-assisted planned surgical movements and osteotomies. The custom TMJ prosthesis is then made using a CAD/CAM wax model. The components of the prosthesis are designed to be patient-fitted, which improves long-term stability and safety. This also allows the prosthesis to fit anomalous glenoid fossa and mandibles. Osteotomy sites and osseous resection for condylar as well as temporal fossa components of the prosthesis can also be planned virtually using CAD/CAM technology. This improved accuracy in osteotomies subsequently allows for greater accuracy in predicted concurrent orthognathic movements.

## Clinical considerations

(See Video 9.1).

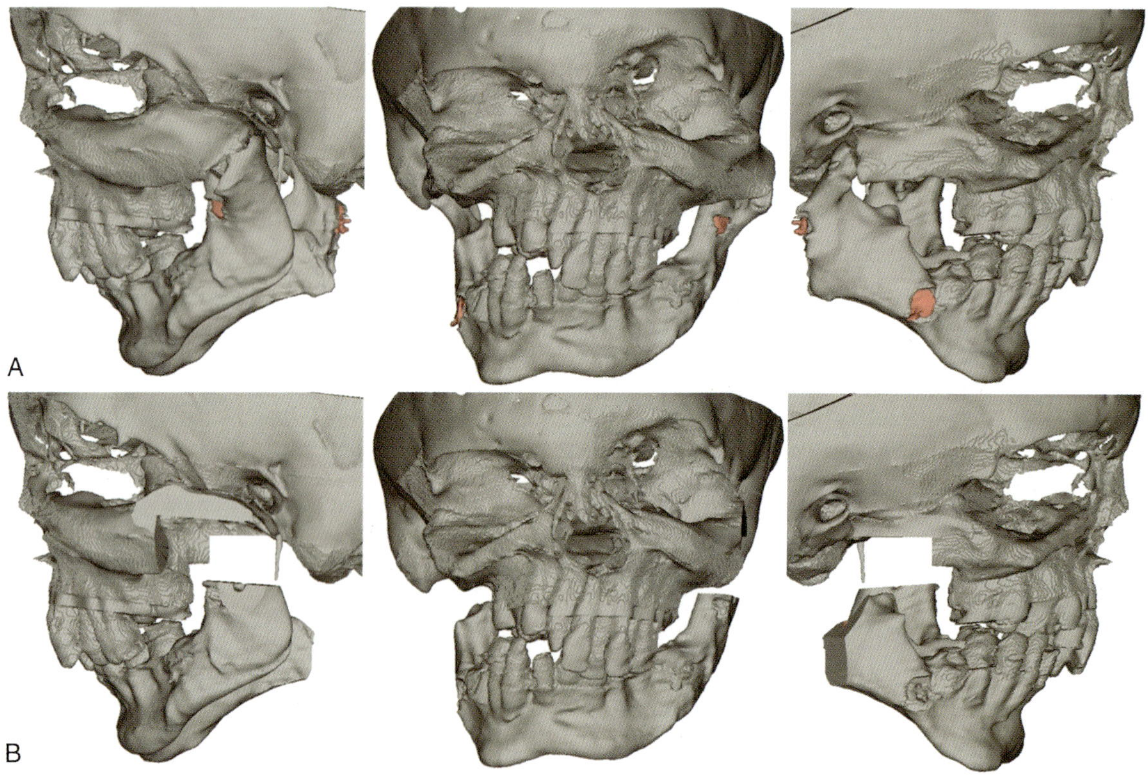

**Fig. 9.1** A 17-year-old male patient born with severe Treacher Collins syndrome developed severe bilateral temporomandibular joint (TMJ) ankylosis as a complication of early mandibular distraction osteogenesis as an infant. This patient underwent bilateral TMJ replacement using custom alloplastic implants designed by computer-assisted surgical planning with computer-assisted design/computer-assisted manufacture technology. The preoperative position (A) and planned movements (B) are shown.

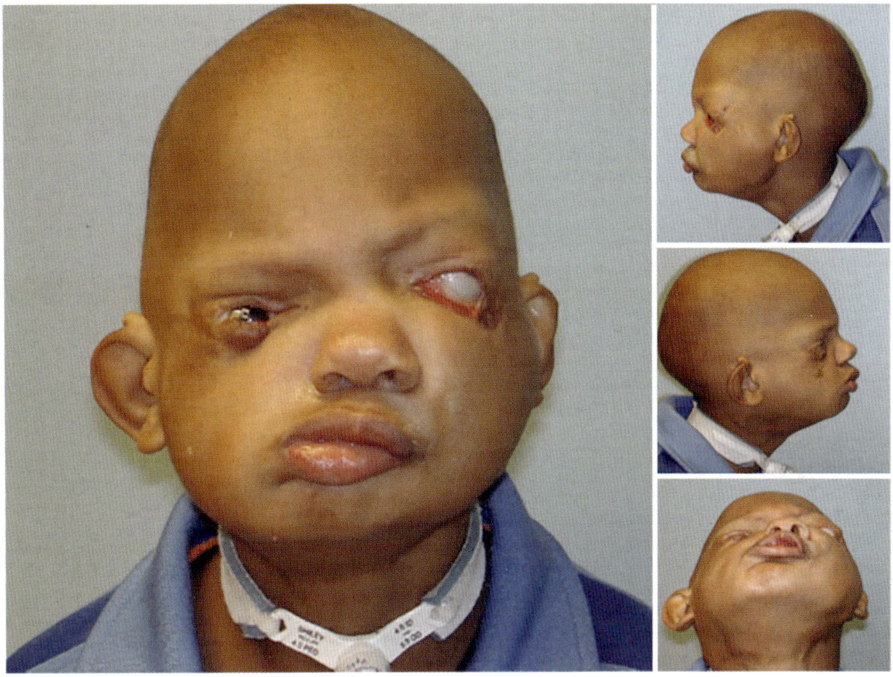

**Fig. 9.2** Preoperative clinic photos of the patient.

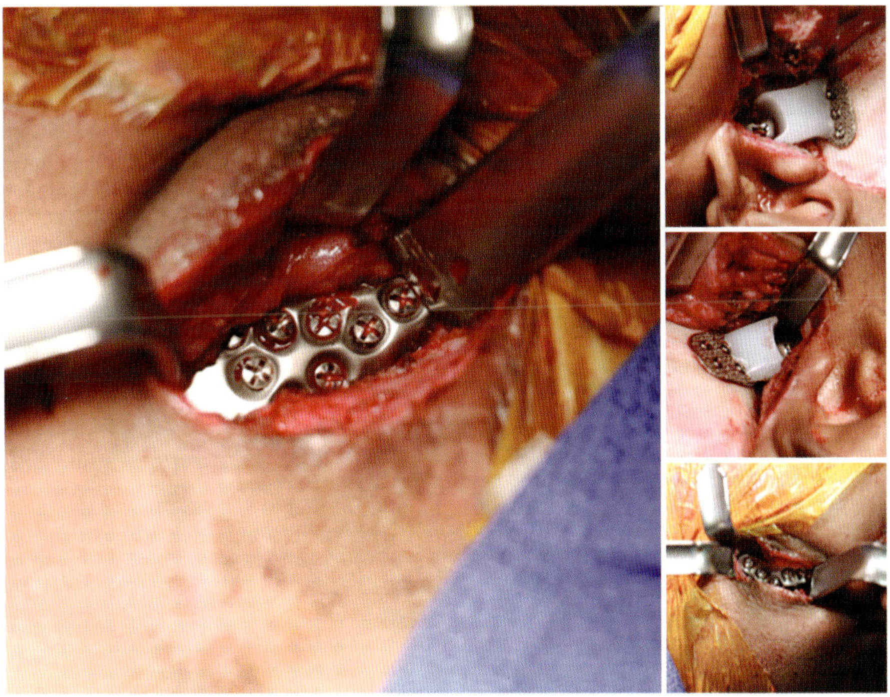

**Fig. 9.3** Bilateral temporomandibular joint replacement with custom alloplastic implants, which were designed using computer-assisted design/computer-assisted manufacture.

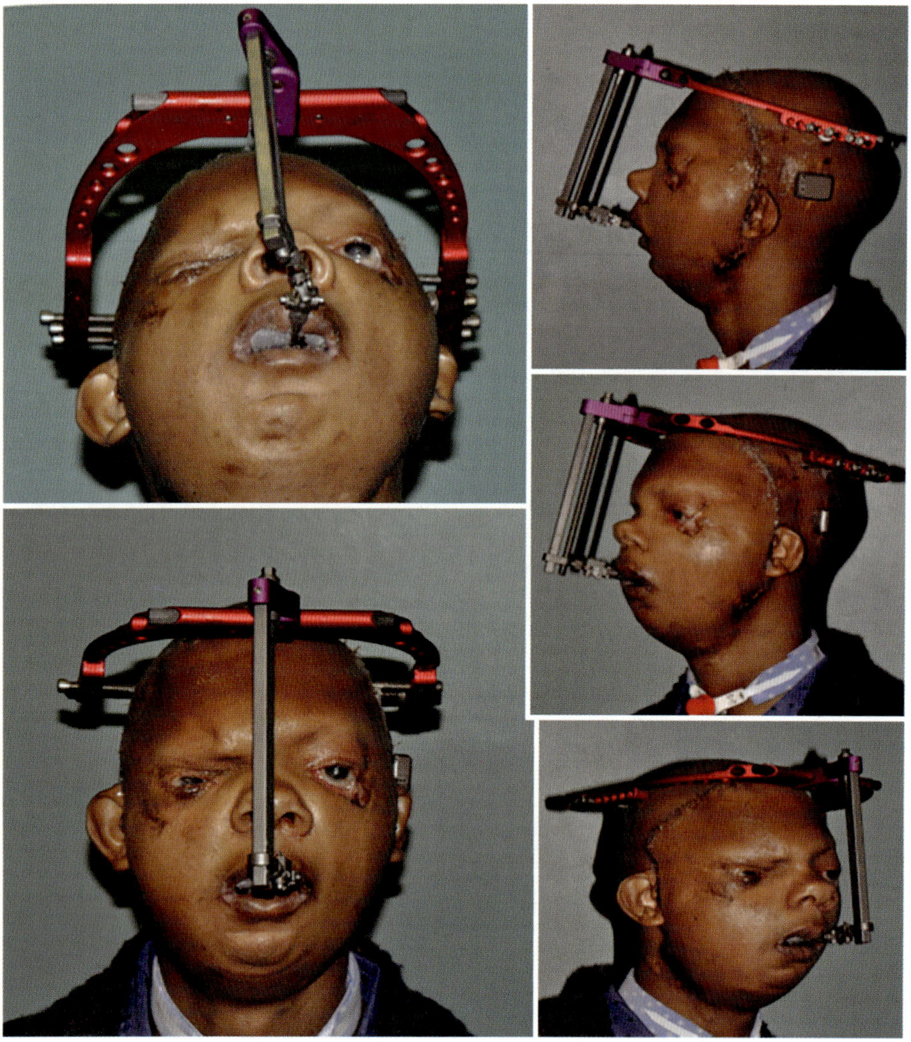

**Fig. 9.4** The patient was fitted with a rigid external distraction halo device during the final stage of his mandibular reconstruction with bilateral temporomandibular joint replacement.

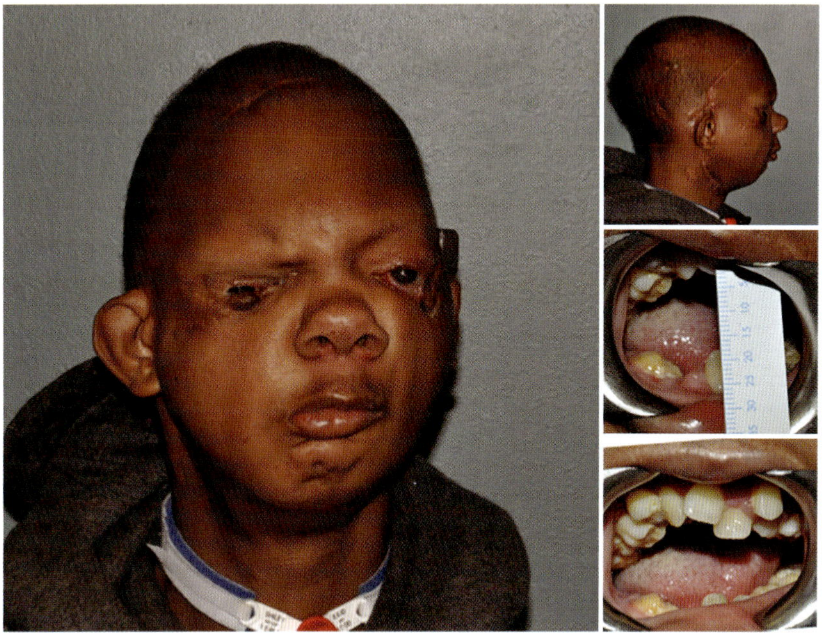

Fig. 9.5 Postoperative clinical features immediately following the removal of the rigid external distraction halo device, 3 months after distraction and consolidation.

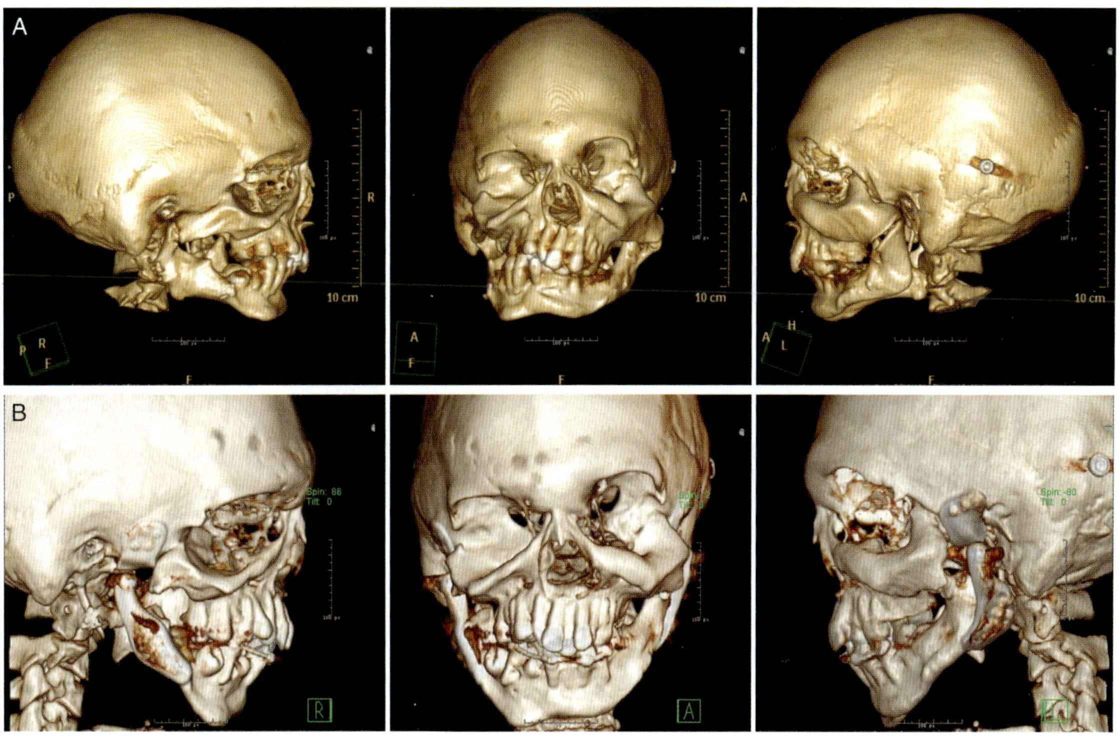


Fig. 9.6 Three-dimensional computed tomography imaging preoperatively (A) at 17 years and postoperatively (B) at 19 years and 2 months.

## Fidelity/verification

Although CAD/CAM technology allows for more accurate and efficient perioperative planning and design, intraoperative assessment, and judgment during any procedure are necessary.

Occlusal splints are used in much the same way that they are used for traditional orthognathic surgery. Proper splint seating is necessary to confirm appropriate bone resection, positioning of the implants, and seating of the mandibular component within the temporal component. An early postoperative CT scan is obtained to assess results and confirm proper positioning of the prosthesis.

The patient's occlusion is monitored in the postoperative period, and reinforcement of proper occlusion is accomplished with the use of postoperative guiding elastics.

## Pearls/pitfalls

- The surgeon should ensure good bone quality, not just depth, at the planned screw sites.
- The course of the mental nerve should be identified and assessed for functionality.
- Intraoperative changes to the plan are not possible; this remains true even in the case of unanticipated intraoperative findings.
- The temporomandibular joint prosthesis should be assessed for stability in situ.
- Malpositioning of the contralateral joint should be avoided.

## Outcomes/complications

Applied to the correct patient, TMJR can improve factors affecting quality of life. A 20-year follow-up shows that TMJR can achieve long-term improvements in pain, function, and eating.[5] Furthermore, the accuracy of custom-fitted TMJR devices has been well studied and verified.[4,6] Studies have shown that preoperative and postoperative distances of movements were consistent, supporting the notion that the outcomes of computer-assisted surgical planning (CaSP) and the use of custom TMJR are reproducible.

CAD/CAM technology and custom TMJR has led to improved outcomes. Lee et al. looked at the outcomes of TMJR as compared to those undergoing costochondral grafts for TMJ reconstruction.[7] In comparison to costochondral grafts, custom TMJR had fewer nonacceptable outcomes.

Although CAD/CAM technology has led to improved accuracy and efficiency of TMJR, complications still occur. Less than 3% of the time, patients experience TMJR complications such as infection, heterotopic ossification, persistent pain, and hypersensitivity.

## Conclusion

Total TMJR has come a long way from its initial techniques. Autologous tissue reconstruction has high rates of complications such as ankylosis. Alloplastic TMJR has multiple benefits, including ease in conforming to the given anatomy, less susceptibility to systemic disease, no need for a donor site, and the ability to start early physical therapy.

The use of CAD/CAM has increased surgical accuracy and efficiency when performing alloplastic TMJR. CT scans can be used to create anatomic models that allow for preoperative CaSP, leading to more precise design of osteotomies and resections. This allows for larger, more predictable, orthognathic movements and custom prosthesis creation and implantation in anatomically complex patients.

Intraoperative changes to the surgical plan are not possible in the case of unanticipated findings, and complications still occur with the use of CAD/CAM planned TMJR. However, good surgical assessment and judgment, anatomical identification of important structures (i.e., the mental nerve), and aseptic techniques can minimize these pitfalls.

In correctly selected patients, CAD/CAM-planned TMJR can dramatically improve outcomes and patient quality of life.

## Take-home points

- CAD/CAM technology has led to the development of custom TMJR.
- Osteotomies and cutting guides designed with CAD/CAM technology improve operative efficiency and accuracy.
- Custom TMJR allows for treatment of patients with complicated anatomy or the need for large concurrent orthognathic movements.
- Even with the use of CAD/CAM technology, TMJR surgery must be performed meticulously and aseptically.

## References


1. Mercuri LG, ed. *Temporomandibular Joint Total Joint Replacement – TMJ TJR – A Comprehensive Reference for Researchers, Materials Scientists, and Surgeons*. Switzerland: Springer International Publishing; 2016.
2. Awal DH, Jaffer M, Charan G, et al. Costochondral grafting for paediatric temporomandibular joint reconstruction: 10-year outcomes in 55 cases. *Int J Oral Maxillofac Surg*. 2018;47(11):1433-1438. doi:10.1016/j.ijom.2018.06.004.
3. Upadya VH, Bhat HK, Rao BHS, Reddy SG. Classification and surgical management of temporomandibular joint ankylosis: a review. *J Korean Assoc Oral Maxillofac Surg*. 2021;47(4):239-248. doi:10.5125/jkaoms.2021.47.4.239.
4. Mercuri LG. Alloplastic temporomandibular joint replacement: rationale for the use of custom devices. *Int J Oral Maxillofac Surg*. 2012;41(9):1033-1040. doi:10.1016/j.ijom.2012.05.032.
5. Wolford LM, Mercuri LG, Schneiderman ED, Movahed R, Allen W. Twenty-year follow-up study on a patient-fitted temporomandibular joint prosthesis: the Techmedica/TMJ Concepts device. *J Oral Maxillofac Surg*. 2015;73(5):952-960. doi:10.1016/j.joms.2014.10.032.
6. Sembronio S, Tel A, Costa F, Isola M, Robiony M. Accuracy of custom-fitted temporomandibular joint alloplastic reconstruction and virtual surgical planning. *Int J Oral Maxillofac Surg*. 2019;48(8):1077-1083. doi:10.1016/j.ijom.2019.01.024.
7. Lee WY, Park YW, Kim SG. Comparison of costochondral graft and customized total joint reconstruction for treatments of temporomandibular joint replacement. *Maxillofac Plast Reconstr Surg*. 2014;36(4):135-139. doi:10.14402/jkamprs.2014.36.4.135.

Chapter | 10 |

# Syndromic craniosynostosis—intracranial/frontofacial reconstruction

Howard Wang, Edward Davidson, Anand Raj Kumar

CHAPTER OUTLINE



## Introduction

Hypertelorism is defined as increased bony interorbital distance (IOD) and is measured by the interdacryon distance, which is the distance between the most medial osseous aspect of the orbits. Orbital hypertelorism is distinct from telecanthus, which refers to the lateral displacement of the medial canthal tendon. Similarly, interpupillary distance is an inappropriate measure of hypertelorism as it can be significantly impacted by the presence of exotropia. Tessier classified orbital hypertelorism into three categories based on IOD as mild (30–34 mm), moderate (35–40 mm), or severe (>40 mm).[1,2] Surgical correction of orbital hypertelorism is possible because in most cases, the distance between the optic canals is thought to be within the normal range, thus allowing mobilization of the orbits and orbital contents without compromising ocular function.[1]

Syndromic craniosynostosis or median facial clefts are conditions commonly associated with hypertelorism.

Surgical options for correction of hypertelorism include orbital box osteotomies and facial bipartition. In a broad sense, these techniques allow for movement of the orbits relative to each other and relative to the skull base, either with the orbits as independent units in the case of orbital box osteotomy or combined with the midface as a monobloc/bipartition osteotomy.[3]

Box osteotomy of the orbits was first described by Tessier as a two-stage procedure and later modified to a single-stage operation.[4] Unlike facial bipartition, orbital box osteotomy allows independent movement of the orbit and thus is an effective technique to correct asymmetric deformities and multiplanar orbital deformities, such as in cases of neurofibromatosis or craniofacial microsomia. Modifications to facial bipartition have also been described that allows for correction of asymmetries in certain cases, but the effect on occlusion limits the degree of freedom in the orbital movements.[5]

Facial bipartition, first described by van der Meulen,[6] has been refined to incorporate modern techniques such as distraction osteogenesis in select patients with sagittal deficiency. In addition to hypertelorism, the indications for facial bipartition include narrowed and high-arched palate and concaved midface such as seen in Apert syndrome. The resection of a bony wedge from the central frontal-nasal region and subsequent rotation of the hemifacial segments flattens the maxillary occlusal plane, corrects the downward vector of the lateral canthi, and increases midface height. Thus, facial bipartition allows medialization and rotation of the orbits while simultaneously achieving expansion and leveling of the maxillary arch.

## Clinical considerations

The choice of operation depends on a number of factors, including the alignment of the maxillary dental arch, the axis of the orbits, the width of the nasal fossa, and the severity of hypertelorism. Facial bipartition has the potential to address abnormalities in the maxillary dental arch and adjust the orbital axis simultaneously. Therefore, it is preferred for patients with narrow and inverted maxillary dental arch or significant downward slanting orbital axis. Facial bipartition is also the preferred choice for large movements compared to box osteotomies.

In patients with syndromic craniosynostosis such as Apert syndrome, monobloc facial bipartition with distraction osteogenesis performed in the mixed dentition stage is a powerful technique to address not only the hypertelorism but also the forehead and midface retrusion that are frequently seen in this patient population.[7-9] Although this constellation of facial deformities is frequently associated with Apert syndrome, it can also be seen in patients with other syndromic synostosis.

Orbital box osteotomy allows correction of orbital dystopia through translational movements of the orbits in multiple dimensions. Thus, the box osteotomy is an excellent operation for patients with well-aligned occlusion and orbits as it can be performed without alteration of the maxillary occlusion or canthal axis. Further refinements of the orbital box osteotomy include segmentation and addition of internal orbital reconstruction to address external orbital dimension and internal volume asymmetries.[10]

In cases of maxillary arch constriction, facial bipartition can address both the orbital deformity and widen the palate and maxillary arch at the same time. The midline palatal division will create a gap between the central incisors and possible vertical discrepancy if asymmetric facial bipartition is performed. These occlusal alterations will spontaneously correct in most cases during the mixed dentition stage within 3 to 6 months but may need additional orthodontic diastema correction if the patient is in adult dentition. Excessive soft tissue is usually present over the nasal dorsum which frequently will improve over time without resection and can be further contracted using techniques such as soft tissue bolsters, internal plication sutures, or the K-stitch as popularized by Henry Kawamoto MD, DDS.[11] Furthermore, excessive resection along the nasal dorsum can result in unsightly scarring and may interfere with nasal development, leading to the need for subsequent nasal lengthening.[12]

The optimal age for hypertelorism correction remains controversial as surgeons and families must weigh the psychosocial benefits of early correction with the risk of skeletal relapse and growth disturbances. Although infant monobloc and early hypertelorism correction had been proposed in the past,[12] we prefer to opt for a later timepoint after the age of 6 years to perform facial bipartition to achieve more durable results.[13-15] At this age, the permanent central incisors have erupted, thus decreasing the risk of injury to permanent teeth during midpalatal splitting. In a study of long-term follow-up after surgical correction of hypertelorism, Wan et al. identified age younger than 6 years and preoperative severity as risk factors for relapse requiring repeat correction.[16] Other studies have also found higher rates of relapse in patients with more severe preoperative phenotypes and raised concerns about growth disturbance with early timing of surgery.[17] The senior author (ARK) prefers to operate between 8 and 10 years of age to minimize risk of dental injury to the central incisors and allow for adequate permanent canine descent out of the osteotomy path of a typical orbital box osteotomy. Further delay after 10 years of age would necessitate additional treatment to manage the developing frontal sinuses such as a cranialization procedure.

## Workflow for computer-assisted design/computer-assisted manufacturing (methods)

(See efigure 10.1 and 10.2)

## Computer-assisted design

### Orbital box osteotomy

Planning for orbital box osteotomy can start with mirroring the contralateral, unaffected orbit. An analysis of the external orbital contour in terms of the vertical position of the superior and inferior orbital rims is then performed to determine the amount of translation and rotation required to correct the specific orbital deformity of the individual patient (Fig. 10.1). The orbital shape should be assessed to determine whether segmentation of the orbit is required (Fig. 10.2). Next, the internal orbital shape and

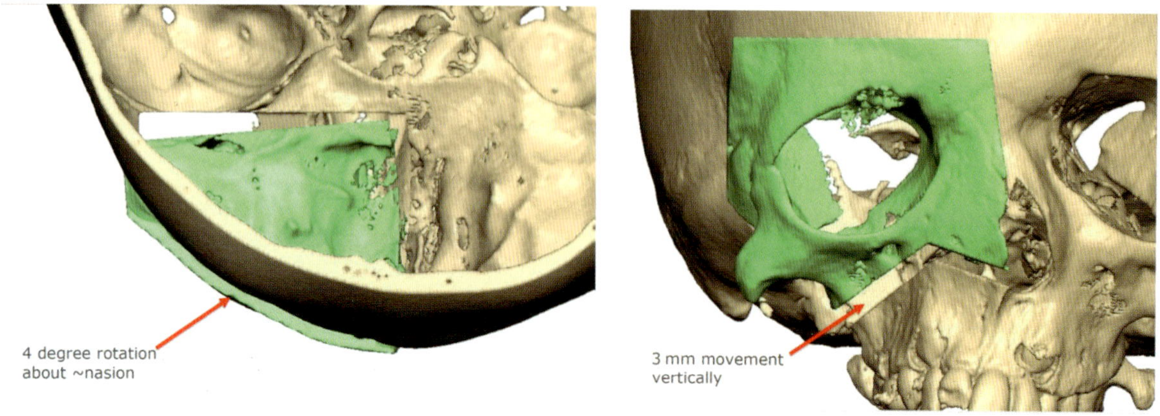


**Fig. 10.1** Computer-assisted surgical planning for translational and rotational movements of the orbit after box osteotomy.

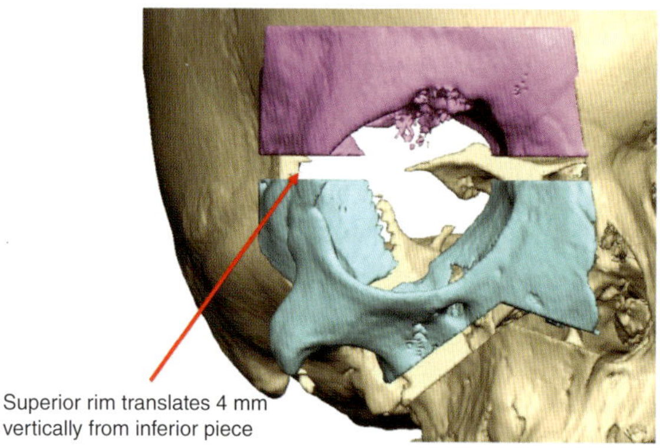


**Fig. 10.2** Segmentation and vertical expansion of the orbit to improve orbital symmetry in a case of severe craniofacial microsomia.

volume is evaluated to determine which orbital walls may require reconstruction, and internal orbital implants can be designed to improve the orbital volume and address enophthalmos or hypoglobus (Fig. 10.3).

## Facial bipartition

In facial bipartition cases, computer-assisted surgical planning (CaSP) can be utilized to determine the appropriate width and angle of the midline bony resection that can be safely performed to achieve the desired IOD and orbital orientation (Fig. 10.4). Normal IOD varies based on the age of the child, but a general guideline is to reduce the interdacryon distance to less than 20 mm. Furthermore, it allows the surgeon to visualize the associated changes that would occur at the occlusal level and to anticipate any

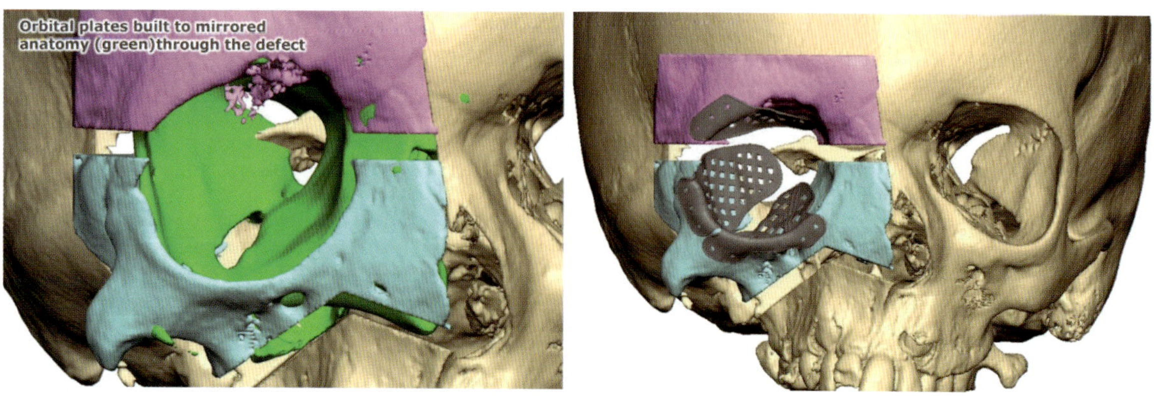


**Fig. 10.3** Mirroring of the contralateral orbit is used to design internal orbital implants to address orbital volume asymmetry in an orbital box osteotomy case.

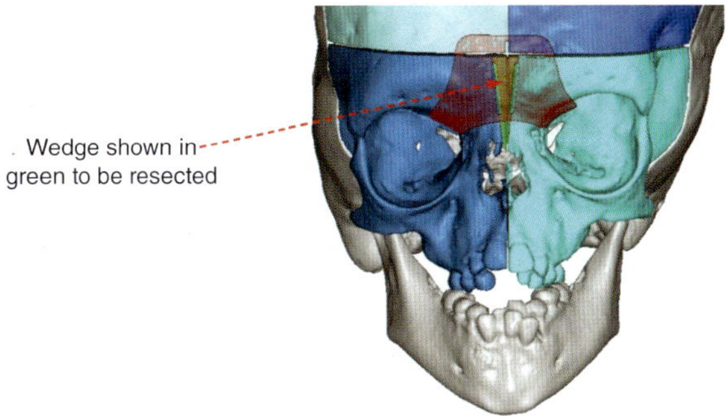


Fig. 10.4 Computer-assisted surgical planning to design the central bony resection and osteotomy marking guide for a facial bipartition case. (Adapted from Hopper RA, Kapadia H, Susarla SM. Surgical-Orthodontic Considerations in Subcranial and Frontofacial Distraction. *Oral Maxillofac Surg Clin North Am*. 2020;32(2):309-320.)

bony interferences that may be encountered with the planned movements (Fig. 10.5). As the degree of narrowing at the nasofrontal region translates to the magnitude of expansion at the palatal level, the amount of palatal widening must also be considered when planning the size and shape of central bony resection.

In cases that will be combined with a monobloc/facial bipartition advancement via distraction osteogenesis, CaSP can be helpful to design the distraction vector based on Frankfurt Horizontal and distractor placement location based on bony and soft tissue anatomy (Fig. 10.6). While the endpoint for advancement is contingent upon achieving an appropriate relationship between the orbital rim and the cornea, CaSP using an estimated advancement of 12 to 18 mm can help the surgeon visualize the expected relationship between

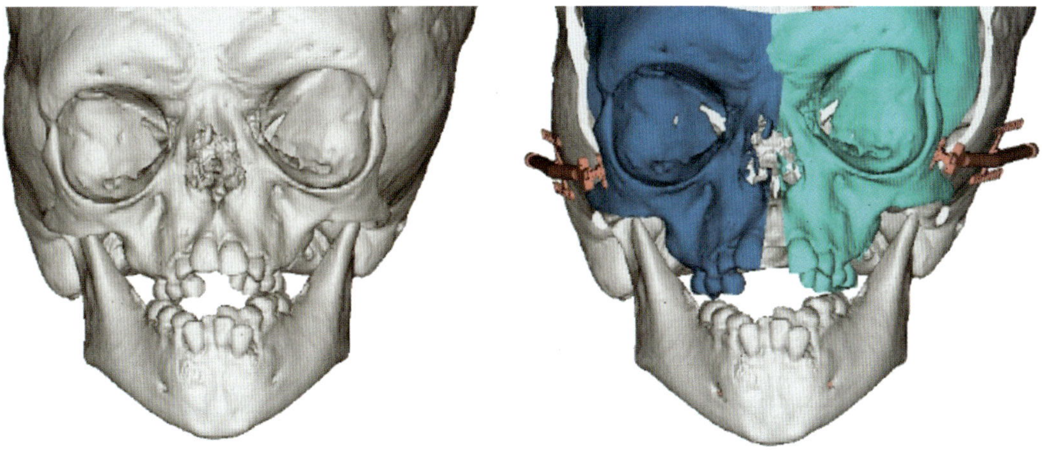

Fig. 10.5 Preoperative and final position of the monobloc facial bipartition segment.

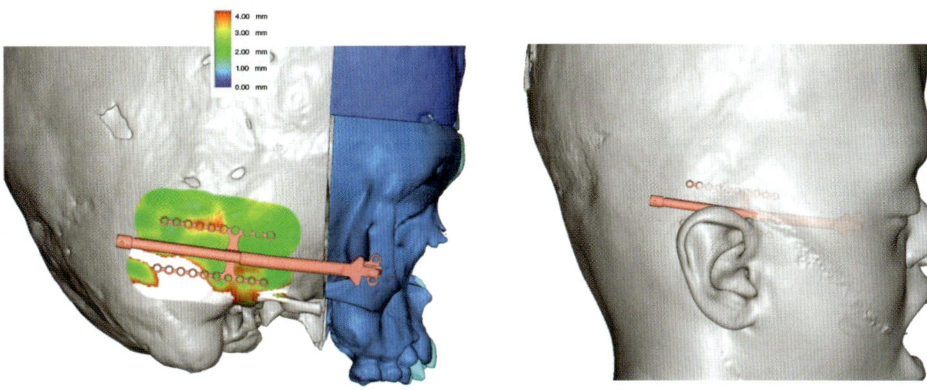


Fig. 10.6 Device placement for monobloc facial bipartition can be planned based on bony contour and thickness and soft tissue anatomy.

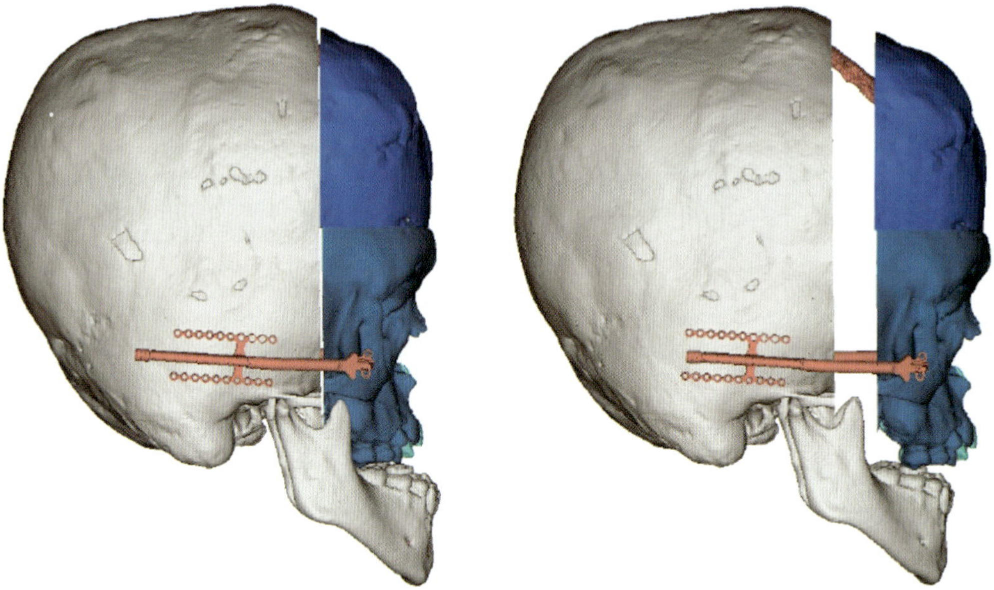

Fig. 10.7 Estimated final distracted position of a monobloc facial-bipartition distraction case. The actual distraction endpoint is determined by the relative position of the cornea and orbital rim. (Adapted from Hopper RA, Kapadia H, Susarla SM. Surgical-Orthodontic Considerations in Subcranial and Frontofacial Distraction. *Oral Maxillofac Surg Clin North Am*. 2020;32(2):309-320.)

forehead and midface projection relative to the mandible (Fig. 10.7).

## Computer-assisted manufacturing

### Orbital box osteotomy

Stereolithographic skull models can be manufactured to demonstrate the intermediate and final positions (Fig. 10.8). They can also be used to help with marking and executing the planned osteotomies intraoperatively (Fig. 10.9). In cases where internal orbital reconstruction is to be performed, patient-specific orbital implants can be designed and fabricated to correct orbital volume or reconstruct bony defects (Fig. 10.10).

### Facial bipartition

Similar to the orbital box osteotomy operation, skull models can be manufactured to visualize the planned osteotomies and intermediate positions. Once the midline bony resection for facial bipartition has been planned, a marking guide can be manufactured to help with executing the central osteotomy at the frontonasal region intraoperatively to improve precision of the bony movements (Fig. 10.11).

## Operative technique

### Orbital box osteotomy

- Exposure to the frontal-orbital region, temporal fossa, and zygomatic arches are obtained through a coronal approach, and an upper gingivobuccal sulcus approach is used to expose the pyriform aperture and the maxilla.
- Care must be taken to avoid detachment of the medial canthal tendons.
- The neurosurgery team then performs frontal craniotomy to gain access to the orbital roof, sphenoid, and cribriform plate.
- Osteotomy of the orbital roof is then performed through a transcranial approach with the frontal lobe and orbital contents retracted.
- Osteotomy of the lateral orbital wall, medial orbital wall and zygomatic arch are then performed.
- Orbital osteotomies need to be performed posterior enough to achieve adequate translocation of the orbital contents while avoiding injury to the optic nerve. The inferior orbital fissure serves as a landmark for starting point of osteotomies.
- Osteotomy of the anterior maxilla is performed through the upper gingivobuccal sulcus incisions high enough

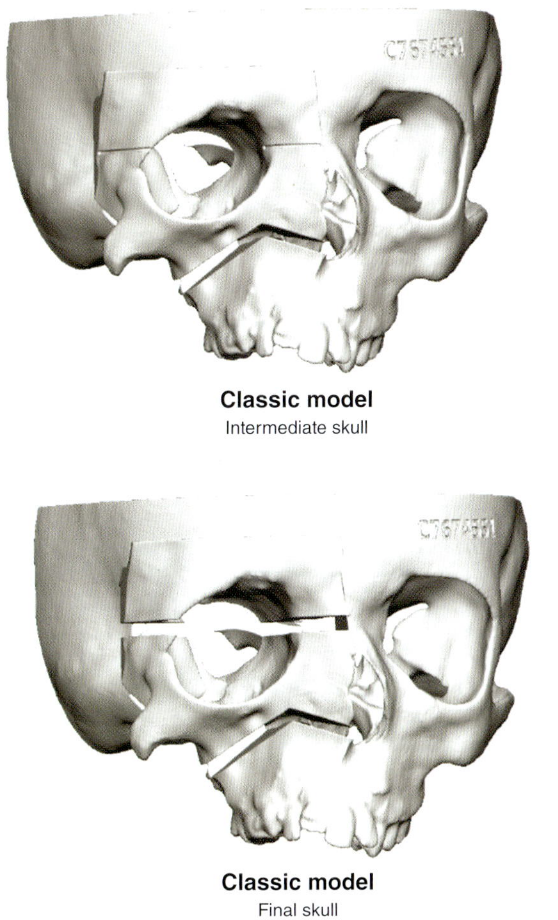


Fig. 10.8 Examples of skull models for intermediate and final position of an orbital box osteotomy case.

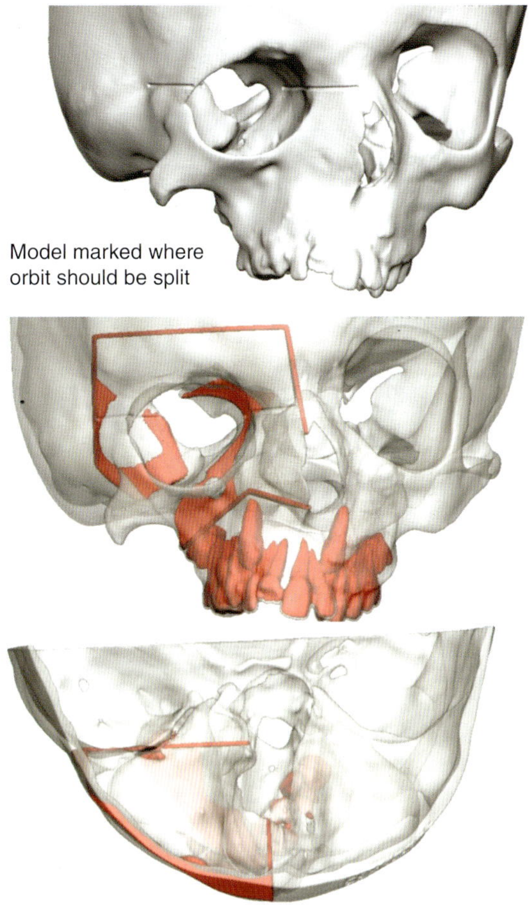


Fig. 10.9 Skull models with the planned osteotomy for orbital box osteotomy outlined.

to avoid injuring the roots of the permanent dentition and taking care to not transect the infraorbital nerve.

- The orbital segment is then mobilized using a laminar spreader.
- A wedge of naso-ethmoid bone centrally, anterior to the cribriform plate is then removed to allow for medial translocation of the orbits.
- Fixation is applied at the midline to the frontal bone superiorly, and along the nasomaxillary and zygomaticomaxillary buttress inferiorly.
- Bone grafts are used to address any bony gaps based on the direction of orbital movement.

## Facial bipartition

- Exposure to the frontal-orbital region, temporal fossa and zygomatic arches is obtained through a coronal

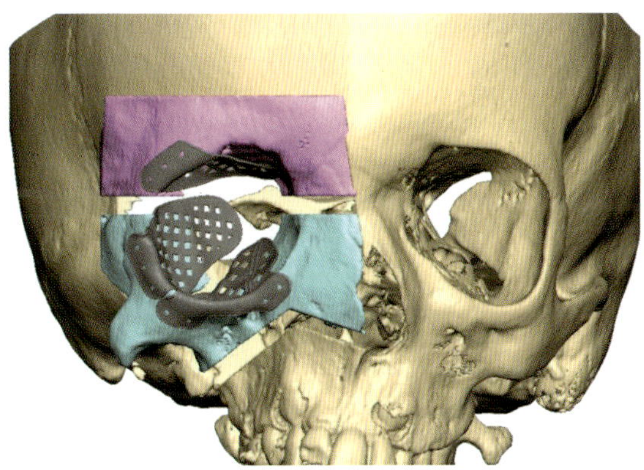

Fig. 10.10 Patient-specific orbital implants are designed to improve symmetry of orbital volume in a segmental orbital box osteotomy case.

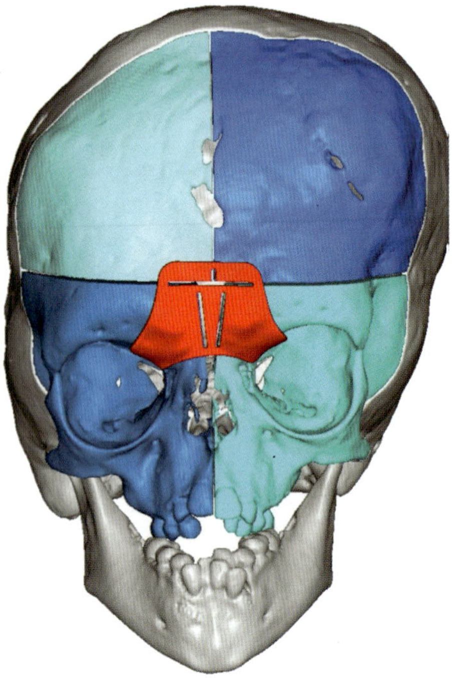

Fig. 10.11 Osteotomy marking guide for central bony resection for a facial bipartition case.

approach, and an upper gingivobuccal sulcus approach is used to expose the pyriform aperture and the maxilla.

- A bifrontal craniotomy is then performed by the neurosurgery team to gain access to the anterior and middle cranial fossa.
- The zygomatic arch osteotomy is completed with a reciprocating saw.
- The lateral orbital wall osteotomy is then made starting at the inferior orbital fissure directing superiorly while protecting the middle cranial fossa.
- Next, the orbital roof osteotomies are carried out through a transcranial approach taking care to remain anterior to the crista galli centrally.
- The orbital floor and medial orbital wall osteotomies are completed with osteotomes.
- Pterygomaxillary osteotomy is then performed through intraoral incisions.
- The monobloc segment is then downfractured using Rowe disimpaction forceps.
- Septal disjunction is then performed with a thin osteotome during the down-fracturing process with a double-guarded osteotome.
- The frontofacial segment is then fully mobilized prior to performing bipartition.
- A central wedge of frontonasal ethmoid bone is removed based on preoperative planning anterior to the cribriform plate.
- The ethmoid air cells are removed to allow medialization.
- The palate is then split between the central incisors through an intraoral incision.
- The two hemifacial segments are then rotated to close the interorbital gap and fixation is applied.
- The anterior cranial fossa is sealed with a pericranial flap.
- The frontal bone is then replaced and may require adjustment to fit the narrowed orbits.

## Fidelity/verification

Verification of the computer-assisted design/computer-assisted manufacturing (CAD/CAM) surgical plan is performed intraoperatively by measuring the size of bony resection and measurement of interdacryon distance. Comparison of postoperative computed tomography imaging with planned final position can be performed to verify the accuracy of the surgical bony movements compared to CaSP.

## Pearls/pitfalls

- In cases where translocation of the orbital contents is the goal, orbital osteotomies should be performed posterior enough (centrum of the globe) to mobilize the orbital contents.
- In patients with significant exorbitism, orbital wall osteotomies need to be just posterior enough to avoid unplanned fracturing of the orbital rims. This is easily avoided by using the centrum of the globe to determine the lateral and posterior position of the osteotomy usually guided by the inferior orbital fissure as the starting point.
- Prediction of periorbital soft tissue changes remains limited using CAD/CAM technology. Minimizing stripping of the soft tissue to ensure adequate visualization for a safe osteotomy execution but leaving midfacial attachments (McGregor's Patch) and the medial canthus attachments intact is critical.
- Medially, the osteotomy of the orbital roof should be tapered anteriorly to avoid injury to the olfactory bulbs by staying within the window between the frontal crest and the crista galli. Care should be taken to avoid or cauterize the anterior communicating venous drainage of the anterior sagittal sinus.

- Glabellar skin and soft tissue excess will result after correction of severe hypertelorism and should be addressed at the time of bony correction with transnasal soft tissue bolsters or internal plication sutures such as the K-stitch.

## Outcomes/complications

Complications of frontofacial surgery, such as facial bipartition and orbital box osteotomy, include bleeding, cerebrospinal fluid (CSF) leak, infection related to communication with sinuses, postoperative seizures, ophthalmological complications, and insufficient correction related to bony positioning or soft tissue relaxation.[18,19] Surgery performed at a younger age is associated with a higher rate of relapse.[15,16] Blood loss can be significant, and the need for blood transfusion is common. Facial bipartition and orbital box osteotomies are major operations. While mortality is rare, it does occur in less than 1% of cases, and the family must be warned about the potential for major morbidity and mortality.[1,14,19] Long-term review of complication rates at the Great Ormond Street Hospital center revealed an 11% rate of major complications and overall infection rate of 25%.[3]

These significant complications must be weighed against the major benefits in terms of functional improvement of the airway, vision, and occlusion. Similarly, few operations have the same potential for appearance improvements in these complex facial deformities (Fig. 10.12–10.15). Secondary soft tissue correction surgeries including midline skin resection, nasal reconstruction with bone or cartilage grafts, and epicanthal fold correction are frequently required.[14] However, long-term follow-up has shown that the results of hypertelorism correction is generally well-maintained if adequate correction is achieved during the initial operation.[14]

## Conclusion

Frontofacial surgery involves complex osteotomies and movements of the orbits and midface. Application of CAD/CAM technology has immense potential to improve precision of the bony movements in all three dimensions. Furthermore, the use of patient-specific guides and implants can facilitate execution of the

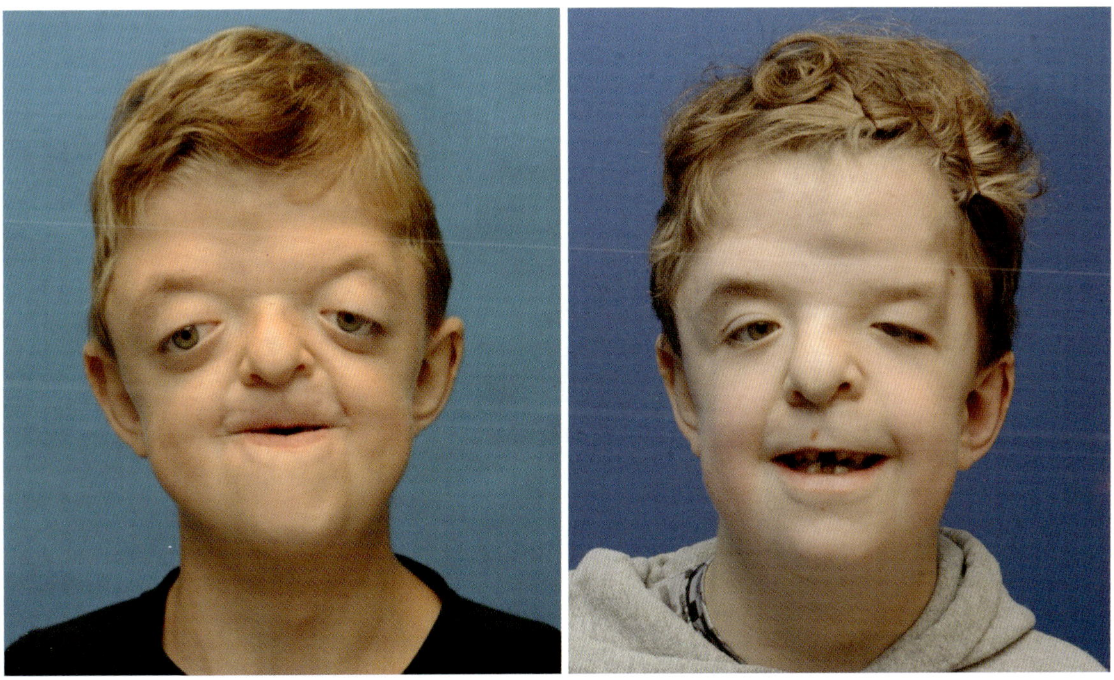

**Fig. 10.12** Clinical photographs of pre- and postoperative appearance after monobloc facial bipartition distraction osteogenesis in a patient with Apert syndrome.

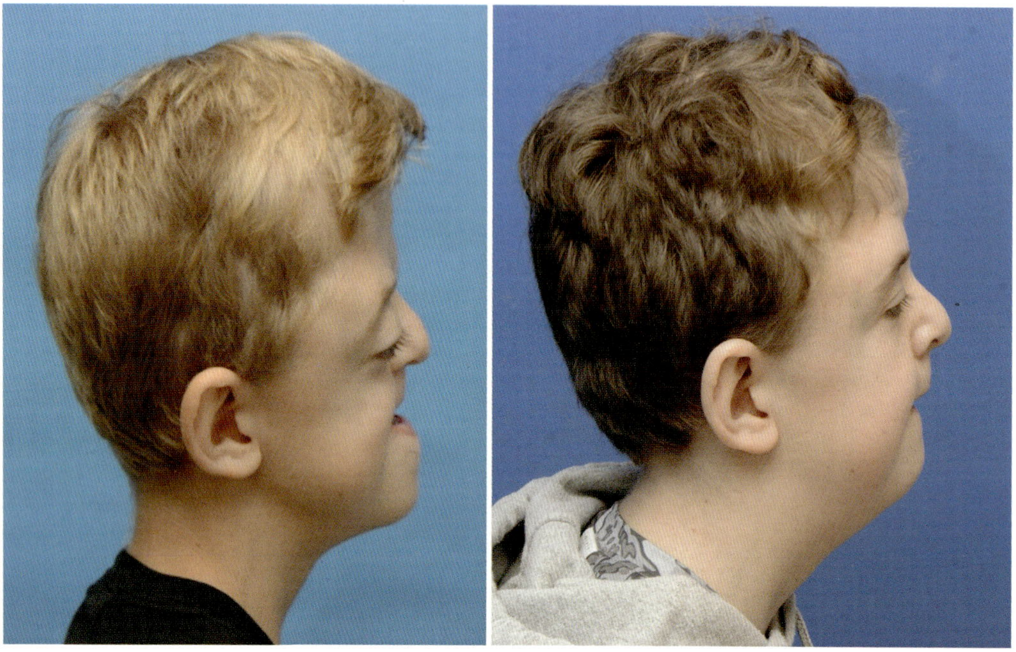

**Fig. 10.13** Profile photographs of pre- and postoperative appearance after monobloc facial bipartition distraction osteogenesis in a patient with Apert syndrome.

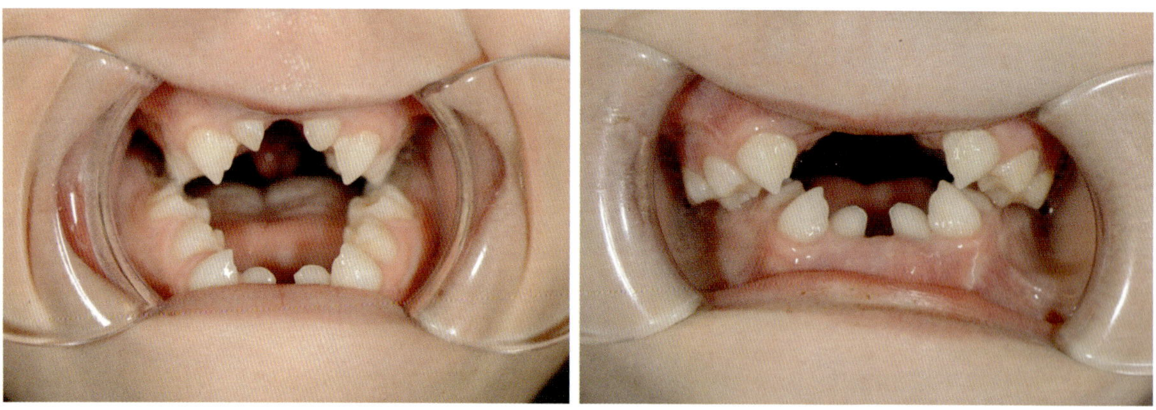

**Fig. 10.14** Intraoral photographs of pre- and postoperative appearance after monobloc facial bipartition distraction osteogenesis demonstrating change at the occlusal level in a patient with Apert syndrome.

surgical plan and help achieve increased accuracy and improved symmetry. For example, a manufactured cutting guide for the central nasal osteotomy can help to precisely translate the surgical plan during the operation. Patient-specific implants such as fixation hardware and internal orbital implants have the potential to improve both efficiency and accuracy.

## Take-home points

- Facial bipartition can achieve medialization of the orbits while simultaneously widening the maxilla and improving facial convexity. In contrast, orbital box osteotomy mobilizes the orbits independent of

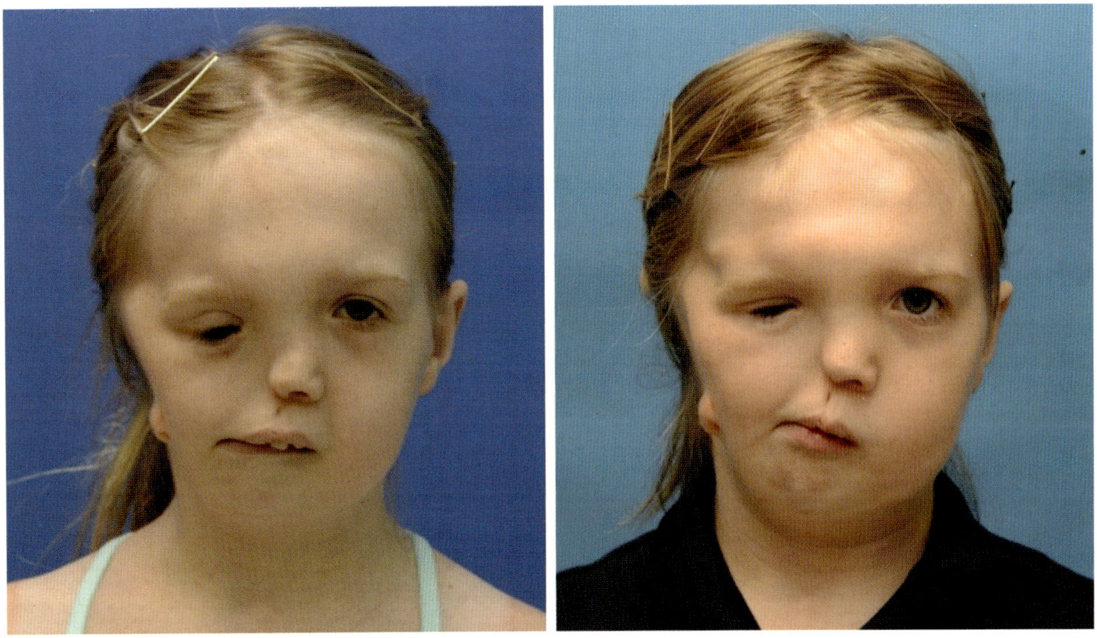

Fig. 10.15 Clinical photographs of pre- and postoperative appearance after right segmental orbital box osteotomy in a patient with right craniofacial macrosomia.

the occlusion and allows for movements in multiple planes.
- CAD/CAM technology provides precise planning of osteotomies and bony movements.
- Cutting guides and patient-specific implants assist the surgeon to execute the computer-assisted surgical plan intraoperatively.
- Detailed preoperative analysis of the patient's bony and soft tissue anatomy allows the surgeon to plan ideal locations for osteotomies and implants.
- Orbital box osteotomy and facial bipartition are complex operations, and the application of CAD/CAM technology has the potential to increase surgical precision and reduce morbidity and operative time.

## References


1. Tessier P. Experiences in the treatment of orbital hypertelorism. *Plast Reconstr Surg*. 1974;53:1-18.
2. Tessier P. Orbital hypertelorism. I. Successive surgical attempts. Material and methods. Causes and mechanisms. *Scand J Plast Reconstr Surg*. 1972;6:135-155.
3. Britto JA, Greig A, Abela C, Hearst D, Dunaway DJ, Evans RD. Frontofacial surgery in children and adolescents: techniques, indications, outcomes. *Semin Plast Surg*. 2014;28:121-129.
4. Tessier P, Guiot G, Rougerie J, Delbet JP, Pastoriza J. [Cranio-naso-orbito-facial osteotomies. Hypertelorism]. *Ann Chir Plast*. 1967;12:103-118.
5. Kawamoto HK, Heller JB, Heller MM, et al. Craniofrontonasal dysplasia: a surgical treatment algorithm. *Plast Reconstr Surg*. 2007;120:1943-1956.
6. van der Meulen JC. Medial faciotomy. *Br J Plast Surg*. 1979;32:339-332.
7. Kumar AR, Steinbacher D. Advances in the treatment of syndromic midface hypoplasia using monobloc and facial bipartition distraction osteogenesis. *Semin Plast Surg*. 2014;28:179-183.
8. Bradley JP, Levitt A, Nguyen J, et al. Roman arch, keystone fixation for facial bipartition with monobloc distraction. *Plast Reconstr Surg*. 2008;122: 1514-1523.
9. Greig AVH, Britto JA, Abela C, et al. Correcting the typical Apert face: combining bipartition with monobloc distraction. *Plast Reconstr Surg*. 2013;131:219e-230e.
10. Davidson EH, Khavanin N, Grant M, Kumar AR. Correction of complex neurofibromatosis

orbital and globe malposition using the orbital box segmentation osteotomy with patient-specific internal orbit reconstruction. *J Craniofac Surg*. 2019;30:1647-1651.
11. Urrego AF, Garri JI, O'Hara CM, Kawamoto Jr HK, Bradley JP. The K stitch for hypertelorbitism: improved soft tissue correction with glabellar width reduction. *J Craniofac Surg*. 2005;16:855-859.
12. McCarthy JG, La Trenta GS, Breitbart AS, Zide BM, Cutting CB. Hypertelorism correction in the young child. *Plast Reconstr Surg*. 1990;86:214-225; discussion 226-228.
13. Marchac D, Arnaud E. Midface surgery from Tessier to distraction. *Childs Nerv Syst*. 1999;15: 681-694.
14. Marchac D, Sati S, Renier D, Deschamps-Braly J, Marchac A. Hypertelorism correction: what happens with growth? Evaluation of a series of 95 surgical cases. *Plast Reconstr Surg*. 2012;129:713-727.
15. Raposo-Amaral CE, Raposo-Amaral CM, Raposo-Amaral CA, Chahal H, Bradley JP, Jarrahy R. Age at surgery significantly impacts the amount of orbital relapse following hypertelorbitism correction: a 30-year longitudinal study. *Plast Reconstr Surg*. 2011;127:1620-1630.
16. Wan DC, Levi B, Kawamoto H, et al. Correction of hypertelorbitism: evaluation of relapse on long-term follow-up. *J Craniofac Surg*. 2012;23: 113-117.
17. Mulliken JB, Kaban LB, Evans CA, Strand RD, Murray JE. Facial skeletal changes following hypertelorbitism correction. *Plast Reconstr Surg*. 1986;77:7-16.
18. Raposo-Amaral CE, Denadai R, Zanco GL, Ghizoni E, Raposo-Amaral CA. Long-term follow-up on bone stability and complication rate after monobloc advancement in syndromic craniosynostosis. *Plast Reconstr Surg*. 2020;145:1025-1034.
19. Dunaway DJ, Britto JA, Abela C, Evans RD, Jeelani NU. Complications of frontofacial advancement. *Childs Nerv Syst*. 2012;28:1571-1576.

Chapter | 11 |

# Computer-assisted surgical planning for midfacial surgery in syndromic craniosynostosis

Anna R. Carlson, Jesse A. Taylor

CHAPTER OUTLINE



## Introduction

The care of children with syndromic craniosynostosis is complex and multifaceted, and surgical interventions are a critical component of treatment and an opportunity to provide significant functional and aesthetic improvements in these patients. The use of computer-assisted design and computer-assisted manufacturing (CAD/CAM) in surgery for children with syndromic craniosynostosis has aided in the performance of increasingly complex operations, and while improved functional and/or aesthetic outcomes directly attributed to the use of computer-assisted surgical planning (CaSP) has not been definitively identified, many experienced craniofacial surgeons would agree that accuracy, precision, and speed of an operation are increased with the use of CAD/CAM. CaSP can be especially valuable in patients with syndromic craniosynostosis due to multivector distortion of bony craniofacial anatomy, variation of anatomy between individual patients, and abnormalities due to previous operations. There are multiple operations frequently performed in children with syndromic craniosynostosis that, in most settings, do not typically warrant the use of CaSP (frontoorbital advancement, posterior cranial vault distraction, single-piece Le Fort II and Le Fort III osteotomies). However, a more complex subset of "customized" operations for children with syndromic craniosynostosis is well-suited for digital planning, including multipiece, multilevel, multivector midfacial or frontofacial surgery. The ability to design these customized, complex osteotomies and surgical plans represents one of the strengths of CaSP, perhaps extending the "completeness" of correction of each individual's dysmorphic anatomy.

In this chapter, we provide an overview of the use of CAD/CAM in syndromic craniosynostosis, and specifically of its role in planning and executing multipiece midfacial and cranial operations. Considerations in the choice of frontofacial osteotomy and specific procedures will be discussed, along with steps for CaSP and considerations for selecting custom cutting guides, plates, and splints. Operative technique, pearls, and outcomes are summarized, and specific scenarios in which the authors recommend the use of computer-assisted surgical planning are reviewed.

## Clinical considerations

The choice of midfacial operation in children with syndromic craniosynostosis is complex and dependent upon the anatomical and functional goals of an operation in an individual patient. High-level considerations for each individual patient include the relative necessity for (1) expansion of the cranium to prevent or treat increased intracranial pressure and (2) correction of abnormal anatomy of the midface, orbits, and frontal skull.[2] With these two overarching goals in mind, specific features to consider that can be addressed in a single operation include the position of the frontal bar, presence of exorbitism, need for rotation of the orbits, degree of hypertelorism, need for expansion of the cranium, extent of central versus peripheral hypoplasia of the midface, nasal length, degree of anterior open bite, maxillary dental arch width, and presence of obstructive sleep apnea.[2,3] The presence of certain single anatomic features may dictate the necessity of a single operation; for example, only a facial bipartition can achieve midfacial advancement and closure of a V-shaped anterior open bite in a single operation. Other features such as palpebral fissure rotation, midface lengthening, and cranial expansion can be achieved by one of several osteotomy designs, and the choice of specific operation will be dependent upon any given patient's anatomy and surgeon's experience and comfort level. The expected clinical alterations of each level and design of midfacial osteotomy are shown in Fig. 11.1. The following workflow and technique discussions are intended to be applicable to patients in whom a multipiece frontofacial operation is chosen (i.e., monobloc advancement with or without facial bipartition). Le Fort III and Le Fort II with zygomatic repositioning, while included in the algorithm shown in Fig. 11.1, are discussed elsewhere in this textbook.

## Workflow for computer-assisted design/computer-assisted manufacturing

Prior to a CAD/CAM session CT imaging is obtained, and the patient's CT scan is transferred to the surgeon's vendor of choice for upload into their planning software and preparation for manipulation by the vendor's engineers. Specific CT protocols have been previously described in the literature regarding the imaging characteristics required for CAD/CAM, but ultimately vary dependent upon the vendor chosen for CaSP; thus, these specific requirements should be reviewed prior to obtaining imaging. While dental models or scans are typically required for patients in adult dentition and/or at skeletal maturity, they are not typically required for patients undergoing midface surgery prior to skeletal maturity. They may be utilized in settings in which addressing the maxilla-mandibular bony relationship and occlusion are the primary goals of an operation even with a patient in mixed dentition (i.e., rib graft for hemifacial microsomia in a child).

Multiple items are available for commercial production and are of varying utility for specific cases. In midfacial surgery in syndromic synostosis, cutting guides are generally the most useful item available via computer-assisted surgical planning (CaSP), and can be used to guide bony resections, design osteotomies in specific configurations and with specific goals (i.e., customized movement of the orbits, zygomas, and so forth), or to place distractors at a predetermined vector. Custom plates are available but less frequently used for patients at skeletal immaturity and undergoing distraction osteogenesis. In a situation in which a patient is undergoing an acute midfacial movement, custom plates can be considered and may be helpful to have produced in order to confirm a specific degree or distance of movement. Finally, acrylic skull or midfacial models can be fashioned to mirror a patient's preoperative or postoperative intended position. Postoperative acrylic models can be useful to prebend stock titanium plates to fit a patient's intended postoperative bony position, which can be used as an alternative to custom-milled plates. Resorbable fixation can also be bent to fit an acrylic skull model for patients considered too young for titanium fixation.

## Operative technique

Midfacial operations are performed under general anesthesia with an orotracheal tube secured to the midline of the mandible with wire or suture. A bicoronal incision is marked, and the incision and the periorbital regions are infiltrated with a solution of lidocaine, epinephrine, and low-dose steroid solution (institutional protocol adapted from Neil-Dwyer et al.[4]). A standard bicoronal exposure is performed in the subgaleal plane, followed by the elevation of an anteriorly based pericranial flap. The extent of exposure required is dependent upon the osteotomies planned, but in general, the maximal exposure permitted via bicoronal incision (including the body of the zygoma, the zygomatic arch, and inferior to the nasofrontal junction) is required. An intraoral upper buccal sulcus incision is generally used only for placement of anchoring plates and transcutaneous pins for the halo distraction device, which is performed at the completion of the osteotomies via the bicoronal exposure. The exception to this rule is when a high Le Fort I osteotomy is being performed in conjunction with frontofacial surgery, and in that case, a more extensive upper gingivobuccal sulcus incision is utilized to separate the dentoalveolar maxilla from the upper midface.

After completion of bicoronal exposure, cutting guides are placed and temporarily fixated with titanium screws. Osteotomies are marked, and if drill hole guides are

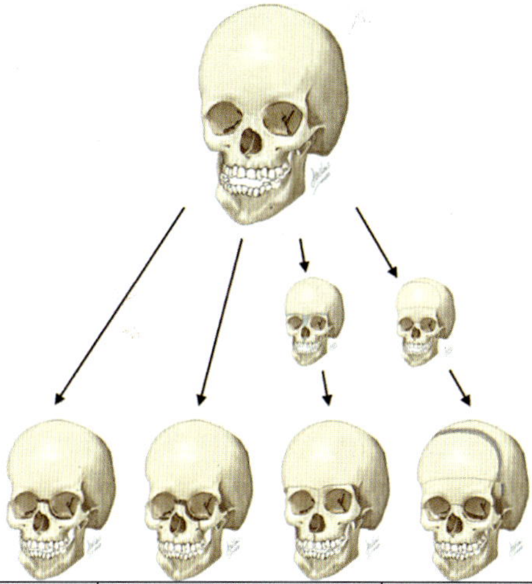

| | Le Fort III | Le Fort II + ZR | Facial bipartition | Monobloc |
|---|---|---|---|---|
| Levels palpebral fissure | −− | ++ | ++ | −− |
| Expands cranium | No | No | Yes | Yes |
| Nasal lengthening | −− | ++ | −− | −− |
| Lengthens midface | −− | ++ | ++ | −− |
| Differential advancement: central vs peripheral | −− | ++ | ++ | −− |
| Close anterior open bite | −− | ++ (level) | ++ (V-shaped) | −− |
| Correct hypertelorism | −− | −− | ++ | −− |
| Decrease bi-zygomatic width | −− | −− | ++ | −− |
| Morbidity profile | Lower | Lower | Higher | Higher |

**Fig. 11.1** Options for midface osteotomy in children with syndromic craniosynostosis, which include Le Fort III, Le Fort II with zygomatic repositioning, monobloc, and monobloc with facial bipartition. The table provides a comparative assessment of the various options. (Adapted with permission from Taylor JA, Bartlett SP. What's new in syndromic craniosynostosis surgery? *Plast Reconstr Surg.* 2017;140(1):82e–93e.)

included within the cutting guide, pilot holes are drilled. At this point, cutting guides are typically removed. If a specific cutting guide also includes a flange to guide angulation of an osteotomy (for example, at the nasofrontal junction with angulation guide provided to avoid transcranial passage of the saw blade) the cutting guide may be left in place for marking, initiation, or performance of the osteotomy. After completion of the custom and noncustom osteotomies, midfacial segments are confirmed to be freely mobile. Any necessary bony fixation is performed, with custom milled or pre-bent stock plates. Internal or external distraction devices are placed, with the scalp closed after placement (internal devices) or before placement (external halo device).

## Case 1: Facial Bipartition

A 9-year-old female with Apert syndrome and a history of frontoorbital advancement presented with ongoing facial deformity including midface hypoplasia, frontal retrusion,

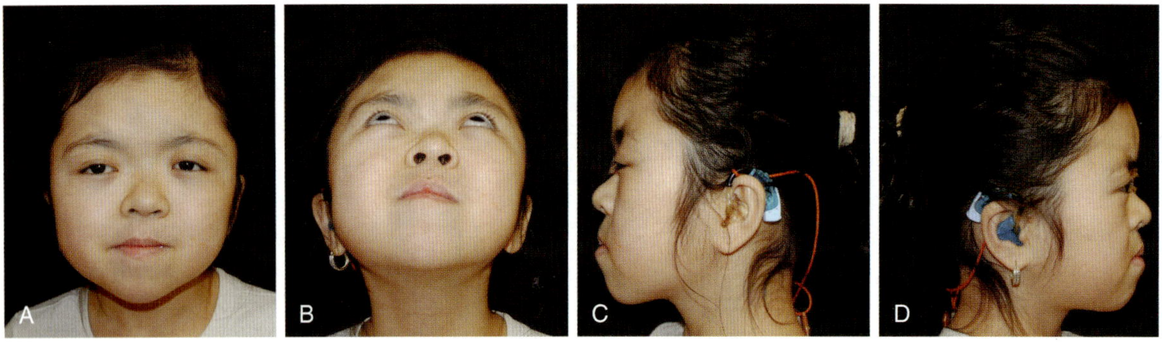


**Fig. 11.2** A 9-year-old female with Apert syndrome (Case 1) and facial deformity including midface hypoplasia, frontal retrusion, orbital hypertelorism, and a V-shaped anterior open bite. A, frontal view; B, worm's eye view; C-D, lateral views.

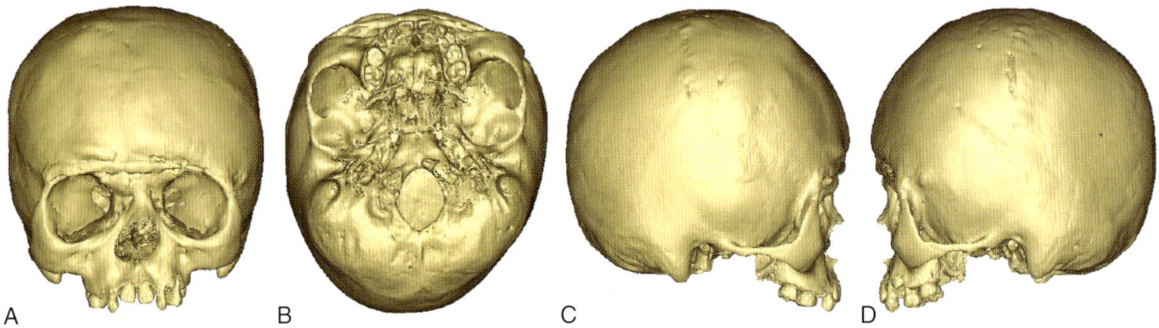


**Fig. 11.3** Computed tomography scan of 9-year-old female with Apert syndrome (Case 1); clinical photos shown in Fig. 11.2. A, frontal view; B, submental view; C-D, lateral views.

orbital hypertelorism, and a V-shaped anterior open bite. For single-stage correction of the identified anatomic features, the patient was determined to be an appropriate candidate for facial bipartition with advancement performed via external distraction (Figs. 11.2 and 11.3).

In this setting, CaSP was used to determine the width of the interorbital wedge resection that would provide optimal interorbital distance, closure of the anterior open bite (Fig. 11.4), and the degree of advancement required for appropriate frontal-midfacial-lower facial relationships. A cutting guide was designed for placement on the frontal bar and nasofrontal junction to dictate the wedge resection to be performed intraoperatively (Fig. 11.5). The expected distances of bony interference between the midfacial and cranial segments (occurring after the midface was rotated anteriorly and inferiorly) were identified in order to facilitate accurate bony resection (i.e., adequate for necessary midfacial rotation and to allow distraction without bony interference) (Fig. 11.6). Custom titanium fixation was not used in this case, and an external halo distractor was used for distraction postoperatively. The final frontofacial position as determined by CaSP is seen in Fig. 11.7; while measurements from this portion of the planning session can be helpful and are generally performed, distraction is typically continued to a clinical endpoint rather than a previously determined specific measurement. The patient is seen two years postoperatively in Fig. 11.8.

## Case 2: Monobloc + Le Fort II

An 11-year-old female with Apert syndrome and no previous craniofacial surgical history presented with headaches, frontoorbital retrusion, an inverted left lower eyelid from severe exorbitism, midface hypoplasia, and a level anterior open bite (Figs. 11.9 and 11.10) and was determined to be an appropriate candidate for a combined monobloc/Le Fort II frontofacial advancement. This specific and customized osteotomy design has been previously described by the senior author for single-stage treatment of the Apert midfacial phenotype,[5] and permits differential advancement of the frontoorbital and midfacial segments, along with midfacial lengthening, nasal lengthening, and closure of an anterior open bite. Initial osteotomy design and

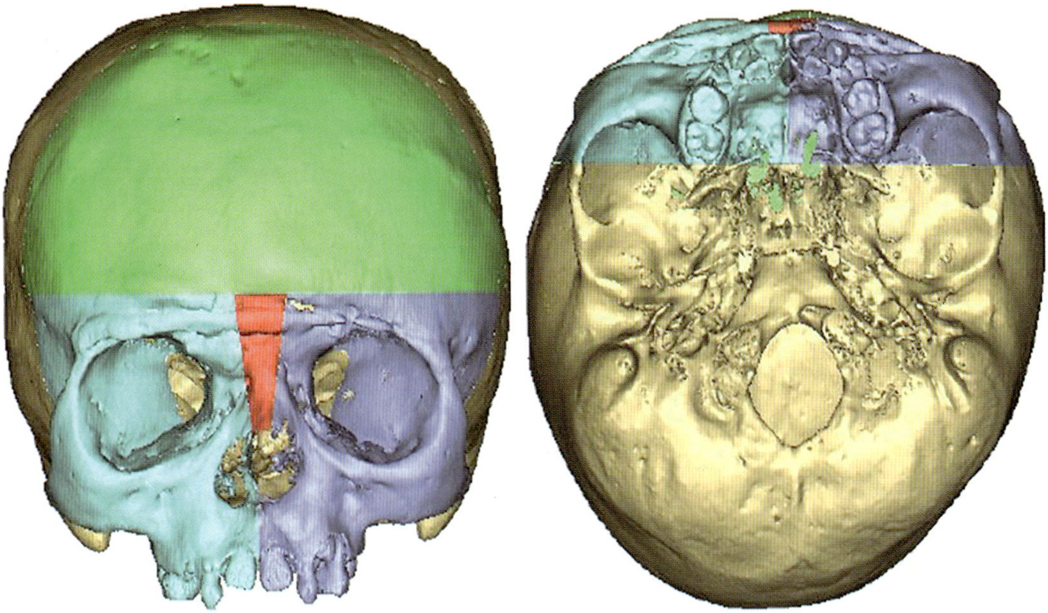

**Fig. 11.4** Computer-assisted surgical planning was used to determine the width of the interorbital wedge resection *(red)* that would provide optimal interorbital distance and leveling of the anterior open bite.

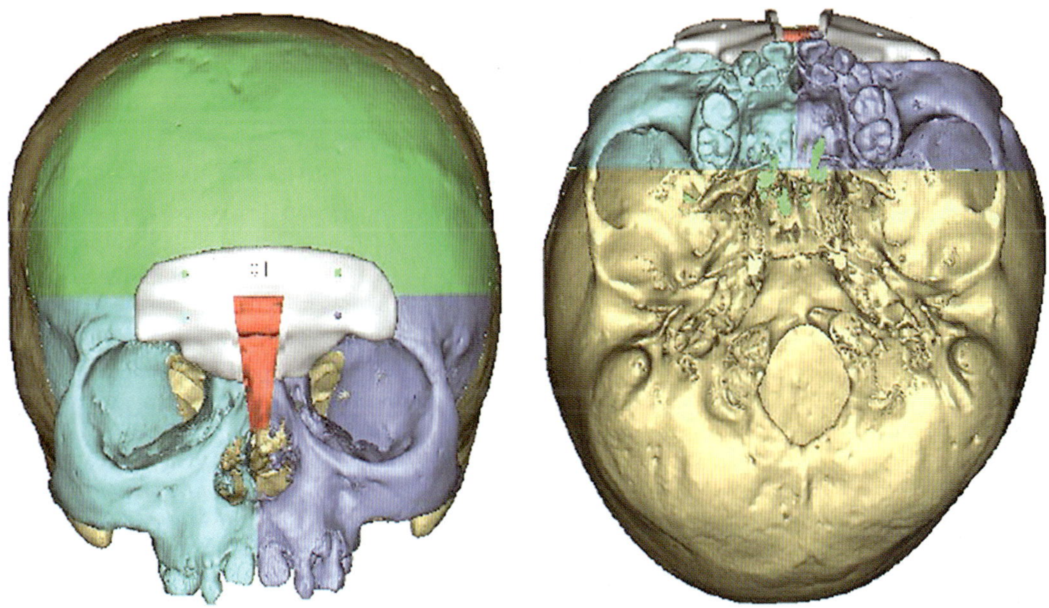

**Fig. 11.5** A cutting guide was designed for placement on the frontal bar and nasofrontal junction to dictate the interorbital wedge resection to be performed intraoperatively.

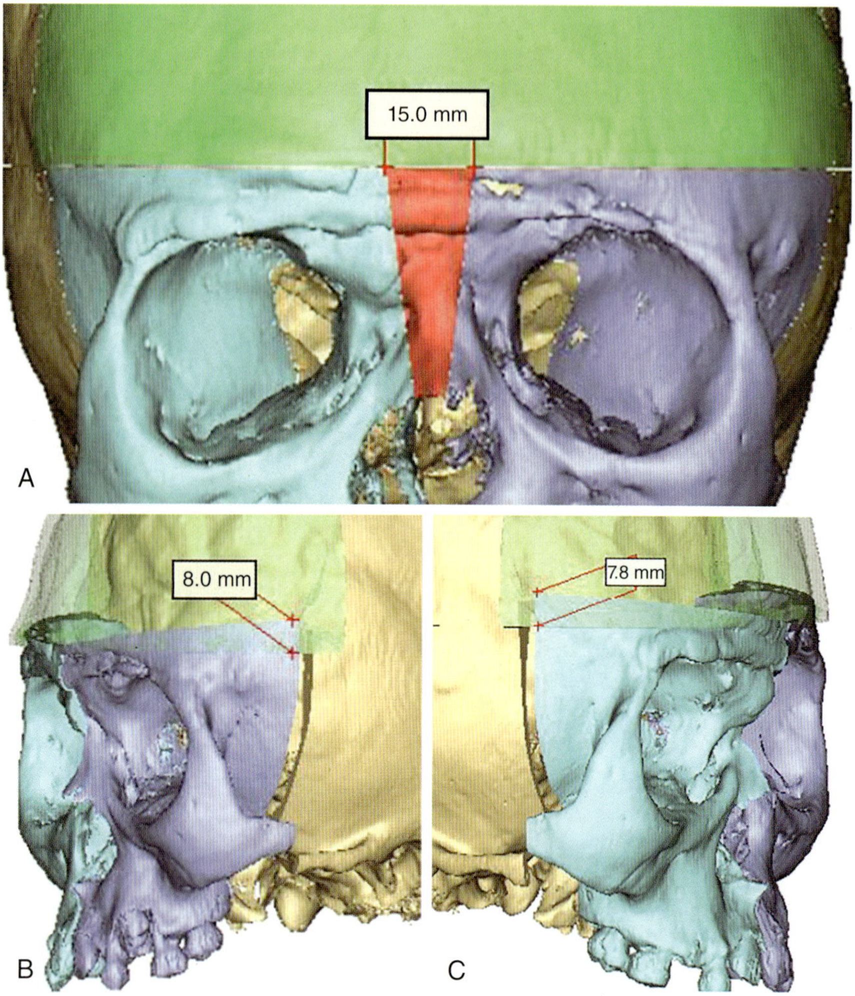


**Fig. 11.6** The expected distances of bony interference between the midfacial and cranial segments (occurring after the midface was rotated anteriorly and inferiorly) were identified to facilitate accurate bony resection (i.e., adequate for necessary midfacial rotation and to allow distraction without bony interference).

planned final position as established via CaSP are shown in Figs. 11.11 and 11.12. In this design, the monobloc segment was intended to be advanced 16 millimeters, correcting the position of the forehead and frontal bar, and the Le Fort II segment intended to be advanced 22 millimeters and rotated 4 millimeters clockwise at the central incisors.

To achieve differential advancement of the multiple segments in this case, the decision was made to perform the frontoorbital component of distraction via an internal distraction device and the LeFort II component of distraction via an external halo distractor. To both ensure the desired vector of advancement and ensure the absence of bony interference with distraction, a distractor placement and vector guide was developed (Figs. 11.13–11.15.) Nasofrontal cutting guides were also developed in this case (Fig. 11.15) and are seen in situ in Fig. 11.16. Internal and external distraction was performed simultaneously and to a clinical endpoint of frontoorbital and occlusal correction. CT scan obtained after removal of internal distractors is seen in Fig. 11.17. The patient is seen two years postoperatively in Fig. 11.18, and seven years postoperatively in Fig. 11.19.

## Case 3: Monobloc + Le Fort I

A 9-year-old male with Antley-Bixler syndrome and no previous craniofacial surgical history presented with

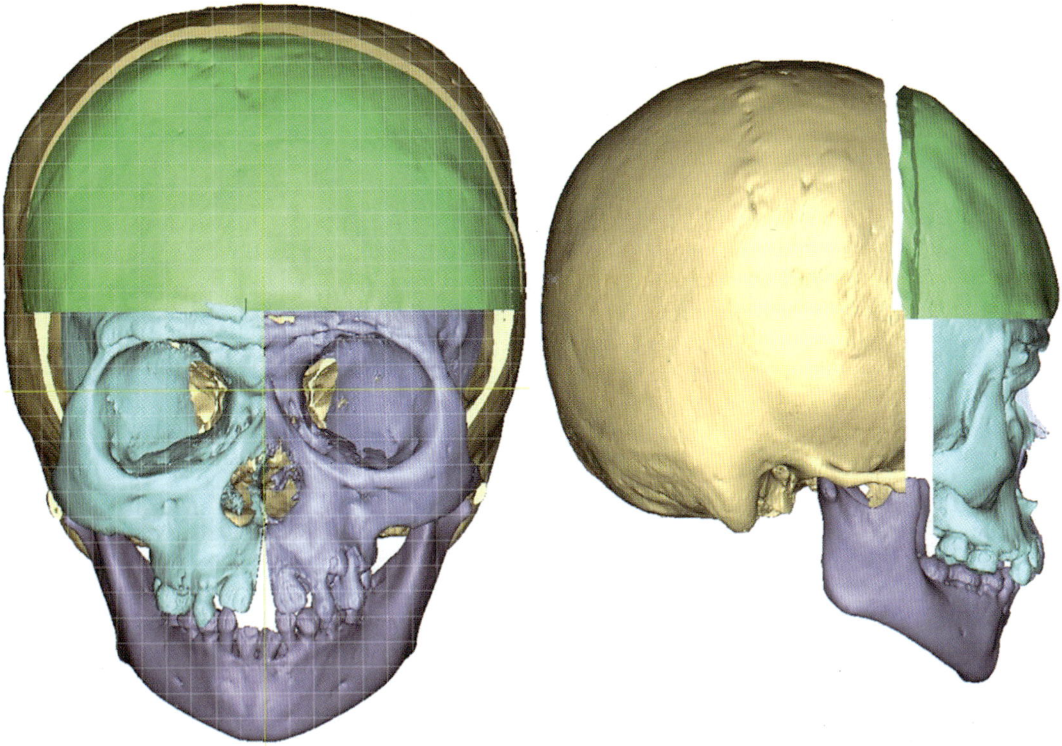

Fig. 11.7 The final frontofacial position as determined by computer-assisted surgical planning.

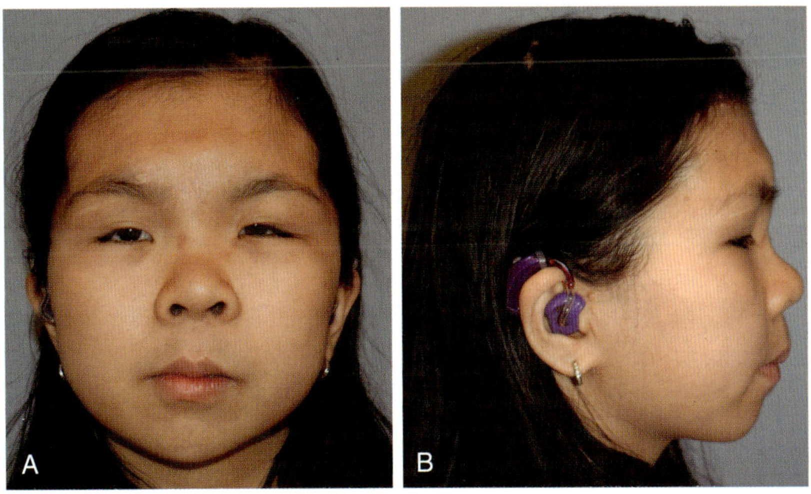


Fig. 11.8 Patient from Case 1 seen 2 years postoperatively.

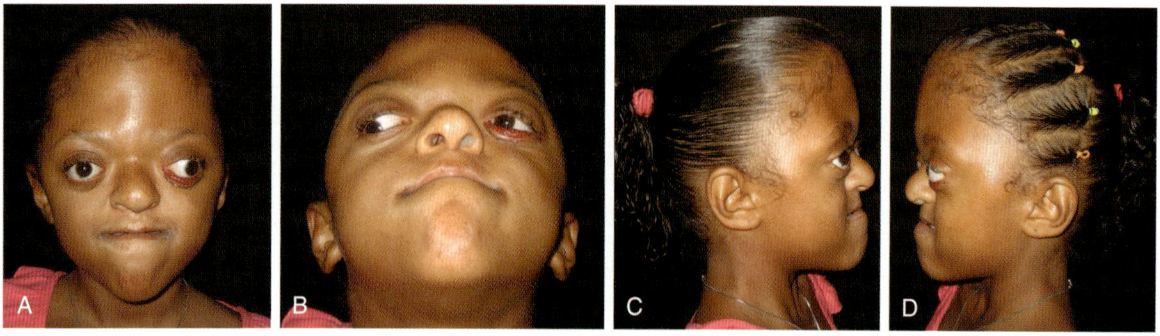


**Fig. 11.9** An 11-year-old female with Apert syndrome (Case 2) and facial deformity including frontoorbital retrusion, an inverted left lower eyelid from severe exorbitism, midface hypoplasia, and a level anterior open bite. A, frontal view; B, worm's eye view; C-D, lateral views.

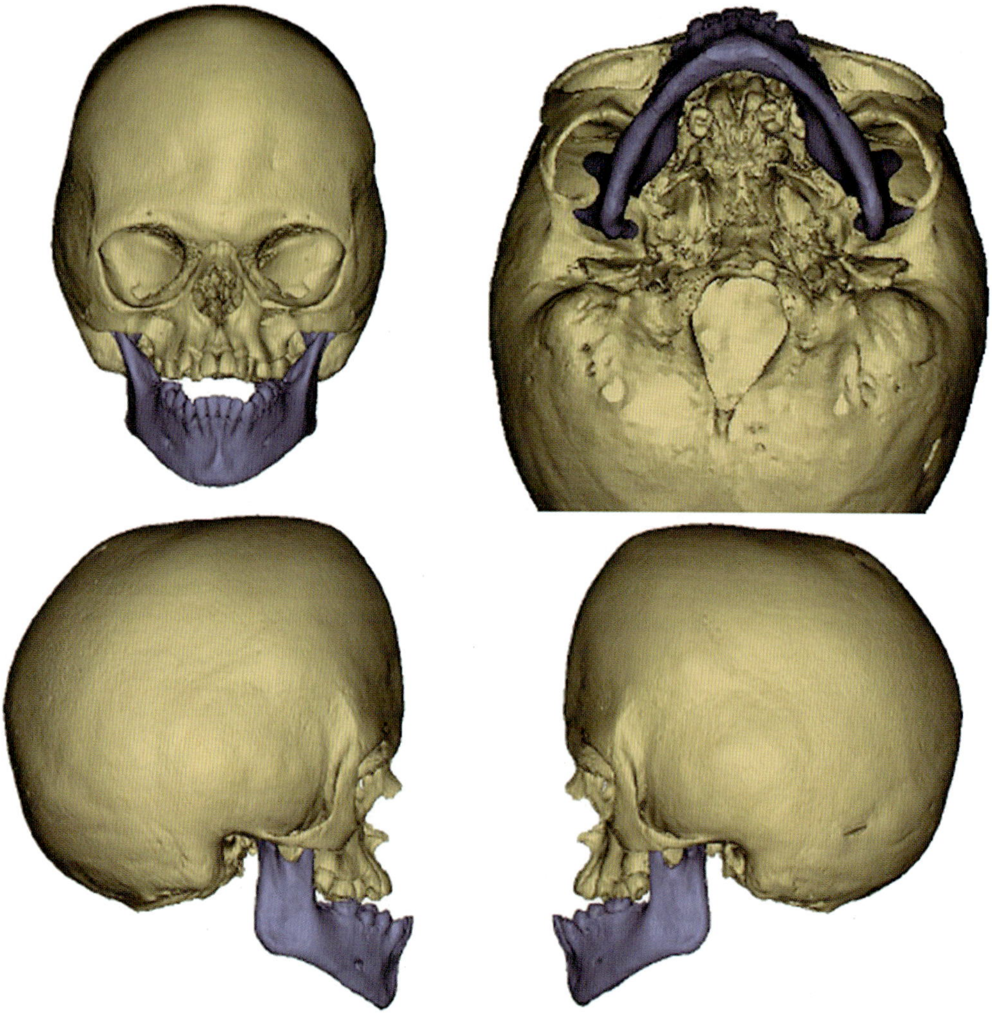

**Fig. 11.10** Computed tomography scan of 11-year-old patient with Apert syndrome (Case 2); clinical photos seen in Fig. 11.9.

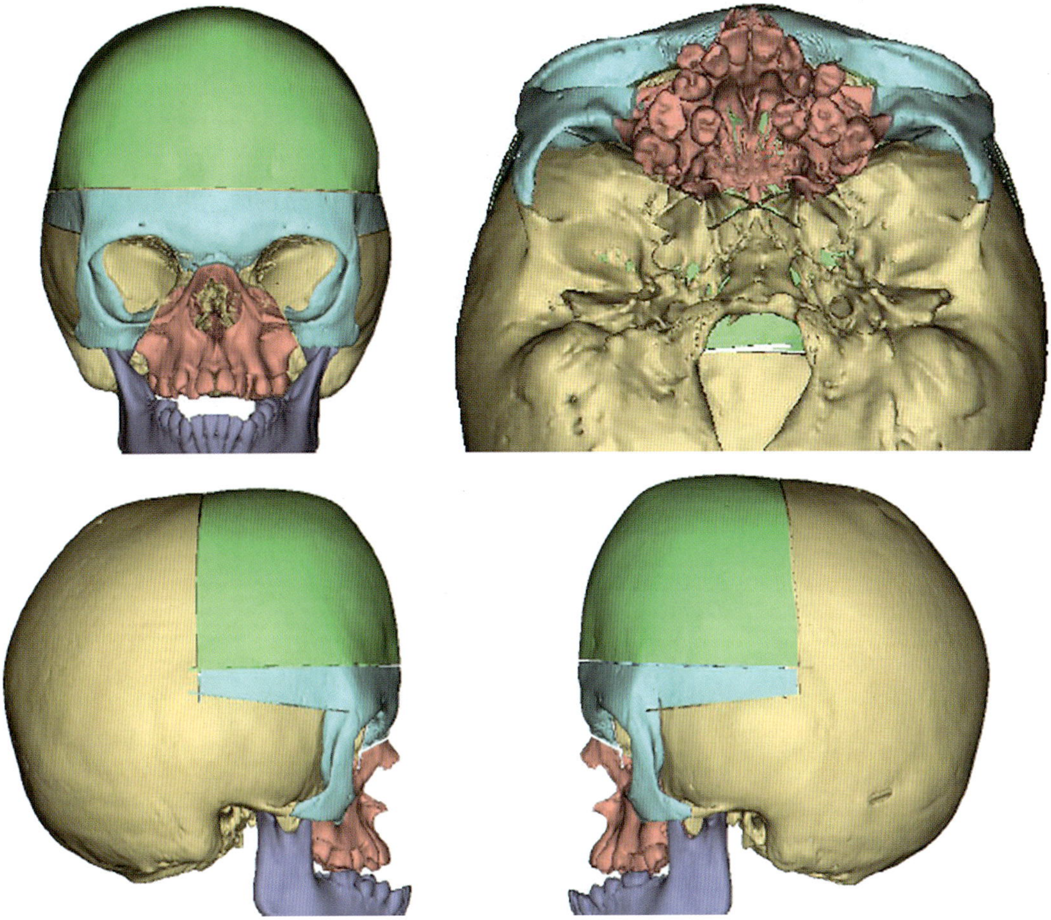

**Fig. 11.11** Initial osteotomy design as established via computer-assisted surgical planning.

multisuture craniosynostosis and midface hypoplasia, with complaints of headaches and clinical findings of obstructive sleep apnea and neurodevelopmental delay (Figs. 11.20 and 11.21.) The patient was determined to be in need of both intracranial expansion and midfacial correction, with relatively more midfacial correction required as compared to frontal advancement. The decision was made to perform a monobloc + LeFort I osteotomy to allow for differential advancement of the tooth-bearing maxilla and the frontal-upper midfacial segment.

The initial osteotomy design for a monobloc + LeFort I is shown in Fig. 11.22. In this operative plan, particularly note the tongue-in-groove osteotomies in the bilateral temporal skull, included to provide added surface area of bony contact and stability of osteotomized segments. The planned distance of distraction and added clockwise rotation of the LeFort I segment is shown in Fig. 11.23 and 11.24. In this case, distraction was performed via external halo device, with frontal and maxillary points of fixation allowing for differential advancement of the bony segments. Again, measurement of expected distraction distance was performed via CaSP, but distraction ultimately continued to a clinical endpoint of appropriate frontal and maxillary correction. The patient is seen postoperatively after halo removal in Fig. 11.25.

## Fidelity/verification

Intraoperative CT-guided navigation systems can be utilized in frontal or midfacial surgery in children with craniosynostosis. However, in the authors' preferred methodology, intraoperative verification and fidelity is

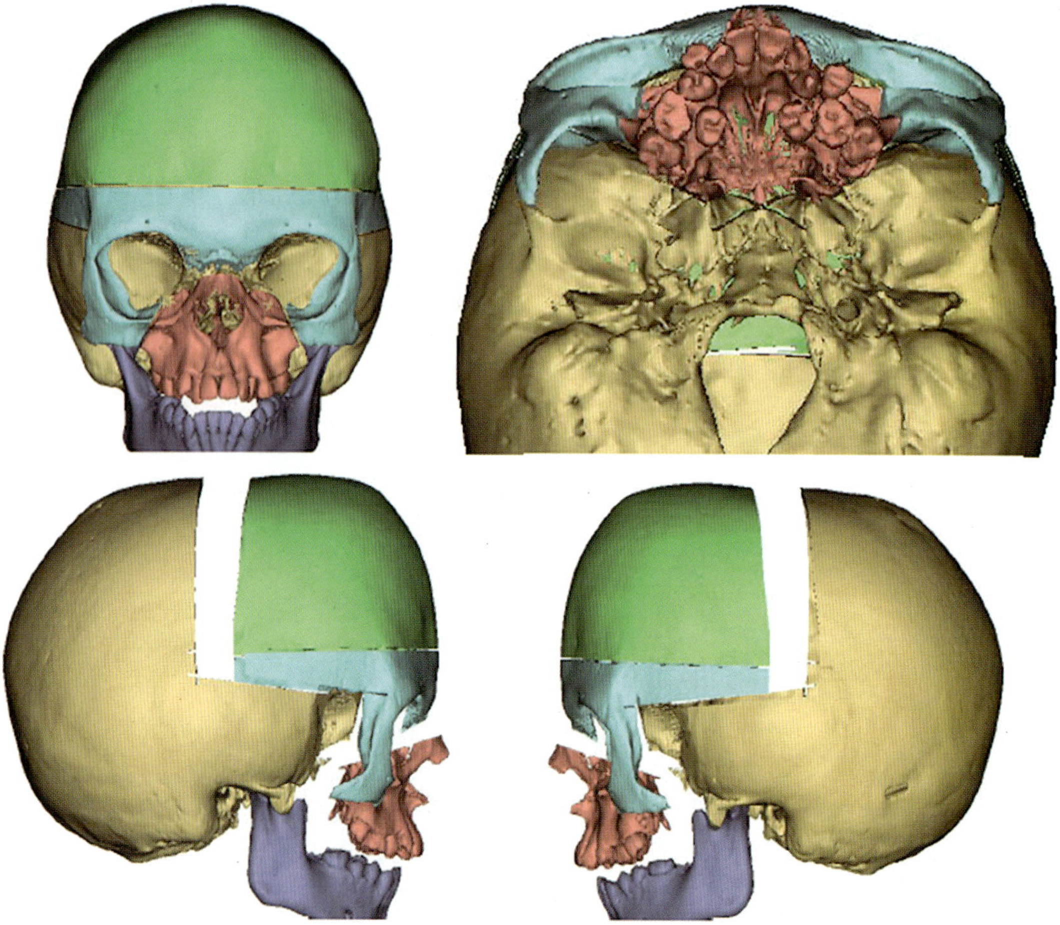

**Fig. 11.12** Planned final frontofacial position as established via computer-assisted surgical planning.

determined by the surgeon during and at completion of the case via direct visualization. The surgical plan is printed preoperatively and brought to the operating room, where it is used as a reference for operative steps and expected anatomy at the completion of the procedure. In computer-assisted planned orthognathic surgery cases in which distraction osteogenesis is not used, final occlusion can be used to clinically verify operative fidelity. However, establishing definitive occlusion is not the focus of frontofacial distraction in the patient population discussed in this chapter.

## Outcomes/complications

Complications are common in midfacial distraction,[6] particularly in those cases in which a transcranial approach is used (monobloc) rather than a subcranial approach (Le Fort III.) In a retrospective review of 18 years of midfacial surgery procedures performed at the Children's Hospital of Philadelphia by Zhang et al., a population of 64 patients undergoing 71 midfacial distractions was evaluated for the presence of perioperative and postoperative morbidity following midfacial surgery.[7] In this study, operative time, anesthesia time, and volume of blood transfusion by weight were all significantly greater in the transcranial group compared to the subcranial group.[7] Complications (surgical, hardware-related, infectious) occurred at a rate of 29% in the subcranial group and 58% in the transcranial group (all $p < .05$).[7] A multivariate analysis including gender, age at surgery, multipiece osteotomy, transcranial osteotomy, use of an external halo device, surgeon, and duration of distractors in place identified the only significant variable associated with increased risk for

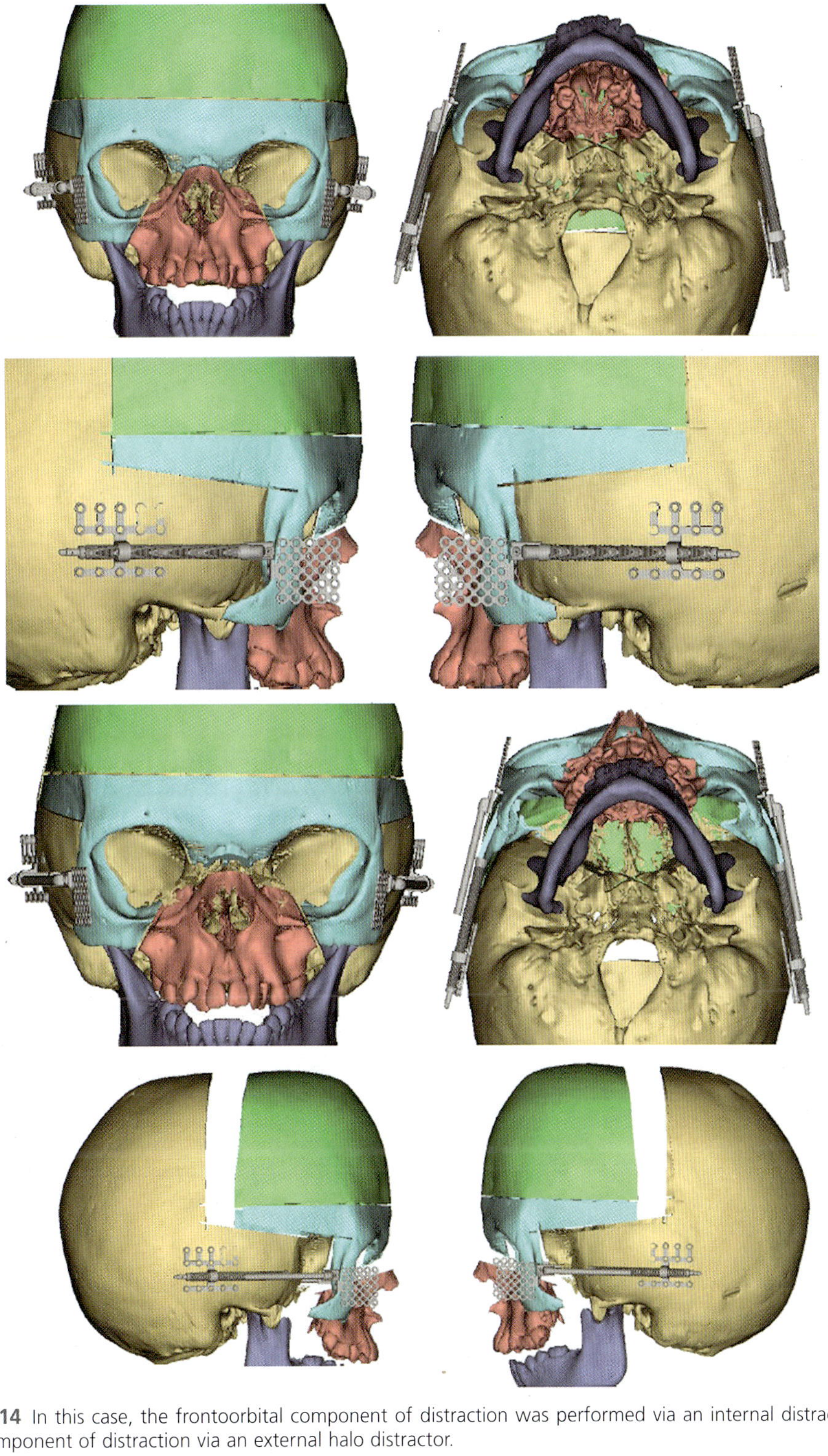

**Fig. 11.13–11.14** In this case, the frontoorbital component of distraction was performed via an internal distraction device and the Le Fort II component of distraction via an external halo distractor.

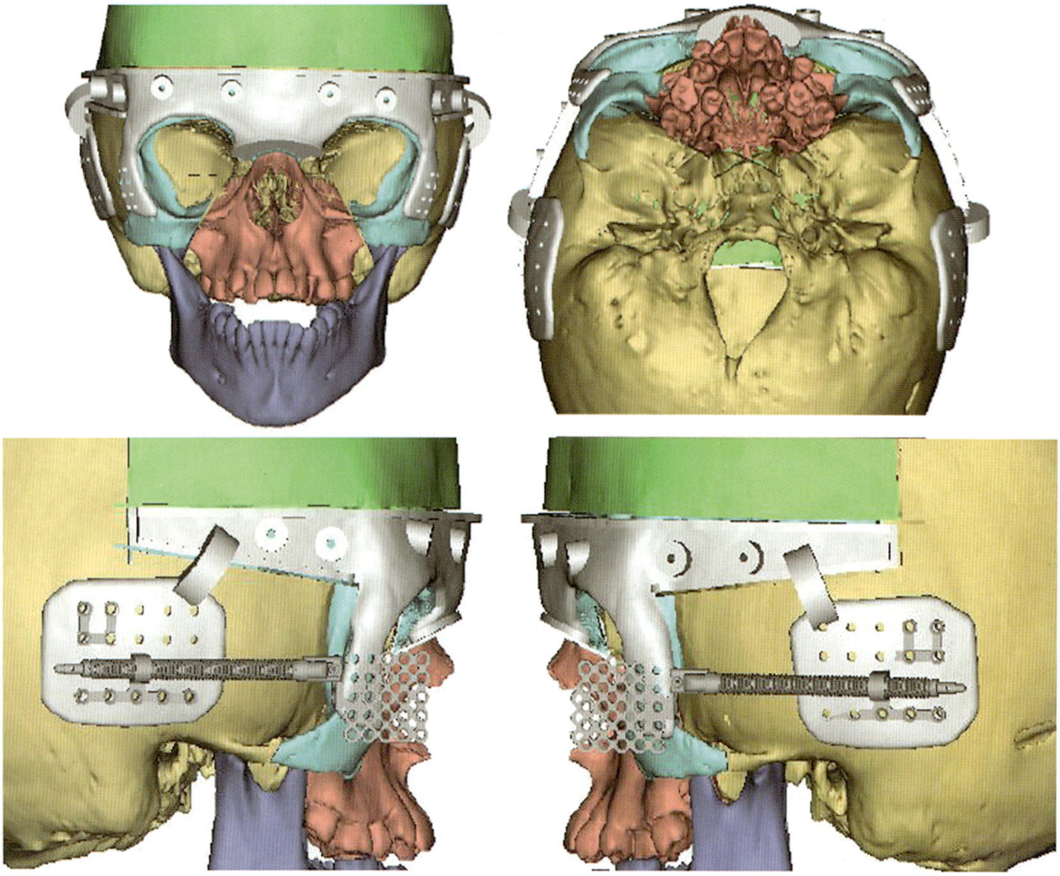

Fig. 11.15 To ensure the desired vector of advancement and the absence of bony interference with distraction, a distractor placement and vector guide was developed. Nasofrontal cutting guides were also fabricated for this case.

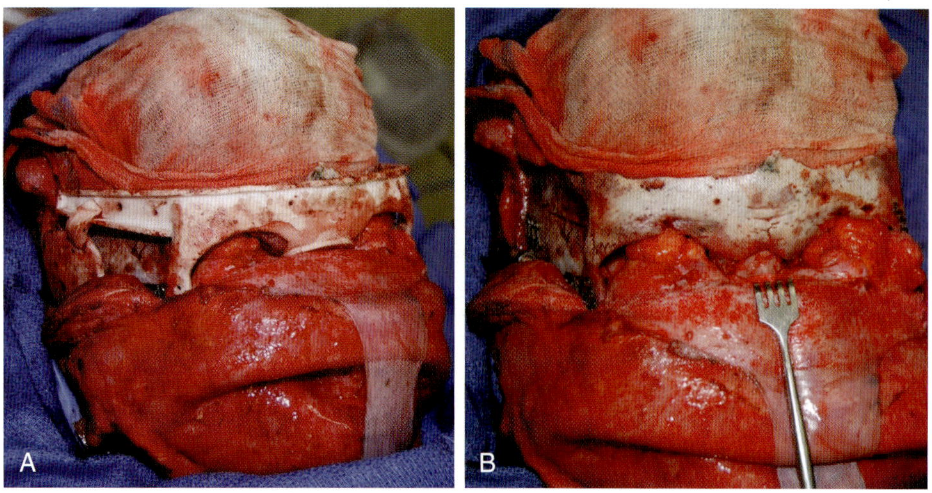


Fig. 11.16 Nasofrontal cutting guide seen insitu.

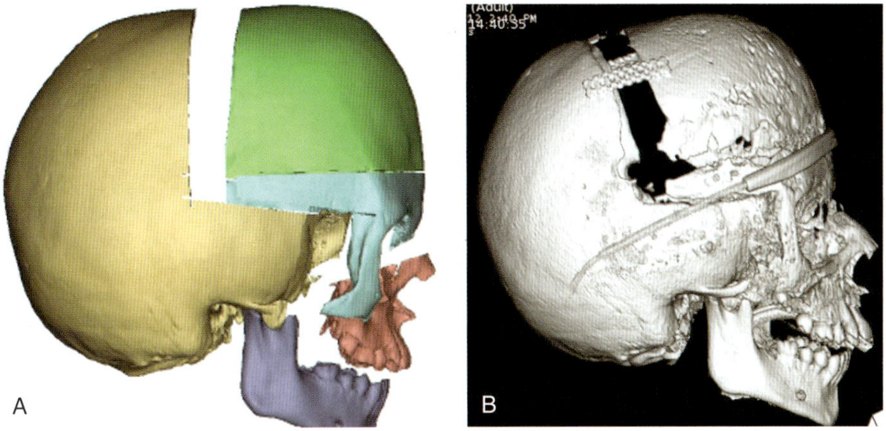


**Fig. 11.17** Computed tomography scan obtained after removal of internal distractors. A, planned frontofacial bony movement; B, frontofacial bony movement seen on computed tomography scan.

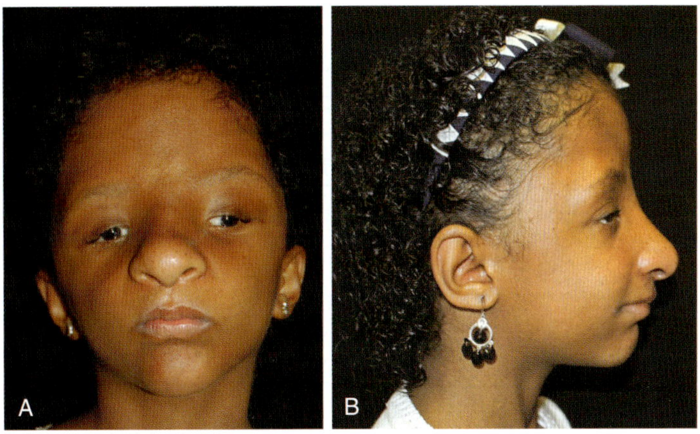


**Fig. 11.18** Patient from Case 2 seen two years postoperatively.

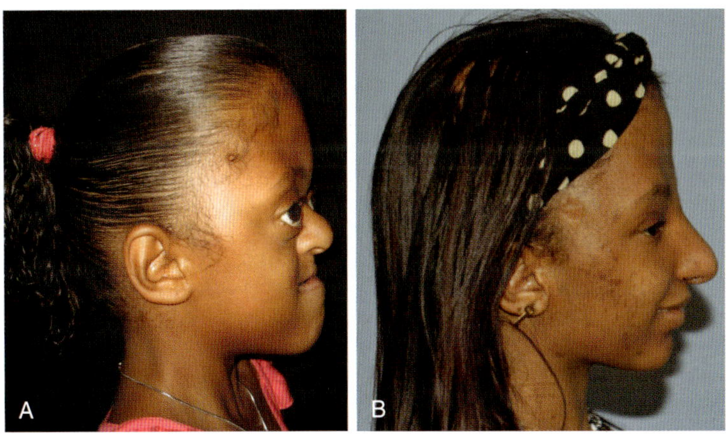


**Fig. 11.19** Patient from Case 2 seen seven years postoperatively.

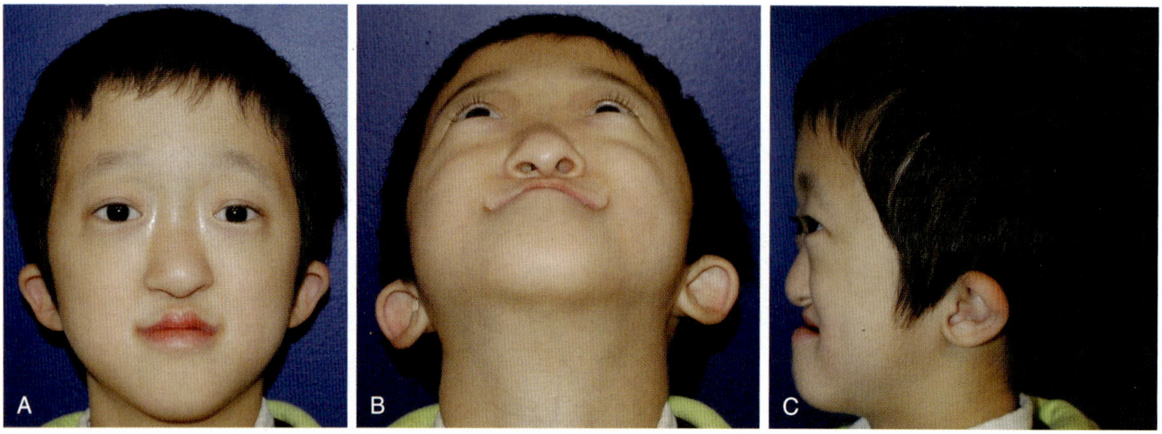


**Fig. 11.20** A 9-year-old male with Antley-Bixler syndrome (Case 3) and facial deformity including frontal retrusion and midface hypoplasia. A, frontal view; B, worm's eye view; C, lateral view.

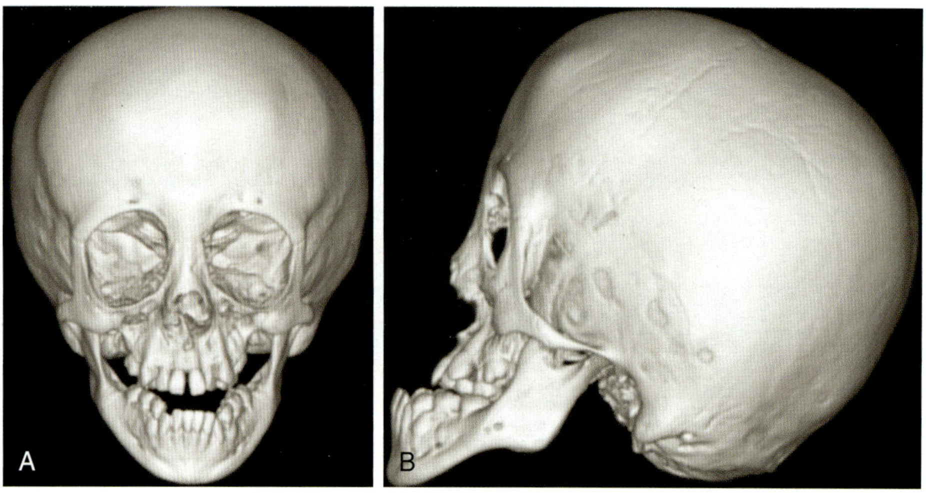


**Fig. 11.21** Computed tomography scan of 9-year-old male with Antley-Bixler syndrome (Case 3); clinical photos seen in Fig. 11.20. A, frontal view; B, lateral view.

complications to be performance of a transcranial osteotomy (odds ratio 5.80, $p$ = .013, confidence interval 1.44–23.29).[7] Similarly-designed studies have corroborated the higher risk of complications in transcranial surgery compared to subcranial surgery.[6,8,9] A 2015 retrospective study by Goldstein et al. of 54 patients with syndromic craniosynostosis undergoing midfacial surgery compared perioperative risks relative to the use of internal, semiburied distractors versus external, halo-type distractors.[8] In this study, 30 midfacial distractions were performed with external distractors (18 Le Fort III, 12 monobloc) and 25 were performed with internal distractors (16 Le Fort III, 9 monobloc).[8] The total number of distractor-related complications was similar between the two groups, with 10 complications occurring in the halo group (18.2%; operative complication in 5 patients or 9.1%) and 9 complications occurring in the internal distractor group (16.4%; operative complication in 6 patients or 10.1%).[8] Patients in the internal distractor group experienced significantly more major infections ($n$ = 8 in internal group versus $n$ = 3 in external group, $p$ = .048), while 7.3% of patients with external halo distractors required operative repositioning after either transcranial pin migration or malposition of pins related to a fall or patient positioning.[8] It should be noted that the complications of semiburied

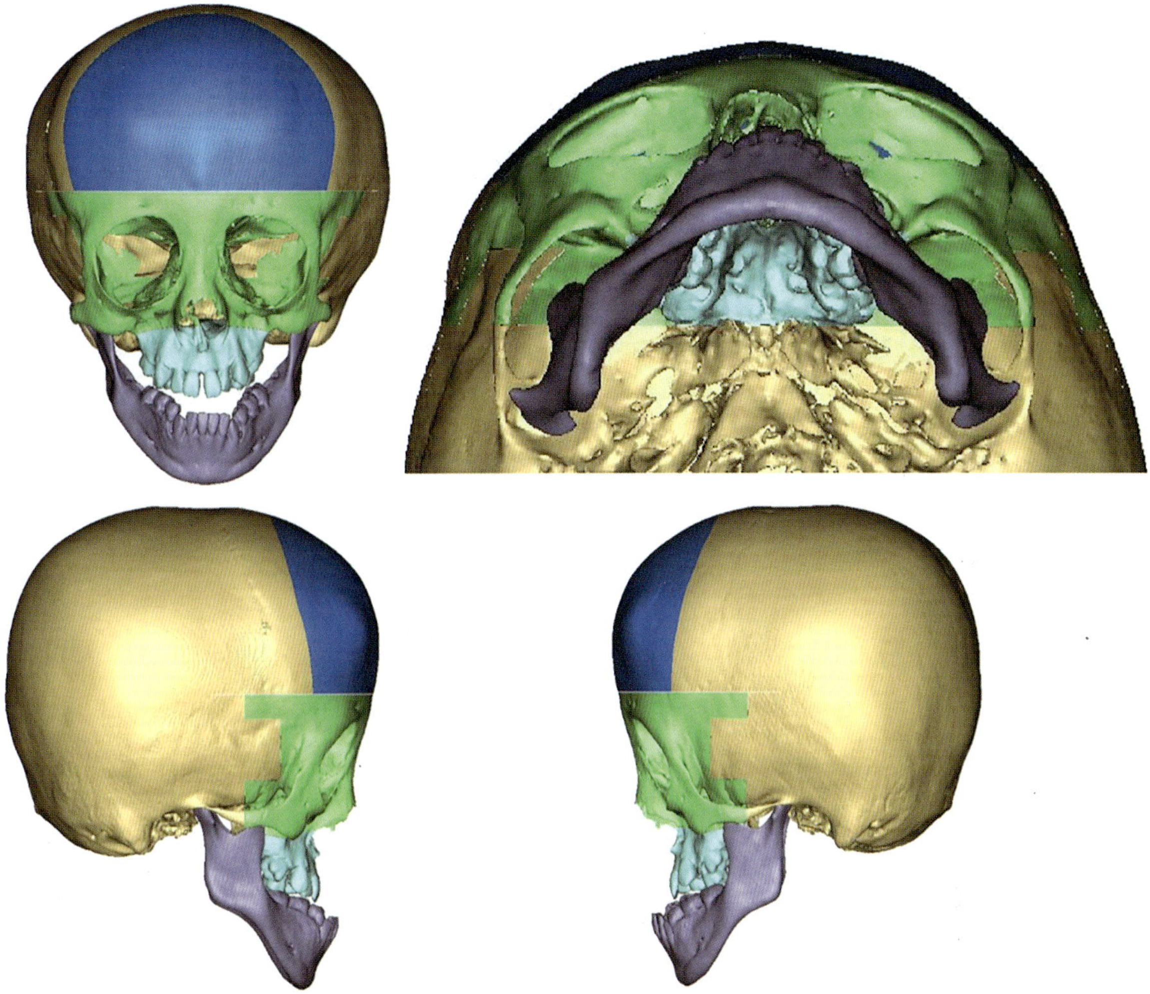

**Fig. 11.22** Osteotomy design for a monobloc + Le Fort I.

or external, halo-type distractors described herein are not specifically known to be associated with the use of CaSP.

Outcome metrics of interest in midfacial surgery in patients with syndromic craniosynostosis include ocular protection, obstructive sleep apnea, tracheostomy status, and intracranial pressure status. The small patient population and unique nature of each individual case creates challenges in performing uniform case-control, cohort, or randomized prospective studies evaluating the metrics of interest in patients with craniosynostosis who have undergone midfacial surgery. Thus, conclusive or high-quality data regarding postoperative outcomes in this group of patients is limited. As surgeons perform more complex, exotic osteotomies in an effort to solve as many problems as possible in a single stage, it will be interesting to see whether complication rates rise, an unintended consequence of this brilliant new technology.

## Conclusion

Computer-assisted surgical planning has been used with increasing frequency in pediatric craniofacial surgery in the last decade, and can be particularly valuable in treating the midface and cranium in select patients with syndromic craniosynostosis. Many operations frequently performed in children with craniosynostosis can be

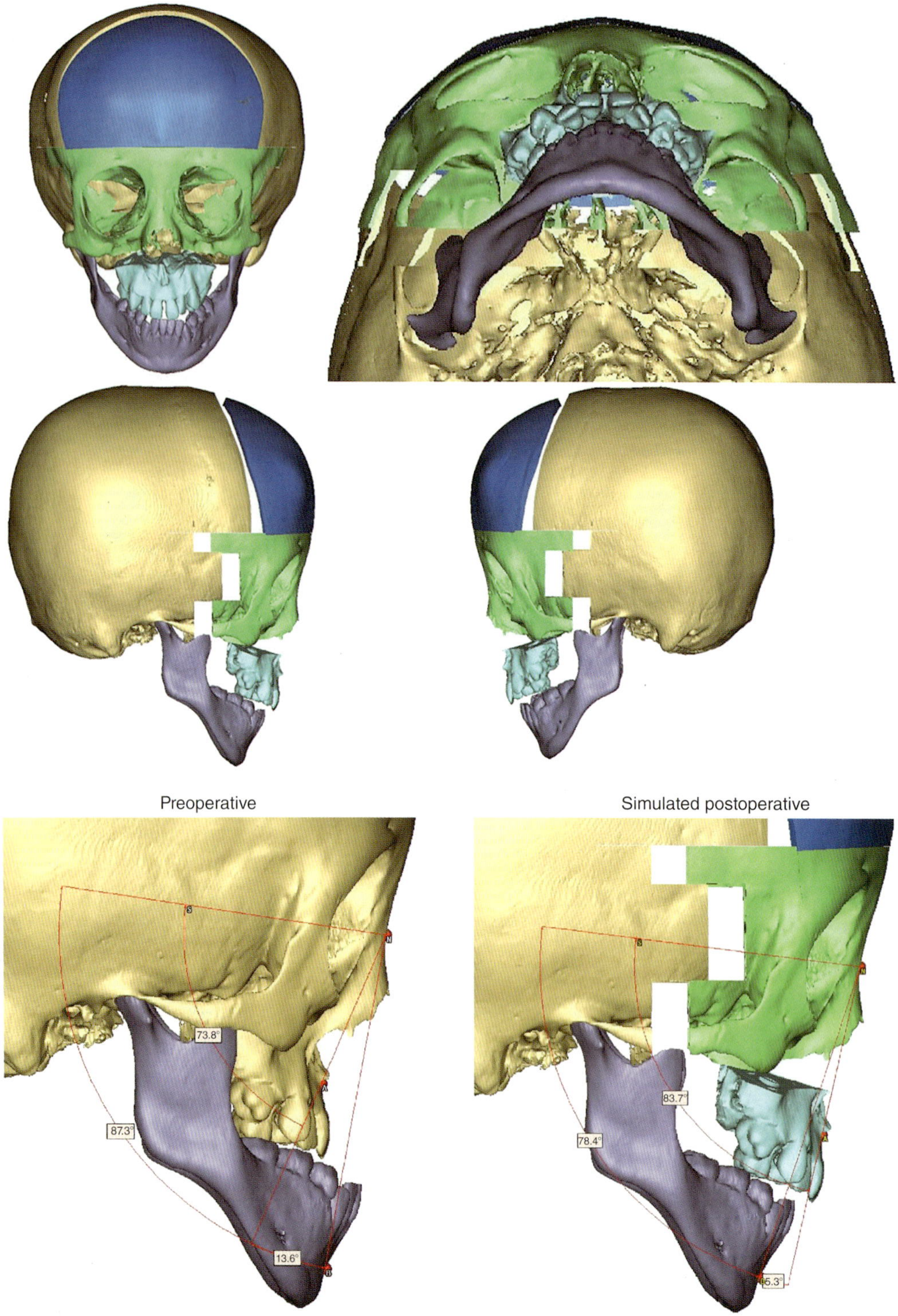


**Fig. 11.23–11.24** The planned distance of distraction and added clockwise rotation of the Le Fort I segment.

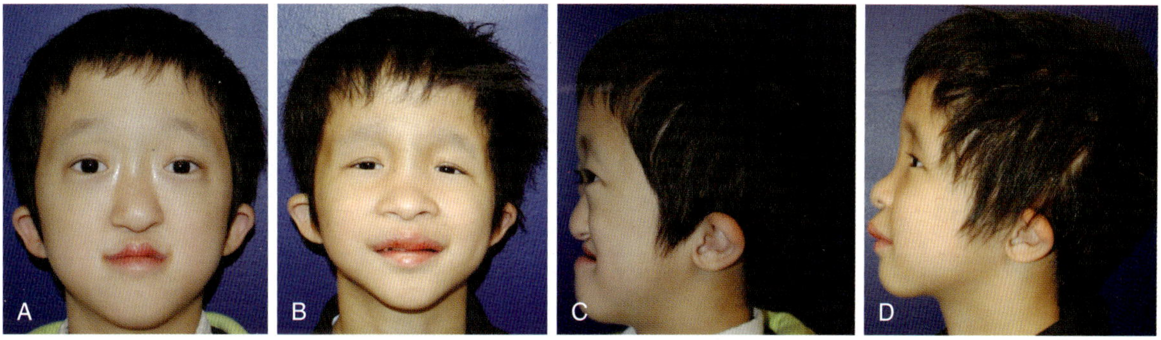


**Fig. 11.25** Patient from Case 3 seen postoperatively after halo removal. A, preoperative frontal view; B, postoperative frontal view; C, preoperative lateral view; D, postoperative lateral view.

reliably performed without the use of CaSP (frontoorbital advancement, posterior cranial vault distraction, single-piece Le Fort II and Le Fort III osteotomies). More complex, multipiece midfacial and cranial operations lend themselves well to CaSP, and this technology is extremely useful in specific facets of design and execution of these operations. Study into the functional and aesthetic benefits provided by CaSP in comparison to those provided by traditionally planned operations will help to financially justify the use of this technology, with the goal of maximizing the improvements in quality of life provided to children with syndromic craniosynostosis via surgical interventions.

## Take home points

- Children with syndromic craniosynostosis generally undergo multiple craniofacial operations throughout the course of their lives. An algorithmic approach to these operative interventions has previously been published[10] and relies upon specific anatomic findings to dictate the choice of osteotomy and surgical plan.
- Frontoorbital advancement, posterior vault distraction osteogenesis, and conventional Le Fort II and Le Fort III osteotomies can typically be performed without the use of CaSP.
- Cutting guides are a common deliverable from digital planning for midfacial surgery in patients with syndromic craniosynostosis. Custom plates and occlusal splints will be used less often given that the vast majority of these patients undergo distraction osteogenesis rather than acute bony repositioning.
- Intraoperative fidelity is typically determined by direct visualization, but intraoperative CT or navigation can be used.
- Complications are common after midfacial distraction procedures, and occur more frequently after transcranial procedures in comparison to subcranial procedures. In our experience, performance of a multipiece osteotomy does not increase the risk of a complication after midfacial surgery.

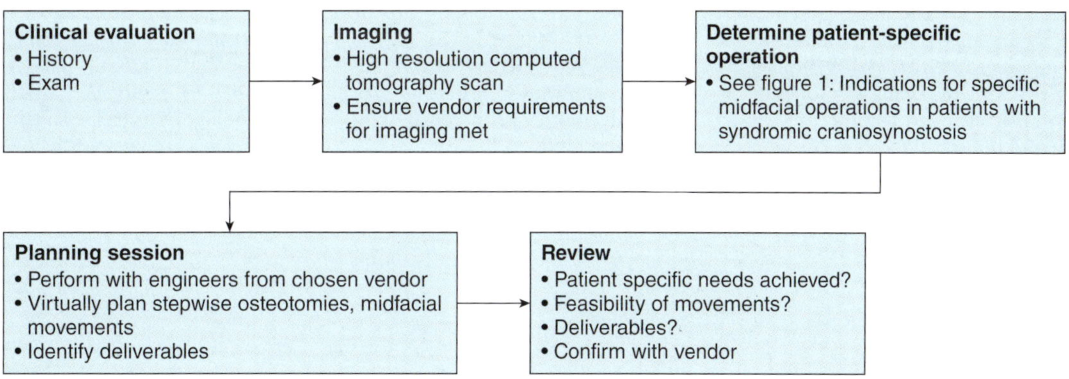

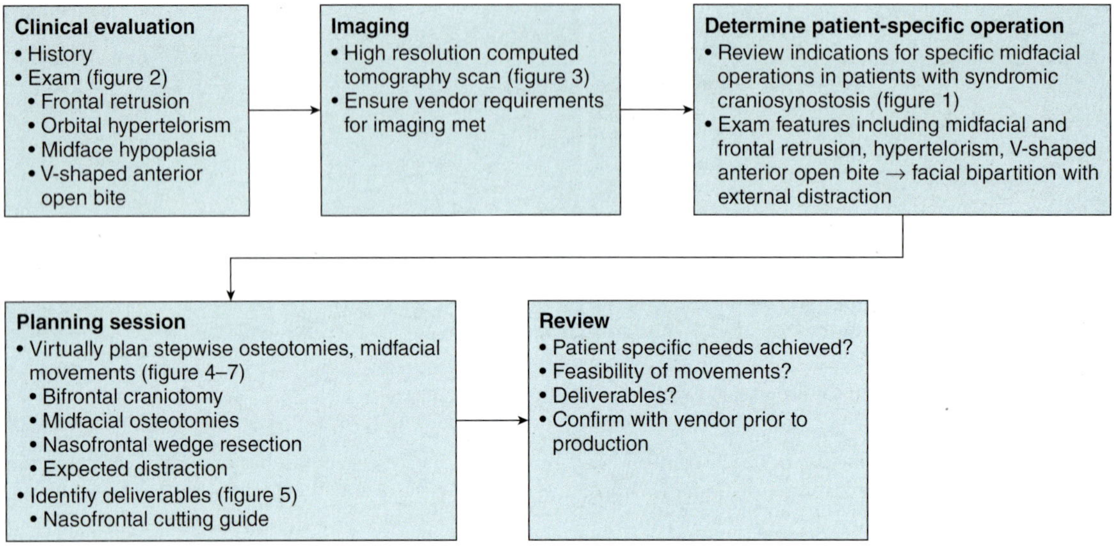


**Disclosure:** Dr. Taylor is co-founder and CMO of Ostiio, LLC. None of the authors has a financial interest in any of the products or devices mentioned in this chapter.

## References


1. Kalmar CL, Xu W, Zimmerman CE, et al. Trends in utilization of virtual surgical planning in pediatric craniofacial surgery. *J Craniofac Surg*. 2020;31(7):1900-1905.
2. Taylor JA, Bartlett SP. What's new in syndromic craniosynostosis surgery? *Plast Reconstr Surg*. 2017;140(1):82e-93e.
3. Posnick JC. The craniofacial dysostosis syndromes. Staging of reconstruction and management of secondary deformities. *Clin Plast Surg*. 1997;24(3):429-446.
4. Neil-Dwyer JG, Evans RD, Jones BM, Hayward RD. Tumescent steroid infiltration to reduce postoperative swelling after craniofacial surgery. *Br J Plast Surg*. 2001;54(7):565-569.
5. Paliga JT, Goldstein JA, Storm PB, Taylor JA. Monobloc minus Le Fort II for single-stage treatment of the Apert phenotype. *J Craniofac Surg*. 2013;24(2):596-598.
6. Hopper RA, Ettinger RE, Purnell CA, Dover MS, Pereira AR, Tuncbilek G. Thirty years later: what has craniofacial distraction osteogenesis surgery replaced? *Plast Reconstr Surg*. 2020;145(6):1073e-1088e.
7. Zhang RS, Lin LO, Hoppe IC, Swanson JW, Bartlett SP, Taylor JA. Retrospective review of the complication profile associated with 71 subcranial and transcranial midface distraction procedures at a single institution. *Plast Reconstr Surg*. 2019;143(2):521-530.
8. Goldstein JA, Paliga JT, Taylor JA, Bartlett SP. Complications in 54 frontofacial distraction procedures in patients with syndromic craniosynostosis. *J Craniofac Surg*. 2015;26(1):124-128.
9. Knackstedt R, Bassiri Gharb B, Papay F, Rampazzo A. Comparison of complication rate between Lefort III and monobloc advancement with or without distraction osteogenesis. *J Craniofac Surg*. 2018;29(1):144-148.
10. Swanson JW, Samra F, Bauder A, Mitchell BT, Taylor JA, Bartlett SP. An algorithm for managing syndromic craniosynostosis using posterior vault distraction osteogenesis. *Plast Reconstr Surg*. 2016;137(5):829e-841e.

Chapter | 12 |

# Computer-assisted surgical planning congenital differences & anomalies: syndromic craniosynostosis – (subcranial) Le Fort III and Le Fort III/I

*Erik M. Wolfswinkel, Katelyn Kondra, Eloise Stanton, Christian Jimenez, Mark M. Urata, Jeffrey A. Hammoudeh*

CHAPTER OUTLINE



## Introduction

Various conditions, congenital and acquired, can limit midface growth resulting in midface hypoplasia. Midface hypoplasia may be a result of developmental maxillary dysplasia, skeletal and dental class III malocclusion, and hard palate narrowing. This can lead to airway obstruction, mastication and speech difficulties, and an altered aesthetic facial cascade.[1,2] Affected conditions include, but are not limited to, patients with cleft lip and palate, congenital skeletal dysplasia, and patients who suffer from craniofacial dysostosis.[3,4,5] Treatment of midface hypoplasia mainly consists of restoring occlusion and optimizing the maxillary position. This can often be achieved at the Le Fort I level alone with maxillary advancement plus/minus rotation of the Le Fort I segment. The treatment of the global midface hypoplasia dysmorphology depends on the extent of hypoplasia and/or deficiency of individual structures of the midface. Therefore, a detailed and thoughtful analysis of the brow position, orbit, periorbital structures, occlusion, and airway is crucial to decide the best treatment option. If the patient has concurrent maxillofacial asymmetries from residual cranial vault dysplasia along with midface deficiency, additional surgical management for these conditions include monobloc, monobloc facial bipartition, box osteotomies, or a Le Fort III osteotomy with or without distraction.[4,5]

The majority of this chapter will focus on treatment of global midface hypoplasia and the use of subcranial Le Fort III and Le Fort III/I procedures, as these interventions may benefit from the use of computer-assisted design and computer-assisted manufacturing (CAD/CAM).

## Clinical considerations

### Evaluations

By analyzing the relative positions of the brow, orbits, periorbital structures, airway and occlusion, one can determine which structures may need corrective surgical intervention. The severity and presentation of these structures can vary greatly based on the etiology. Patients may not be bothered by or realize what structures are anomalous. They typically just want to "look better" and have their "teeth work better." Therefore, there should be a detailed discussion of the patient's and surgeon's goals with this type of operation. Any surgery at the Le Fort III level requires a coronal incision, which can be stigmatizing to patients; consequently, patients will often select for a less optimal aesthetic outcome than undergo a Le Fort III surgery. Less invasive surgeries and camouflage surgeries, such as a high Le Fort I or a modified Le Fort II, are then often performed to achieve similar results.[6,7]

### Le Fort III advancement

The indications for Le Fort III advancement are global midface hypoplasia with hypoplasia in the infraorbital region, airway obstruction secondary to midface retrusion, and skeletal and dental malocclusion.[3,6-8] An isolated Le Fort III surgery is best suited for a patient at skeletal maturity and that requires a small advancement.[9,10] More stable movements and better outcomes are rendered in patients that require approximately 5 mm of advancement or less at the inferior orbits due the degree of soft tissue constraints. If 6 mm or more of movement is required, a Le Fort III distraction is performed during the patient's growth and development followed by a Le Fort I osteotomy procedure performed at the completion of skeletal growth to address malocclusion. As our practice continues to develop, fewer patients seem to benefit from a Le Fort III advancement alone. More often, a Le Fort III distraction or simultaneous Le Fort III/I is required.

### Le Fort III distraction

Le Fort III distractions provide optimal management in children with global midface hypoplasia who require significant advancement ≥6 mm at the inferior orbital rims. This is commonly performed in a growing child to help correct functional impairments, such as orbital exorbitism, to improve airway obstruction, and to decrease the degree of a patient's syndromic appearance.[11] Given that the hardware is removed after completion of the operation, any subsequent midface surgery or orthognathic surgery can be performed. It should be noted that after an initial Le Fort III distraction, the pterygoids have been separated, which may limit future facial growth,[8,11] and it may be more challenging to redo these osteotomies. However, depending on the degree of the surgeon's experience, these operations can consistently be reproduced. Although it has been described, we do not utilize CAD/CAM for distraction procedures as the vector and length of distraction may vary from preoperative plan.[12] Custom-designed footplates, based on CAD/CAM, may be beneficial in specific patients with extremely anomalous anatomy.

### Le Fort III/I

In patients with global midface hypoplasia and class III skeletal and dental malocclusion, a Le Fort III/I procedure can optimize orbital rim positioning while also addressing occlusal adjustments. The Le Fort III/I procedure is especially useful in patients with significant difference in degree of midface hypoplasia between the orbital and dentoalveolar regions.[13] Furthermore, by moving the midface and maxilla simultaneously, less movement is required for each bony segment to reach proper alignment, and the total movement is additive.[3,14] The escalator effect of these movements helps create a more aesthetically pleasing cascade. It should be noted that this procedure is best carried out on patients of skeletal maturity to deter recurrence, relapse, and need for revisional surgery.[10,15] CAD/CAM allows surgeons to move the Le Fort III segment forward and then individually rotate or move the Le Fort I segment to restore functional occlusion as seen in our patient example and video (Video 12.1).

### Considerations in patients with craniofacial dysostosis

Craniofacial dysostosis describes a group of syndromic forms of craniosynostosis. This includes Apert syndrome, Crouzon syndrome, Carpenter syndrome, Pfeiffer syndrome, Saethre-Chotzen syndrome, and other types of craniofacial dysostosis which suffer from craniosynostosis and midface deficiencies. Given the variability of phenotypes, these dysmorphologies can be quite heterogeneous and therefore require attentive individualized treatment sequences based on the specific malformation, growth disturbances, and psychosocial aspects.

There remains no one blanket approach for treatment of these children. The timing of surgery and specific operation chosen at each stage of reconstruction is based on a number of factors, including their prior surgical history and results. For example, when evaluating children with craniofacial dysostosis, we typically begin by evaluating their appearance by age. At three months of age, we assess the amount of brachycephaly, turricephaly, and if they suffer from a Chiari malformation. If any of these are severe, then the patient will often be recommended for posterior distraction followed by a frontoorbital advancement (FOA) and cranial vault remodeling procedure. If not severe, then we proceed with an FOA closer to eight months of age. The patient is then continuously followed and assessed for increased intracranial pressure, unequal hypoplasia, and airway obstruction. This may lead one to perform an early Le Fort III distraction for airway concerns or repeat FOA if the residual cranial vault dysplasia is significant and/or they suffer from increased intracranial pressure. At approximately seven years of age, the patient's hypertelorism is evaluated, and if it requires correction, this can be achieved by facial bipartition or box osteotomies depending on the palatal width restrictions. If hypertelorism is not a concern and the patient's global midface hypoplasia is severe, then the child will most likely undergo Le Fort III distraction. Anecdotally, given the enhanced stability and decreased relapse seen in our FOA surgeries, fewer patients now require monobloc distraction and are receiving Le Fort III distraction at this stage than earlier in the senior author's (MMU) career. Lastly, once the patient achieves skeletal maturity, the patient's hypoplasia and occlusion are assessed and may be treated with Le Fort I, Le Fort III, Le Fort III/I, or any of these with the combination of bilateral sagittal split osteotomies (BSSO) and genioplasty. Given the variable phenotypes of midface hypoplasia, orthognathic surgeons can harness CAD/CAM to address each unique case with customizable interventions. Following orthognathic surgery, patients often require definitive rhinoplasty upon completion of their reconstruction.

A simplified algorithm is presented in Fig. 12.1. Typically, CAD/CAM surgery is not a part of this algorithm until the patient has reached skeletal maturity and is undergoing orthognathic-related surgery.

## Computer-assisted design and computer-assisted manufacturing

Historically, the traditional approach to presurgical planning and operative intervention was rooted in model surgery. This method was time consuming, tedious, and riddled with opportunity for human and material error. CAD/CAM provides precise and predictable movements of the maxillofacial skeleton in 15 to

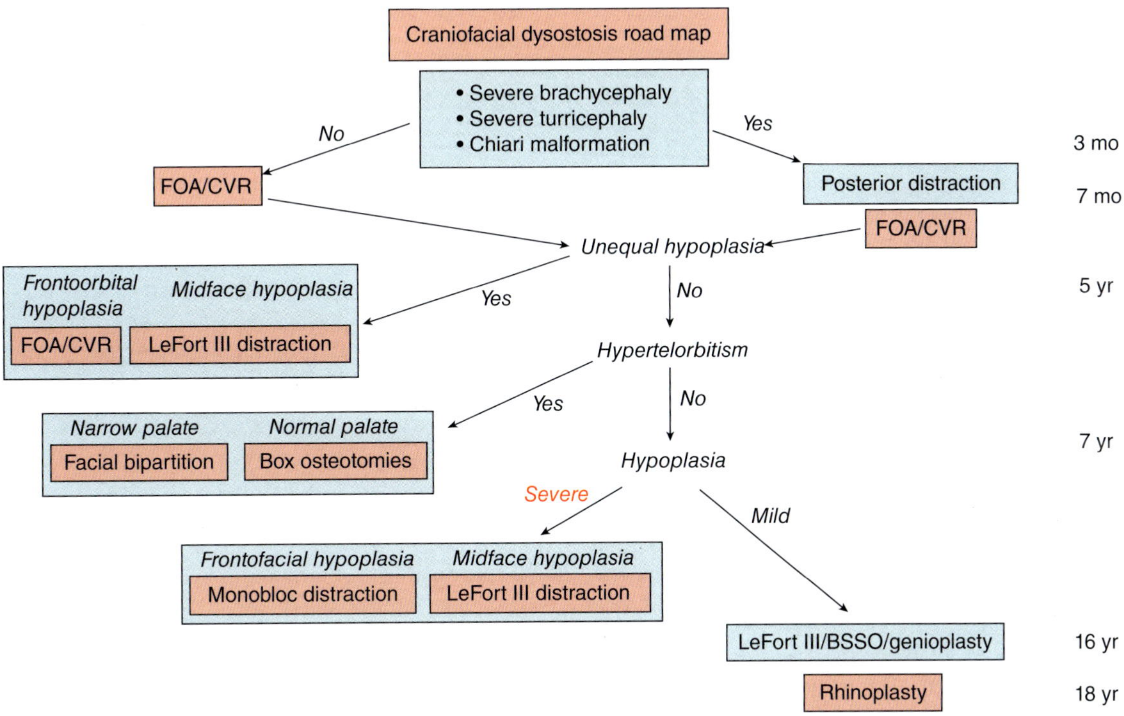


**Fig. 12.1** Simplified algorithm for timing and techniques of interventions for patients with craniofacial dysostosis. *CVR*, Cranial Vault Remoldeling; *FOA*, frontoorbital advancement.

20 minutes of software planning without the need for traditional dental impressions, Frankfort horizontal plane alignment, facebow transfers, or model surgery. There is no destruction of physical models with computer-assisted surgery, allowing for assessment of numerous osteotomies without increasing expense.[16] This results in more accurate splint fabrication[17] with the possibility of adjunct custom plates and cutting guides with predrilled holes, thus mitigating the need for internal and external reference markers, and allowing for more precise osteotomies and fixation in a multidimensional plane, especially in the setting of positing the maxilla in appropriate occlusion. The sum is a predictable and accurate method that allows for more precise surgical outcomes and reduced pre- and intraoperative times, which invites an additional cost-savings benefit.[17-19] This paradigm shift not only has potential to improve patient outcomes, but also provides for further research and development through computer-generated analysis of the virtual reconstructions.

## Workflow for computer-assisted design/computer-assisted manufacturing–based surgery

### Orthognathic team referral

At our institutions, we have created multidisciplinary teams that include numerous subspecialists with expertise in caring for children with significant midface hypoplasia. Once the patient reaches approximately 15 to 16 years of age and it is perceived that orthognathic surgery may be of benefit, the patients are referred to the Orthognathic Team. The Orthognathic Team consists of members from various disciplines, including plastic surgery, oral maxillofacial surgery, orthodontics, dentistry, and psychology, among others. We work closely together and partner with patients and their families to make sure that each child's care is individualized to meet their unique developmental, physical, and psychosocial needs.

There should be a detailed discussion of the patient's and surgeon's goals with this type of operation and a commitment from the patient that they will complete the pre- and postorthodontic treatments associated with this surgery. Once agreed upon, the orthognathic timeline for Le Fort III or Le Fort III/I is initiated. This typically requires a minimum of 6 to 12 months, and often much longer due to presurgical preparation with orthodontia, models to determine surgical readiness, and then preoperative planning. The orthognathic team PowerPoint deck provides a workflow of how this process is accomplished.

### Computer-assisted design

Once the patient is determined ready from an occlusal standpoint, a preoperative visit is scheduled approximately 1 month before the surgery date. At this point, the surgeon determines surgical readiness by confirming the models. A cone-beam computed tomography (CT) scan is obtained. These items are then provided to the bioengineering company for surgical planning. Ultimately, the team meets with the bioengineering company via teleconference to design both the osteotomies and the final movements of each of the segments.

The initial steps of designing the osteotomies and planning final movements of the segments requires referring back to the patient's examination and relative positions of the inferior orbits, midface position, occlusion, and chin position. For stability purposes and tolerance of soft tissue contraction on advancement at the Le Fort III level, the patient's movements in an anterior-posterior advancement between 3 and 6 mm is simulated in the CAD. This newly created skull is saved and used as the new starting point for the movements at the Le Fort I in the planning software. As such, soft tissue prediction in the sagittal plane and anterior portion of the maxilla at the Le Fort I level is possible, but the technology is unable to predict the soft tissue at the Le Fort III/I level because these soft tissue movements cannot be combined.

Next, attention is focused on correcting occlusion at the Le Fort I level and is consistent with maxillary sequence planning performed in previous chapters. This includes correcting the maxillary cant, making maxillary and dental midlines coincident, adjusting the yaw, adjusting the occlusal plane, and then determining the amount of anterior advancement necessary. Given that the Le Fort III segment has already advanced the maxilla forward, the degree of movement at the Le Fort I level will be significantly smaller, as these movements are additive.

Lastly, a BSSO can be used to bring the mandible to the new position of the maxilla, restore functional occlusion, and improve the facial cascade. Throughout this workflow, compared to traditional methodology, CAD/CAM-based surgery provides an accurate, predictable, reproducible, and streamlined technique. The workflow for CAD-based orthognathic surgery for Le Fort III/I is provided.

### Computer-assisted manufacturing

CAM is primarily used for three-dimensional (3D)-printed occlusal-based intermediate and final splints. For the combined Le Fort III/I procedure, the intermediate splint or splints follow the surgical sequence. First, the Le Fort III is performed. We prefer to use sandwich style splints, utilizing the same final occlusal splint throughout. This way, the final splint is wired in for the duration of the procedure

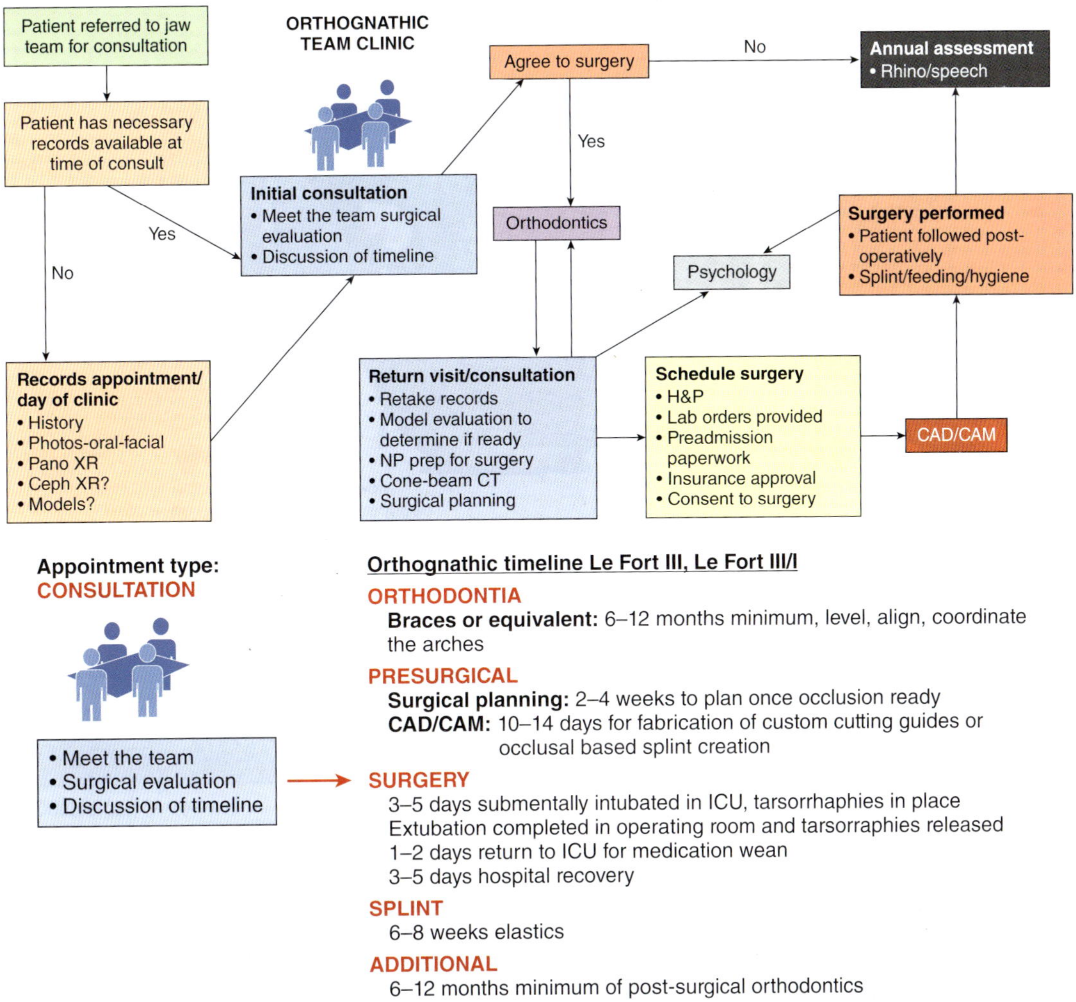


**ppt 12.1** Orthognathic team.

and forms the initial complex with the Le Fort III intermediate splint, and then the Le Fort I intermediate splint, if a BSSO is also being performed. The PowerPoint deck for CAM provides a depiction of the various occlusal-based splints. A palatal strap helps with stability in patients with clefts or in a segmented maxilla. CAD/CAM can also produce custom cutting guides and titanium plates for fixation at the surgeon's request.

## Operative techniques

The operative steps are done in a top-down approach starting at the Le Fort III, then Le Fort I ± BSSO.

Steps:

- Intubation
  - Submental intubation is necessary given the need for maxillomandibular fixation in the setting of coronal exposure.
- Tarsorrhaphy
  - Bilateral tarsorrhaphies are temporarily placed to protect the orbits during postoperative swelling and intubation period.
- Coronal access
  - A "stealth incision" using a zigzag pattern helps conceal coronal scars.
- Le Fort III
  - Performed osteotomies at the nasofrontal junction, zygomaticosphenoid junction carried cephalad up

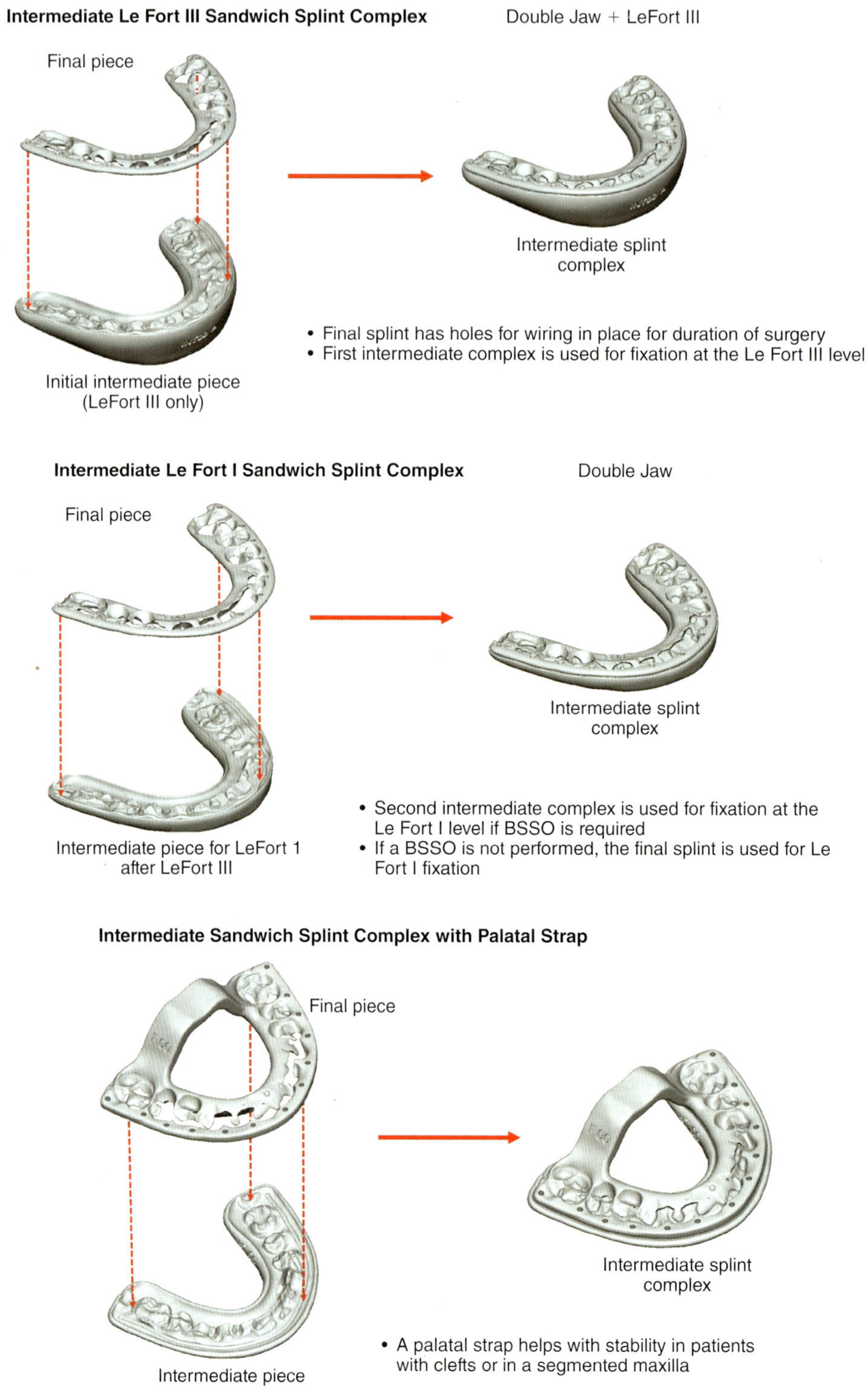


**ppt 12.3** Computer-assisted manufacturing.

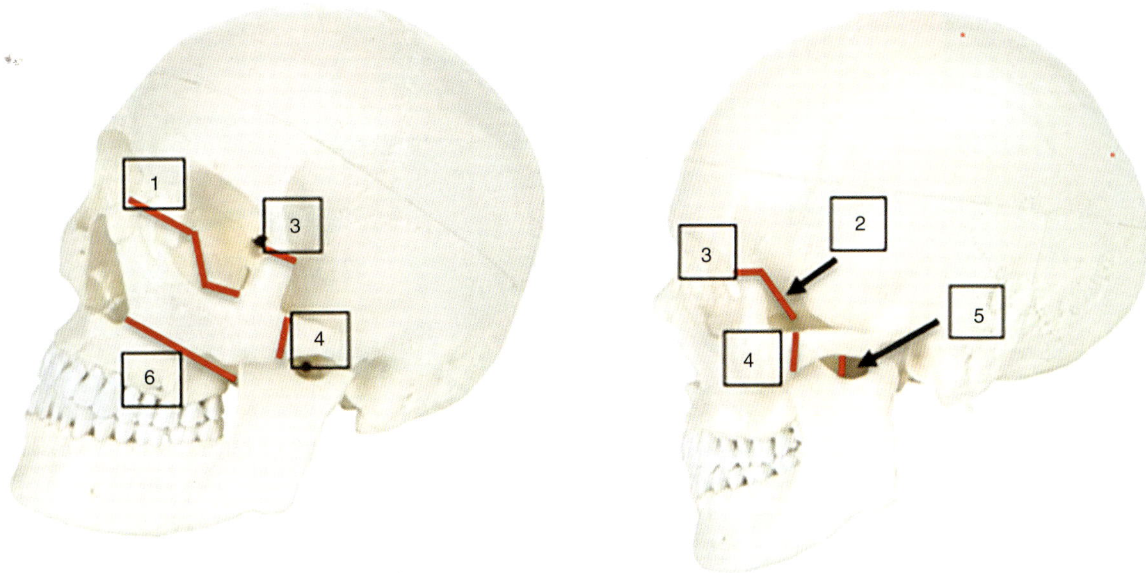


Fig. 12.2 Depiction of osteotomies completed during the combined Le Fort III/I procedure. Le Fort III osteotomies (1–5): 1. nasofrontal osteotomy, 2. zygomaticosphenoid osteotomy, 3. frontozygomatic osteotomy, 4. zygomaticotemporal junction, 5. pterygoid osteotomy, and Le Fort I Osteotomy (6): Osteotomy spanning the nasomaxillary and zygomaticomaxillary buttresses.

- Fixation is achieved along the nasomaxillary and zygomaticomaxillary buttresses for increased stability.

## Case 1: Class III skeletal dysplasia with asymmetric mandibular hyperplasia, severe midface hypoplasia, and Class III dental malocclusion

A 17-year-old male presented with Class III skeletal dysplasia with asymmetric mandibular hyperplasia, severe midface hypoplasia, and Class III dental malocclusion with a negative overjet of 21 mm (Fig. 12.3). Formal recommendations were made for a Le Fort III/I with BSSO based on model surgery with 6 mm of movement for the Le Fort III segment with bone grafting, 8 mm of movement for the Le Fort I segment, and a sagittal setback of 6 mm using three splints (Fig. 12.4). The patient achieved good orthognathic results and ultimately underwent open septorhinoplasty with septal and rib grafts for columellar support and nasal reconstruction (Figs. 12.5 and 12.6).

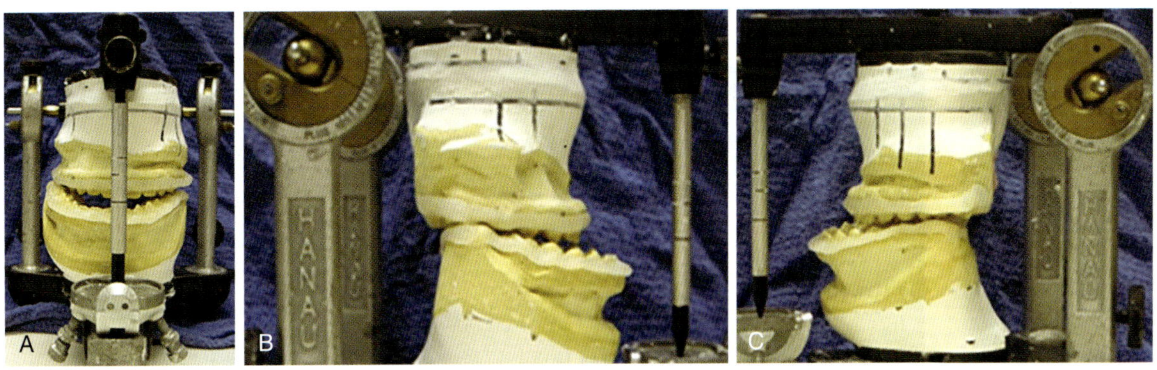


Fig. 12.3 Acrylic and plaster casts employed in model surgery: (A) anterior view, (B) right lateral view, (C) left lateral view.

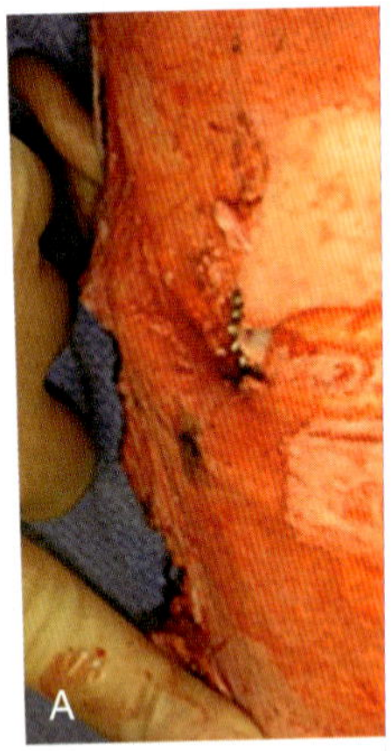

**Fig. 12.4** Le Fort III/I os
osteotomy.

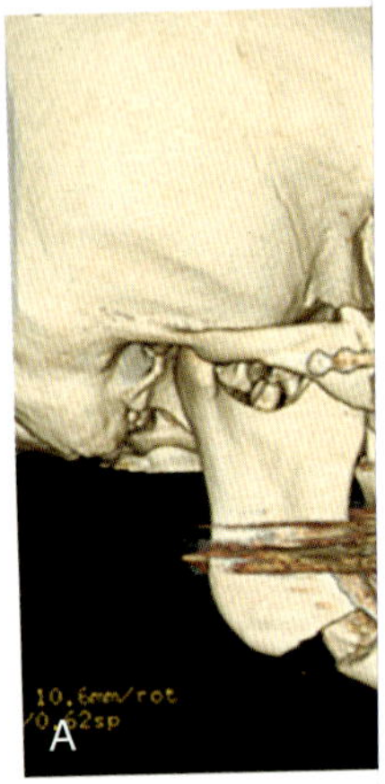

**Fig. 12.5** Postoperati
view, (B) anterior view



Fig. 12



traditional surgical planning.[15] The skeletal changes are often compared with an immediate postoperative CT scan compared to the predicted CAD movement with good accuracy of predicted movements skeletally. The soft tissue changes are harder to confirm as when developing a Le Fort III/I simulation, the current software requires the osteotomies to be performed on two separate mock-ups, which are then overlain to render the completed configuration; at this time, this limitation does not appear to affect outcomes or precision.

There is no question that for this particular surgery, CAD/CAM and full visualization of skeletal complexities in multiple dimensions and perspectives, permits surgeons a less onerous, time-efficient process, with fewer opportunities for error.[17,20]

- Pearls
  - Use of Sonopet Ultrasonic Bone Aspirator (Stryker, Kalamazoo, MI) permits controlled and fine osteotomies.
  - Recommend creation of duplicate final splints, as one may get fractured when advancing the Le Fort I segment with the splint wired in place.
  - In large occlusal discrepancies, several intermediate splints can be made. One in the ideal aesthetic position, and one or two more in slightly less advanced positions. If one is unable to advance the Le Fort passively into the ideal position, the difference can be compensated for in the mandible with one of the less advanced positions.
- Pitfalls
  - Setting patient expectations is key to successful surgery. The patient needs to understand what the expected recovery and incisions for this surgery entails. Representative photos of patients are extremely helpful. Not preparing the patient appropriately can lead to dysphoria.
  - A psychologist is critical for coping before and during this surgery, as well as recovery.

## Outcomes/complications

The combined Le Fort III/I osteotomy is an underutilized tool for aesthetic and functional correction of global midface hypoplasia. This technique should be considered in select patients with total midface retrusion and class III malocclusion. Our experience demonstrates the feasibility of simultaneous Le Fort III and Le Fort I advancement, with or without bilateral sagittal split osteotomy.

Complications are similar to any craniofacial disjunction procedure and orthognathic procedure. Potential complications include bleeding requiring transfusion, infection, brain damage, cerebral spinal fluid leak, blindness, paralysis, nonunion, malunion, fibrous union, unpredictability of bone retention, asymmetry, non-cosmetic result, damage to teeth, need to extract teeth, numbness, need for further surgery, and anesthetic complications. As such, the Le Fort III/I procedure should be performed by experienced surgeons, familiar in both orthognathic surgery and craniofacial surgery, and carried out in an appropriate surgical environment.

## Conclusion

Modern innovations have allowed for the seamless transfer of virtual representation to physical reconstruction. The accuracy and efficiency of computer-assisted surgery renders it an excellent alternative to traditional model surgery in Le Fort III/I presurgical planning and improving the intraoperative experience.

## References


1. Linton JL. Comparative study of diagnostic measures in borderline surgical cases of unilateral cleft lip and palate and noncleft Class III malocclusions. *Am J Orthod Dentofacial Orthop*. 1998;113(5):526-537.
2. Scolozzi P. Distraction osteogenesis in the management of severe maxillary hypoplasia in cleft lip and palate patients. *J Craniofac Surg*. 2008;19(5):1199-1214.
3. Hammoudeh JA, Goel P, Wolfswinkel EM, et al. Simultaneous midface advancement and orthognathic surgery: a powerful technique for managing midface hypoplasia and malocclusion. *Plast Reconstr Surg*. 2020;145(6):1067e-1072e.
4. Posnick JC, Ruiz RL. The craniofacial dysostosis syndromes: current surgical thinking and future directions. *Cleft Palate Craniofac J*. 2000;37(5):433.
5. Posnick JC. The craniofacial dysostosis syndromes. Staging of reconstruction and management of secondary deformities. *Clin Plast Surg*. 1997;24(3):429-446.
6. McCarthy JG, ed. *Craniofacial Distraction*. Cham: Springer; 2017.
7. Tahiri Y, Taylor J. An update on midface advancement using Le Fort II and III distraction

osteogenesis. *Semin Plast Surg.* 2014;28(4):184-192.
8. Mittermiller PA, Flores RL, Staffenberg DA. Craniosynostosis: Le Fort III distraction osteogenesis. *Clin Plast Surg.* 2021;48(3):473-485.
9. Fearon JA. Halo distraction of the Le Fort III in syndromic craniosynostosis: a long-term assessment. *Plast Reconstr Surg.* 2005;115(6):1524-1536.
10. Shetye PR, Davidson EH, Sorkin M, Grayson BH, McCarthy JG. Evaluation of three surgical techniques for advancement of the midface in growing children with syndromic craniosynostosis. *Plast Reconstr Surg.* 2010;126(3):982-994.
11. Patel N, Fearon JA. Treatment of the syndromic midface: a long-term assessment at skeletal maturity. *Plast Reconstr Surg.* 2015;135(4):731e-742e.
12. Fisher M, Medina M III, Bojovic B, Ahn E, Dorafshar AH. Indications for computer-aided design and manufacturing in congenital craniofacial reconstruction. *Craniomaxillofac Trauma Reconstr.* 2016;9(3):235-241.
13. Vachiramon A, Yen SLK, Lypka M, et al. A novel model surgery technique for LeFort III advancement. *J Craniofac Surg.* 2007;18(5):1230-1235.
14. Wolfswinkel EM, Jacob L, Hammoudeh JA, Urata MM. Reply: Simultaneous midface advancement and orthognathic surgery: a powerful technique for managing midface hypoplasia and malocclusion. *Plast Reconstr Surg.* 2021;148(3):504e-505e.
15. Brown MS, Okada H, Valiathan M, Lakin GE. 45 Years of simultaneous Le Fort III and Le Fort I osteotomies: a systematic literature review. *Cleft Palate Craniofac J.* 2015;52(4): 471-479.
16. Westermark A, Zachow S, Eppley BL. Three-dimensional osteotomy planning in maxillofacial surgery including soft tissue prediction. *J Craniofac Surg.* 2005;16(1): 100-104.
17. Wang Y, Zhang Z, Liu Y, Ye B, Luo E, Li J. Virtual surgical planning assisted management for cleft-related maxillary hypoplasia. *J Craniofac Surg.* 2019;30(6): 1745-1749.
18. Toto JM, Chang EI, Agag R, Devarajan K, Patel SA, Topham NS. Improved operative efficiency of free fibula flap mandible reconstruction with patient-specific, computer-guided preoperative planning. *Head Neck.* 2015;37(11): 1660-1664.
19. Resnick CM, Inverso G, Wrzosek M, Padwa BL, Kaban LB, Peacock ZS. Is there a difference in cost between standard and virtual surgical planning for orthognathic surgery? *J Oral Maxillofac Surg.* 2016;74(9):1827-1833.
20. Hua J, Aziz S, Shum JW. Virtual surgical planning in oral and maxillofacial surgery. *Oral Maxillofac Surg Clin North Am.* 2019;31(4):519-530.

Chapter | 13 |

# Computer-assisted surgical planning congenital differences and anomalies—nonsyndromic craniosynostosis: a practical workflow

*Christopher D. Lopez, Amir H. Dorafshar, Robin Yang, Jordan P. Steinberg*

CHAPTER OUTLINE



## Introduction

Nonsyndromic craniosynostosis refers to the premature fusion of cranial sutures in the absence of other congenital anomalies. Fusion typically occurs at only one suture, though in rare nonsyndromic cases, fusion at multiple sutures can occur and is referred to as "complex nonsyndromic craniosynostosis." The order of frequency for single suture fusion has been well characterized; sagittal synostosis is most common, followed by coronal, metopic, and finally lambdoid. The incidence of nonsyndromic craniosynostosis is 0.4 to 1.0 per 1000 births.[1] Sex differences are also clear: sagittal synostosis occurs in a 4:1 male-to-female ratio, whereas unilateral coronal synostosis presents more commonly in females in a 3:2 ratio.[1] Although the complete genetic underpinnings of nonsyndromic craniosynostosis have yet to be fully elucidated, it is now known that *SMAD6, TWIST1, TCF12, ERF, MSX2,* and *FGFR3* genes all play a role in the various single-suture synostoses.[2-5]

## Clinical considerations

### Evaluation

On initial evaluation, all children should undergo a history and physical exam with an emphasis on ruling out nonoperative conditions such as positional plagiocephaly. Virchow's landmark contribution describes the characteristic compensatory changes in skull growth perpendicular to prematurely fused sutures.[6] These compensatory changes serve as the hallmarks for clinical diagnosis of single-suture craniosynostosis. Several studies have shown that clinical features alone can allow for reliable diagnosis in almost all cases, rendering imaging unnecessary on this basis alone.[7] Imaging does, however, provide the foundation for computer-assisted design and computer-assisted manufacturing (CAD/CAM), as reviewed in this chapter. Imaging should include noncontrast craniomaxillofacial computed tomography (CT) with three-dimensional (3D) reconstruction. When operative intervention is decided upon, a family discussion should be initiated that explains the collaboration between plastic surgery and neurosurgery intraoperatively. The question of whether surgery is indicated in mild phenotypic cases is beyond the scope of the present chapter. In such instances, multidisciplinary discussion becomes paramount, and may include input from the specialties of ophthalmology, genetics, and developmental neuropsychology in addition to plastic surgery and neurosurgery.

## Timing of surgery

Although the optimal timing for surgical intervention has yet to be established, certain principles are well understood. Earlier intervention—defined as earlier than 1 year of age—has been shown to reduce the risks for subsequent elevations in intracranial pressure and cognitive deficits.[8-11] Taking advantage of the time period shortly after the infant hematopoietic nadir, between 3 to 6 months, has also been described.[1] This time frame also capitalizes on the rapid expansion of the cranium and dural osteoinductive capacity for optimal open remodeling outcomes. Beyond 1 year of age, open remodeling can prove more difficult due to the stiffer quality and thickness of the cranial bone. Moreover, beyond this age, bony gaps may be less likely to completely heal.[1,12] The benefits of early intervention for open cranial vault remodeling surgery must be balanced by the risks, including significant blood loss. The excellent vascular perfusion of the craniofacial region makes this concern especially pertinent in young children with relatively less reserve due to size. With the above considerations, it has been become common practice to proceed with open surgery in the age range of 6 to 12 months. While open surgery is infrequently performed prior to this time point, more minimally invasive strip craniectomy surgery is, by contrast, performed earlier than 4 months of age. Because the latter procedures rarely involve the use of CAD/CAM approaches, particularly in patients with nonsyndromic craniosynostosis, they are not discussed in this chapter.

## Computer-assisted design and computer-assisted manufacturing

The benefits of CAD/CAM in craniofacial surgery have been well-described.[13-16] Given the complexity of calvarial remodeling, the ability to virtually plan, assess, and modify operative approaches with infinite variation can be an invaluable resource. Advantages have been cited for more atypical cases of craniosynostosis with multiple-suture involvement, older patients with significantly thickened bone not amenable to manual bending, and for craniofacial surgeons with less experience in performing complex on-table manipulations.[16] A recent study showed that less experienced craniofacial surgeons using CAD/CAM may achieve noninferior results when compared with more experienced surgeons using traditional methods.[16] Outcomes such as estimated blood loss, inpatient length of stay, and postoperative complications were not significantly different between the two groups, though less experienced surgeons using CAD/CAM did have longer operative times.[16]

Indications for CAD/CAM in craniofacial surgery includes complex reconstructive procedures such as multi-suture reconstruction, cranial vault revisions, facial bipartitions, box osteotomies, and distraction osteogenesis cases.[15] Although the utility of CAD/CAM in these cases has been demonstrated, the role of these technologies in nonsyndromic, single-suture open craniosynostosis surgery is certainly less clear. It has been argued that, for these cases, the financial cost is too great to justify the optimization of more straightforward reconstructive needs, such as patients with single suture fusion that present early enough to plan intervention well before 1 year of age.

In our experience at a large academic medical center, a key consideration favoring CAD/CAM in nonsyndromic craniosynostosis open surgery is late presentation, particularly after 1 year of age when the cranial bone is less amenable to traditional bending and remodeling techniques. As in many tertiary centers, our experience includes a disproportionately large number of patients with such delayed presentations. The reasons for this may be multiple, and include recent immigration to the US from a country without expertise in surgical management of craniosynostosis, previous absence of a diagnosis, and the presence of other intercurrent medical issues that preclude the timely scheduling of open cranial vault remodeling surgery. Because late presenters may frequently exhibit a more severe, abnormal phenotype and an even greater need for complex manipulation of bony segments to establish an aesthetic outcome, CAD/CAM can be particularly advantageous. The innate osteoinductive capacity of the calvarial skeleton is also diminished with age, as previously noted.[17] This translates into a more precise need for bony segment realignment and contact, without relying on secondary healing processes for open bone fill. CAD/CAM can aid in this aspect as well, and bone gaps can be minimized.

## Workflow for computer-assisted design/computer-assisted manufacturing

When embarking on CAD/CAM for open calvarial remodeling in nonsyndromic, single suture synostosis cases, it is important to recognize that, just as with traditional on-table remodeling approaches, "cookbook" algorithms do not exist. Many surgeons have adapted their basic on-table approaches to CAD/CAM for each of the different types of craniosynostosis. Alternatively, some have found it useful to adopt different techniques that rely on abnormal bone replacement (i.e., "switch" procedures) rather than bone bending or bandeau-centered approaches.[18] "Bending" of cranial bone is perhaps the hardest aspect to model digitally. It is our observation that surgeons who rely predominantly on bone bending, and visual inspection intraoperatively tend to find the technology, with cutting guides, assembly guides, and stereolithographic models, less useful. In this chapter, we have elected to focus on CAD/CAM use in 3 cases of nonsyndromic, single suture, late-presenting craniosynostosis, which we believe to be more representative examples of the advantages of this technology.

On a general level, when planning open reconstructions with CAD/CAM technology, noncontrast CT scan images of the craniofacial skeleton are acquired within 8 weeks of the anticipated surgical procedure. Due to growth of the calvarium and skull base in young patients, particularly those under 1 year of age, it is important to obtain the scan as close as possible to the time of surgery, but also with enough time to allow for digital online planning sessions, modifications of plans by both the engineer and the surgeon, and for delivery of customized products from manufacturers with international production facilities and possible shipping constraints. We have found the 8-week time point to represent a good balance with respect to all of the above factors. In most institutions, scans may be acquired in infants and young children without the need for anesthesia. Once scans have been acquired, Digital Imaging and Communications in Medicine (DICOM) data may be uploaded to the preferred craniomaxillofacial product vendor for online planning. An internet planning session is thereafter scheduled, typically for 1 hour.

As noted, the conduct of online planning sessions for cranial vault remodeling is heavily dependent on individual surgeon preferences and may reflect the typical approaches and visuospatial metrics that one would otherwise use in an actual open case. Of paramount importance for the surgeon is the realization that the biomedical engineer assisting with planning may be unaware of soft tissue constraints, or the difficulty or risk associated with various craniotomies. It is therefore incumbent on the surgeon to direct the engineer to design the osteotomies in practical locations, and to virtually model movements that they feel will be technically feasible and safe to execute during the actual procedure. Superimposition of plans on normal, age-matched control skulls may be of benefit during planning as a check on the modeled shape. In a similar fashion, checking the final cephalic ratio to ensure "normalization" may be of benefit, as well as verification of final "intracranial volume" to ensure net expansion as may be desired. Once again, there are no "cookbook algorithms," and the workflow will often mirror an individual surgeon's approach in a typical "freehand" case. Because contours can be checked and examined, and "swap" movements tested for best fit, there are advantages to spending time either online or "offline" to optimize the final shape (e.g., if a posterior parietal bone segment is used to substitute for the frontal bone in an anterior vault remodeling). "Overcorrection" may be modeled at the discretion of the surgeon. Age is a significant factor in our decision to employ overcorrection, and is commonly performed for frontoorbital surgeries to address the tendency for relapse over time.[19]

## Operative techniques

### Case 1: late-presenting right unilateral coronal craniosynostosis

A 2-year-old male presented with a diagnosis of right unilateral coronal craniosynostosis after recent immigration to the United States. Due to the significant deformity and concern for neurocognitive sequelae, a decision was made to proceed with frontoorbital advancement to best address both aesthetic asymmetry and the need for more anterior intracranial space. CAD/CAM was utilized (Fig. 13.1) to compare several variations of bandeau advancement preoperatively for a subjectively optimized reconstruction with mild overcorrection. For the procedure, the calvarium was accessed in the usual fashion. A bifrontal craniotomy was marked, as well as a bandeau in a three-fourths fashion (Fig. 13.2). Following completion of the osteotomies, the right aspect of the bandeau was made convex and advanced appropriately to achieve symmetry. The pterional region was fixated with an approximate 1-cm advancement using resorbable plates. The cranial bone flap was repositioned to correspond to the new bandeau as per the CAD/CAM (Fig. 13.3). This was secured to the frontal bandeau with resorbable suture. Bone graft was used to fill in any remaining gaps as well as the area of the pterional advancement. The temporalis muscles were resuspended and advanced and the scalp closed in the usual fashion.

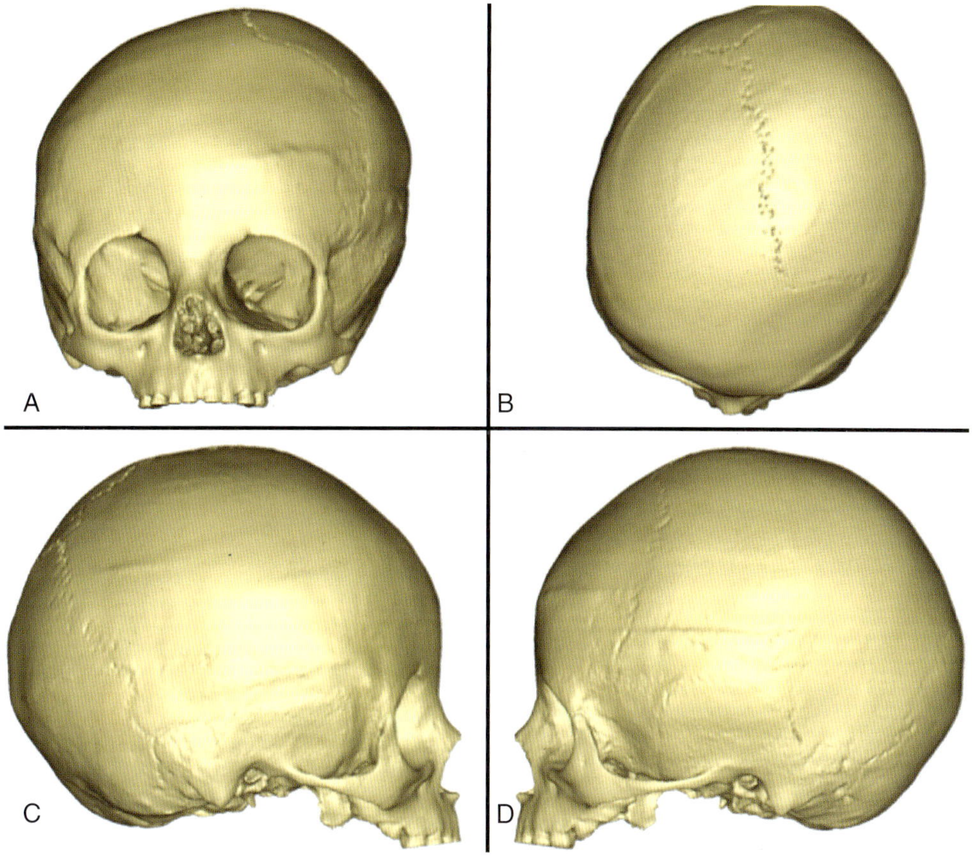


**Fig. 13.1** Preoperative computed tomography. (A) Frontal view. (B) Bird's-eye view with intact left coronal suture and fused right coronal suture. (C) Lateral view demonstrating absence of right coronal suture. (D) Lateral view demonstrates intact left coronal suture.

## Case 2: late-presenting sagittal craniosynostosis

A 2-year-8-month-old male was evaluated for a late presentation of sagittal craniosynostosis. Upon presentation to our craniofacial team, the patient was seen to have overt stigmata of scaphocephaly with sagittal craniosynostosis, which was confirmed with CT scan imaging (Fig. 13.4). Given the patient's significant scaphocephalic deformity and thick bone at this age, total cranial vault reconstruction was planned with a Melbourne-type approach,[17,20] adapted from a modification detailed by Dr. C. Forrest of Toronto, Canada (personal communication). CAD/CAM was performed in order to optimize the surgical approach, to map out the venous sinuses, and to allow for remodeling to include the frontal and occipitál regions.

Approach to the calvarium was performed in a standard fashion. Once the area was dissected sufficiently for placement of premanufactured, customized marking guides, these were brought onto the field and snapped together with right and left halves (Fig. 13.5). A marking pencil was used to outline the area for the frontal craniotomy, occipital craniotomy, and intervening temporal and parietal regions (see Video 13.1). Registration tabs were also marked on the guide and on the skull base, where the occipital bone would be reset to allow proper alignment later. The guides were then removed and the markings for the craniotomies were reinforced. Major craniotomies performed by the neurosurgical team included a single bifrontal piece, a single large occipital bone piece, two large temporoparietal rectangular pieces, and then a midline rectangular block. Additional cuts as per the virtual plan were then performed off the field. Assembly was performed for the anterior and posterior portions as per the CAD/CAM design, using resorbable plates. The anterior and posterior reconstructed bone portions were then brought onto the field and secured in place to the skull base (Figs. 13.6 and 13.7). Intervening gaps were filled with split bone and

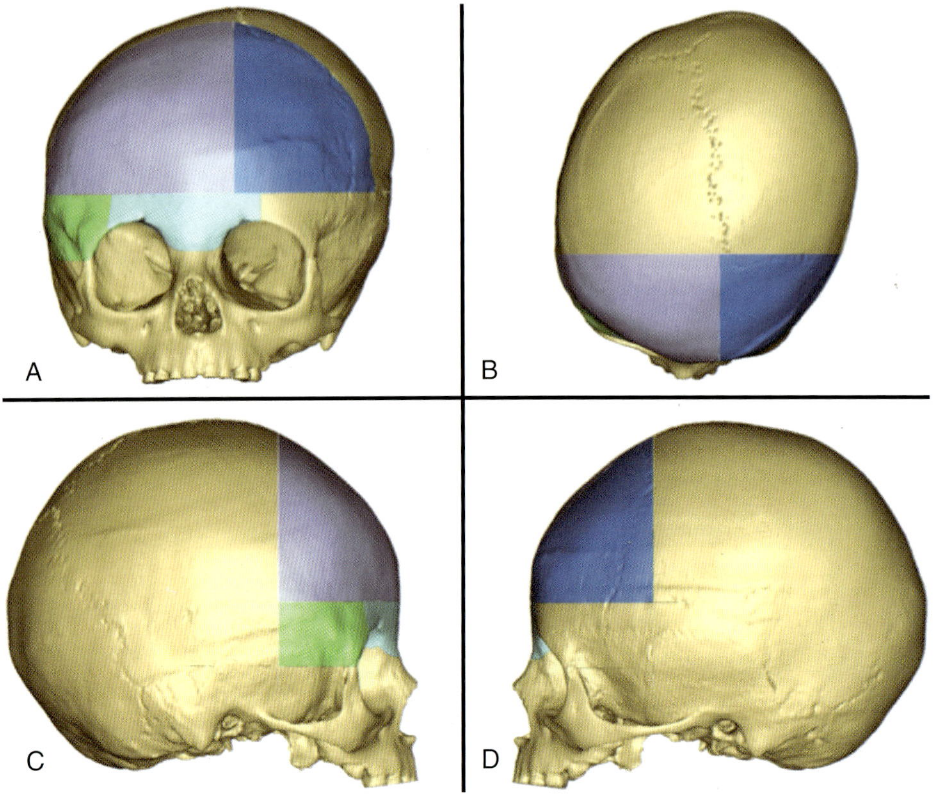


Fig. 13.2 Surgical plan. Osteotomies denoted by different colors. (A) Frontal view. (B) Bird's-eye view. (C) Lateral view of right side. (D) Lateral view of left side.

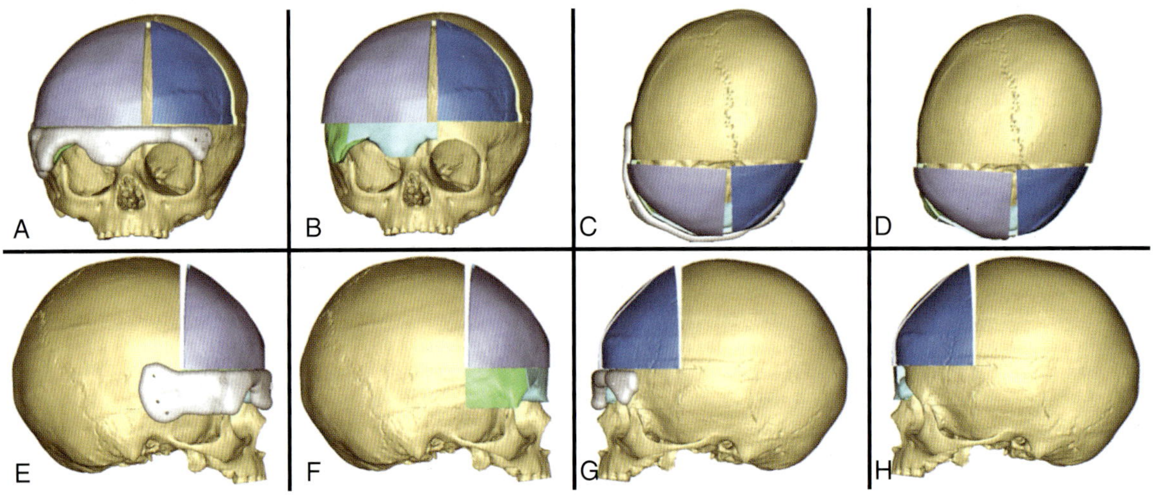


Fig. 13.3 Guide design and final positions. (A) Frontal view with bandeau positioning guide. (B) Final frontal view position with final bandeau position. (C) Bird's-eye view with positioning guide in place. (D) Bird's-eye view with final frontal bone positions and pterion advancement after osteotomies. (E) Right lateral view with positioning guide. (F) Right lateral view with osteotomies at premature fusion site. (G) Left lateral view with positioning guide. (H) Left lateral view with final bony position of frontal bone.

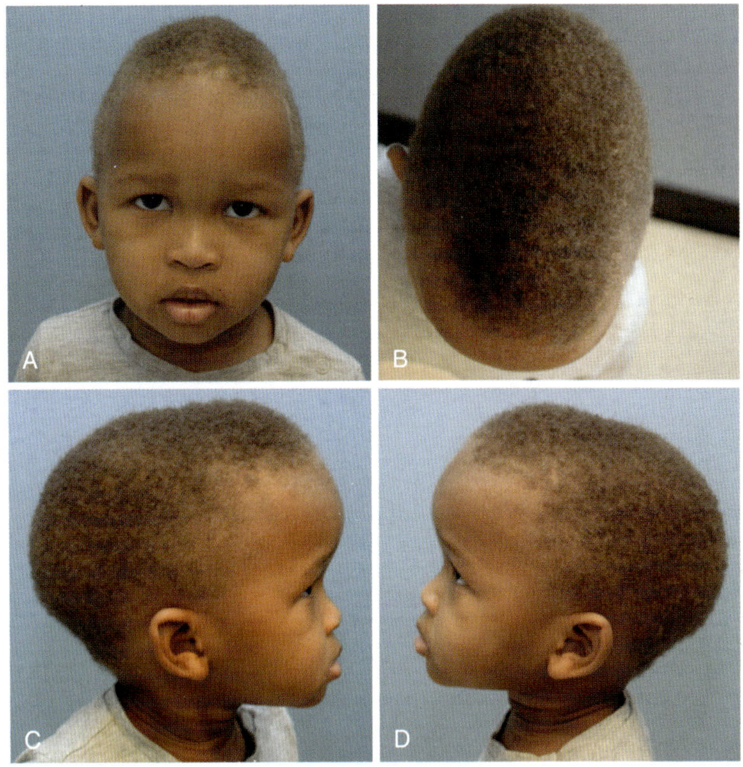


**Fig. 13.4** Preoperative clinical images demonstrating pathogenic sagittal craniosynostosis. (A) Frontal view with narrow head width. (B) Bird's eye view with prominent antero-postero elongation. (C) Right lateral view. (D) left lateral view.

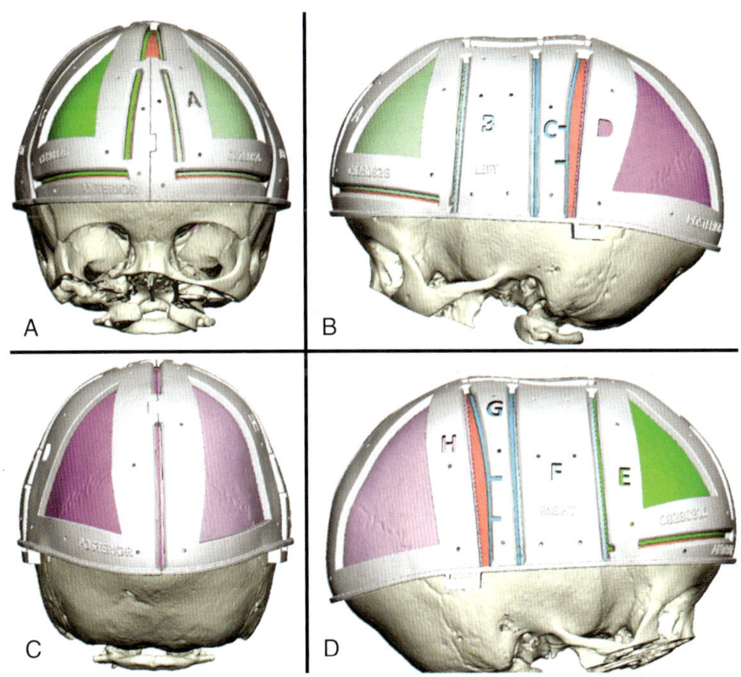


**Fig. 13.5** Cutting guides labeled with letters to avoid dural sinus while optimizing calvarial segment rearrangement after osteotomies and reconstruction. (A) Frontal view. (B) Left lateral view with cutting guides attached together. (C) Posterior view. (D) Right lateral view.

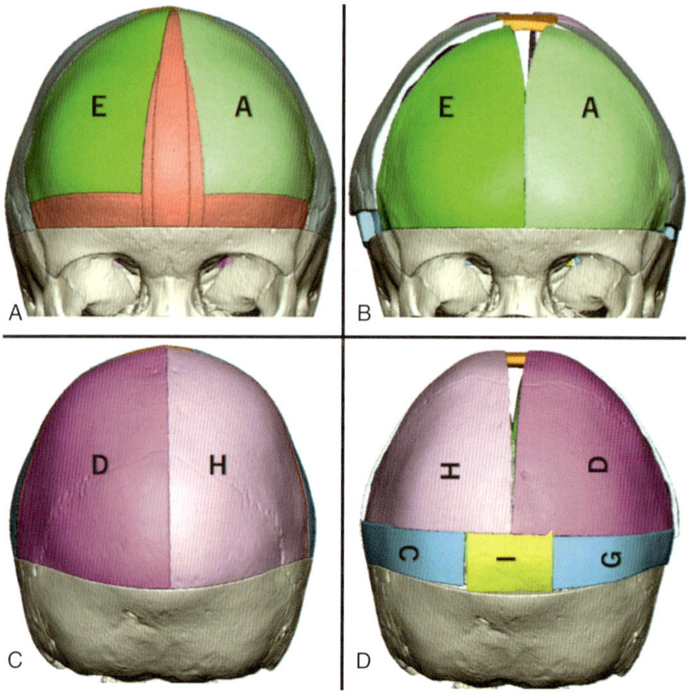


Fig. 13.6 Preoperative and final position of osteotomies in anteroposterior views. (A) Preoperative frontal view with frontal bones that will be adjusted in green, and segment of bone that will be removed in red. (B) Final position of bony segments. (C) Posterior view with preoperative osteotomy lines marked. (D) Posterior view after switch of bony segments D and H with addition of bony segments C, I, and G to address cranial height.

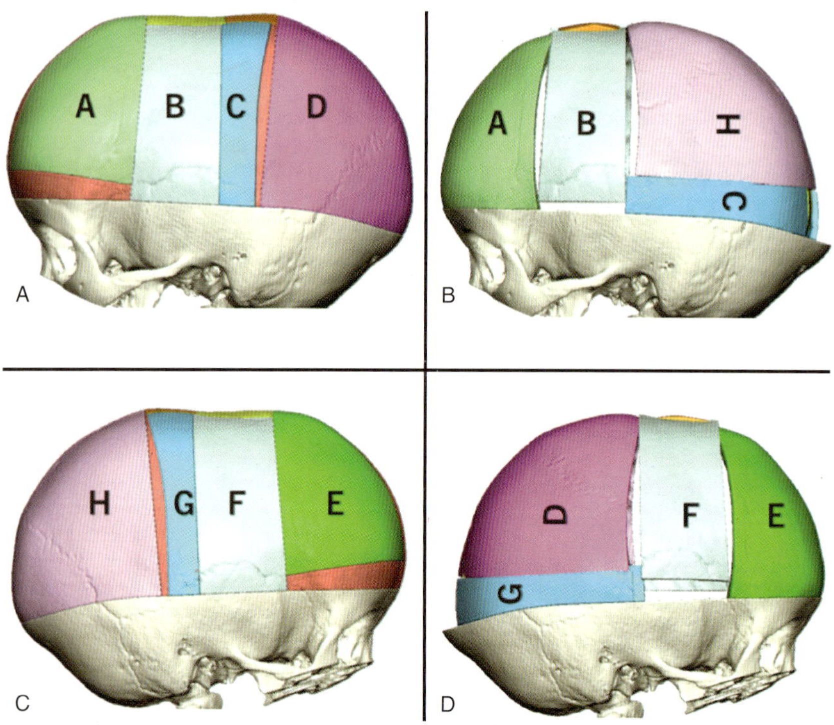


Fig. 13.7 Preoperative and final position of osteotomies in lateral views. (A) Preoperative right lateral view with frontal bones that will be adjusted in green, occipital in purple, parietal in shades of blue, and segment of bone that will be removed in red. (B) Right lateral view with final position of bony segment with segment C moved to address anteroposterior (AP) length and address skull base height deficit. (C) Left lateral view with frontal bones that will be adjusted in green, occipital in purple, parietal in shades of blue, and segment of bone that will be removed in red. (D) Left lateral final position of bony segment with segment C moved to address AP length and address skull base height deficit.

milled bone graft. The scalp was closed in the usual fashion. Follow-up images are seen in Fig. 13.8.

## Case 3: late-presenting lambdoid craniosynostosis

A 13-month-old male was diagnosed with left unilateral lambdoid craniosynostosis. There were no signs of developmental delay or any signs of elevated intracranial pressure, but the patient did present with physical manifestations of lambdoid craniosynostosis, including left posterior flattening with an obvious mastoid bulge and contralateral parietal bossing (Fig. 13.9). CT scan imaging confirmed the diagnosis. In order to address the overt aesthetic issue while simultaneously creating greater intracranial volume, posterior vault reconstruction was recommended. CAD/CAM and cutting guides were utilized (Fig. 13.10) to compare several virtual plans including switch cranioplasty of 180 degrees, 90 degrees, and orthotopic cranioplasty. After comparing several CAD/CAMs, it was determined that the best approach for this case would be a switch cranioplasty with 90 degrees of rotation.

Access to the calvarium was achieved in the standard coronal fashion. The posterior scalp was dissected and the entirety of the posterior calvarium was exposed. Osteotomy markings were aided by the use of 3D-printed cutting guides and the posterior cranial bone was elevated as one piece. This was taken to the back table, at which point bone graft was harvested from the inner lamina. The bone piece was then split in the middle and subjected to the 90-degree switch cranioplasty technique (Fig. 13.11). Resorbable plates were then fashioned

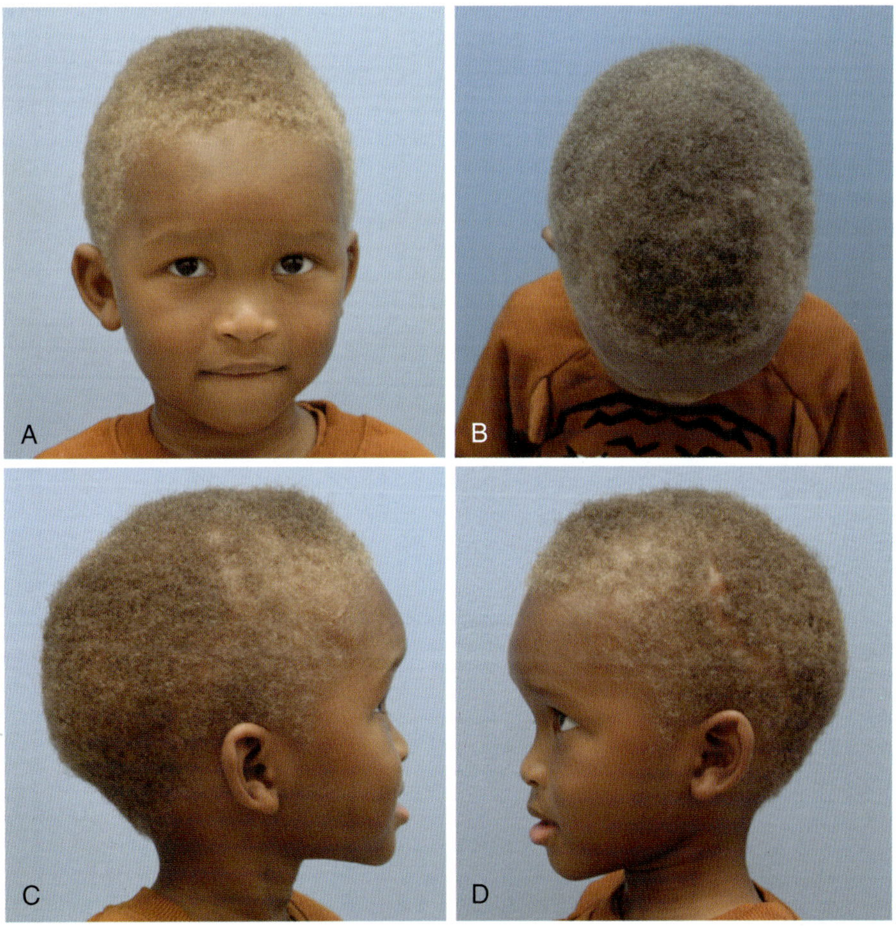


**Fig. 13.8** The 12-month follow-up clinical images demonstrate correction and normalization of temporal narrowing and anterior-posterior length of head. (A) Frontal view. (B) Bird's-eye view. (C) Right lateral. (D) Left lateral.

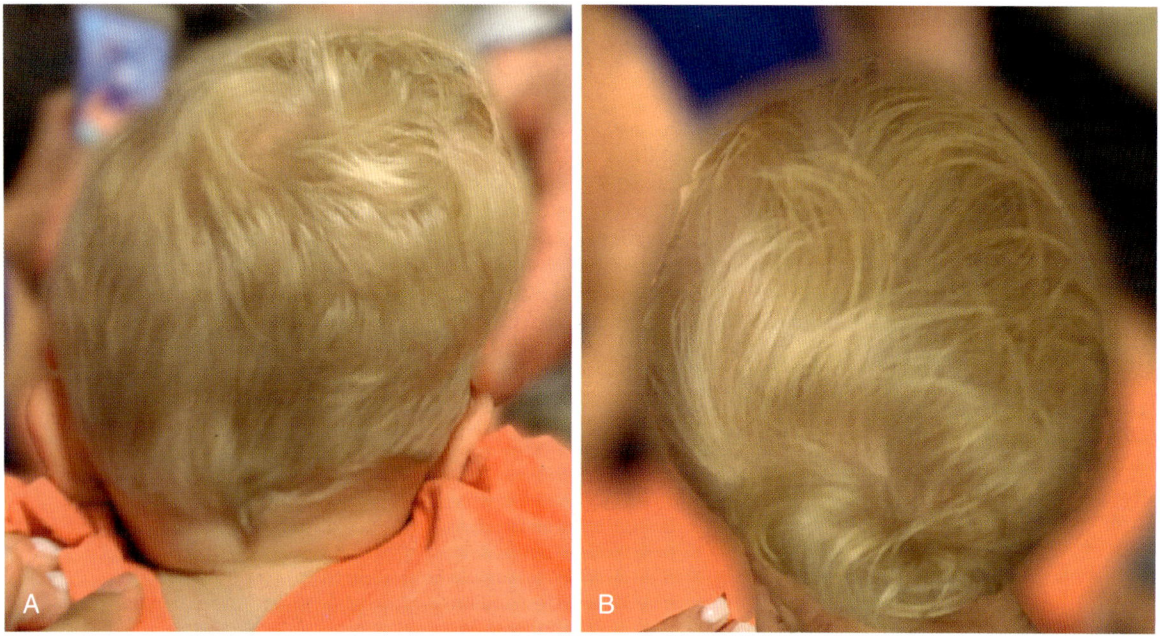


**Fig. 13.9** Preoperative clinical images. (A) Posterior view with prominent asymmetry noted. (B) Bird's-eye view with anterior above and posterior below.

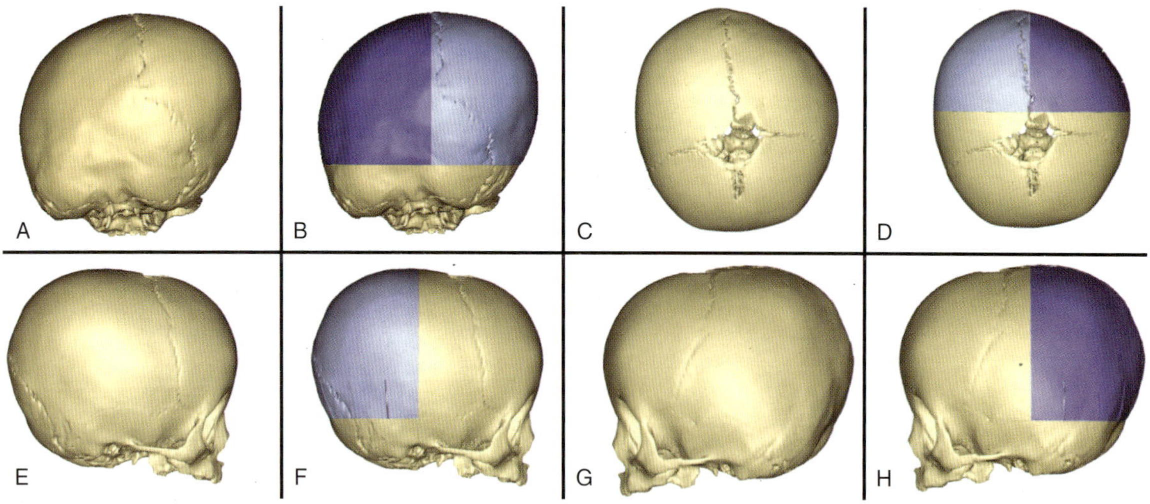


**Fig. 13.10** Preoperative computed tomography and planned osteotomies. (A) Posterior view demonstrating absence of left lambdoid suture. (B) Computer-assisted surgical planning (CaSP) osteotomies include lambdoid suture and partial sagittal suture. (C) Bird's-eye view. (D) CaSP demonstrates inclusion of partial sagittal suture. (E) Right lateral view. (F) Right lateral CaSP with optional barrel staves. (G) Left lateral view. (H) Left lateral view with CaSP including optional barrel staves.

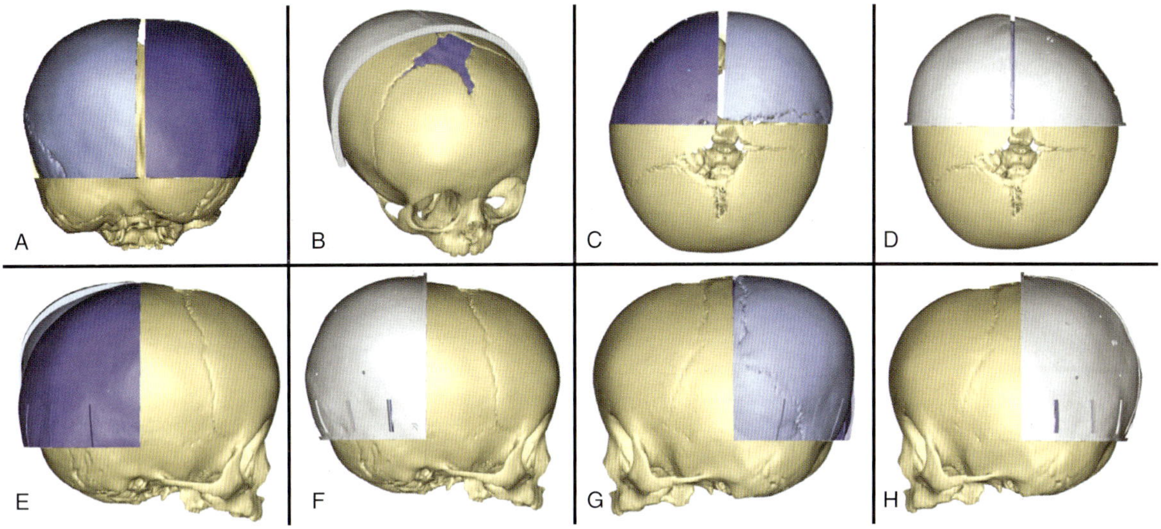


**Fig. 13.11** Postoperative bony segment position and cutting guide position. (A) Posterior view demonstrating switch cranioplasty with each bony segment placed contralateral and rotated 90 degrees. (B) Cutting guide in position. (C) Bird's-eye view of final bony position with expanded intracranial volume. (D) Bird's-eye view of cutting guide. (E) Right lateral view with final bony position and barrel staving. (F) Right lateral view with cutting guide demonstrating barrel stave cutting sites. (G) Left lateral view with final bony placement. (H) Left lateral view with cutting guide in place demonstrates barrel staving osteotomy sites.

appropriately, and the newly positioned bony segments were examined to identify bony margins that sat too proudly relative to the uncut osteotomy/skull base interface and created step-off. These regions were addressed by creating vertical barrel staves to facilitate bending of the prominent bony segments. Resorbable sutures were used to fix the bone into place. Particulate bone graft was then placed into the bone gaps. Closure was performed in the standard fashion. Follow-up clinical images are seen in Fig. 13.12.

## Fidelity/verification

The role of postoperative CT imaging in verifying the accurate execution of a CAD/CAM is controversial. The rationale for assessment of fidelity is self-explanatory, and there are reports of protocols that include postoperative CT imaging, utilized, at least in part, to obtain anthropometric values.[17] However, the risks associated with additional radiation secondary to imaging are not negligible in the pediatric patient and should always be considered by the craniofacial surgeon. In our experience, we disfavor routine postoperative imaging in order to avoid additional radiation, and do not feel this is needed for outcome comparisons in a well-executed, uncomplicated CAD/CAM. Of note, this does not apply to cases with complicated operative courses, or cases with postoperative sequelae concerning for complications.

## Pearls/pitfalls

When utilizing CAD/CAM, it is critical to remember that not all facets of an operative plan can be accounted for virtually, and that CaSP can never substitute for sound surgical judgment. These procedures require flexibility from the operating surgeon, and are ultimately the by-product of both art and science. The surgeon aims to achieve optimal form and function with a simultaneous emphasis on aesthetics. For example, although a primary goal of reconstruction is to address the abnormal head shape and associated symptoms from suture fusion, it is also important to alleviate regions of the skull that are prone to increased pressure. In our experience, failing to account for the latter while executing a virtual plan can result in sequelae such as significant brain parenchymal swelling that is unable to accommodate fixation of the reconstruction assembled at the back table, or the inability to close the original scalp flaps primarily.

Surgical judgment is also critical with respect to soft tissue. This is perhaps the greatest limitation of modern-day CAD/CAM techniques, in that the planning is focused solely on the bone. Engineers on virtual sessions may

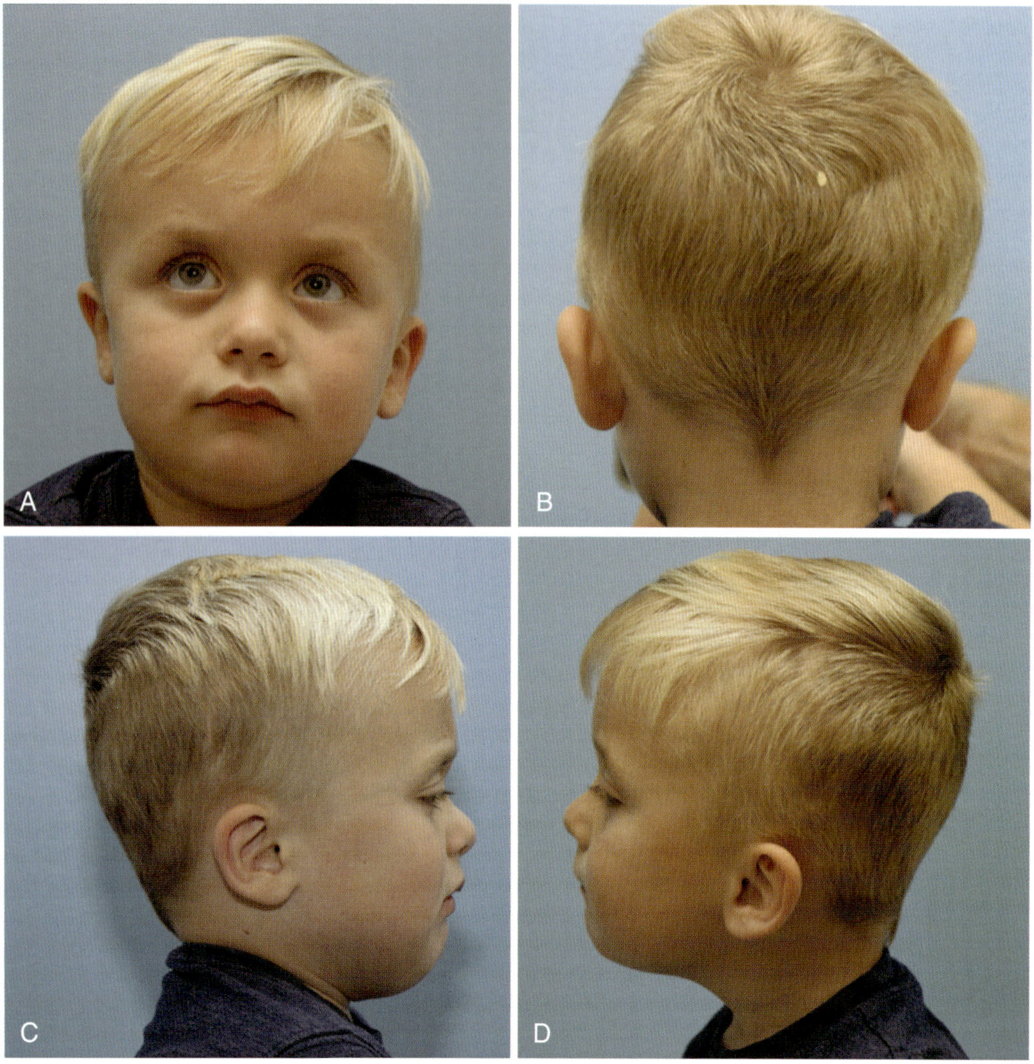

Fig. 13.12 A 24-month follow-up. (A) Frontal view. (B) Posterior view demonstrating improved symmetry. (C) Right lateral view demonstrating absence of previous bossing. (D) Left lateral view demonstrating improved contour from previous flattened region.

frequently underestimate the difficulty of accessing some areas of the craniofacial skeleton under the constraints of the soft tissue. Moreover, it may prove difficult to estimate the degree of overcorrection needed from a bone-only reconstruction, without the ability to see the redraped soft tissues. Redraped tissues may also be put under significant tension when following the bone-only reconstructive plan.

Perhaps the most important consideration in avoiding CAD/CAM pitfalls is, as noted above, surgical design flexibility. While it is always possible to assemble bone virtually to the design of our choice, it is not always so in reality due to complex three-dimensional relationships amongst the dura, bone, and soft tissues. Therefore, it is key to limit constraints as much as possible. For example, in cases of total vault reconstruction, separate and independent design and assembly of anterior and posterior bone segments can allow for "wiggle room" in the center, where adjustments can be made in custom fashion with interposition bone grafts. By incorporating these operative "safety nets" into the original CaSP, the astute surgeon can create fail-safes and avoid potentially catastrophic sequelae.

## Outcomes/complications

Data related to CAD/CAM-specific complications in nonsyndromic craniosynostosis reconstruction are limited, but reports suggest that complications may be similar to non-CAD/CAM groups. Cho and colleagues determined that a non-CAD/CAM reconstruction cohort had a 29% incidence of cases necessitating revision (Whitaker category II, III, or IV) compared to a CAD/CAM group requiring revision in 14.3% of cases.[16] Of note, both postoperative outcomes and hospital length of stay were not significantly different between these groups. Dural tears have been reported even when using CAD/CAM, but this also can occur without CAD/CAM.[17] Further investigation comparing CAD/CAM complications to non-CAD/CAM complications is warranted.

## Conclusion

CAD/CAM is a powerful tool in the craniofacial surgeon's armamentarium. Although it may not confer advantages in all cases of nonsyndromic craniosynostosis, it does appear to offer advantages in cases of high complexity or delayed presentation, where bone is less adaptable on-table.

## Take-Home Points

- Optimal timing for repair of nonsyndromic craniosynostosis has not been elucidated, but beyond 1 year of age open remodeling becomes more difficult due to the stiffer quality and thickness of the cranial bone, and bony gaps are less likely to fully heal.
- The role of CaSP in nonsyndromic craniosynostosis is controversial; however, the technique may be more indicated in settings of late presentation (with intervention after 1 year of age) due to the difficulties associated with delayed repair.
- Not all facets of an operative plan can be accounted for with CaSP—factors such as brain parenchymal swelling may require changes in fixation approaches and soft tissue closure.
- Surgical design flexibility is critical for success. Not all CADs succeed in reality due to complex 3D relationships amongst the dura, bone, and soft tissues. Operative constraints should therefore always be minimized.

## References


1. Persing JA. MOC-PS(SM) CME Article: management considerations in the treatment of craniosynostosis. *Plast Reconstr Surg*. 2008;121:1-11.
2. Jabs EW, Müller U, Li X, et al. A mutation in the homeodomain of the human MSX2 gene in a family affected with autosomal dominant craniosynostosis. *Cell*. 1993;75:443-450.
3. Seto ML, Hing AV, Chang J, et al. Isolated sagittal and coronal craniosynostosis associated with TWIST box mutations. *Am J Med Genet A*. 2007;143A:678-686.
4. Timberlake AT, Choi J, Zaidi S, et al. Two locus inheritance of non-syndromic midline craniosynostosis via rare SMAD6 and common BMP2 alleles. *Elife*. 2016;5:e20125.
5. Timberlake AT, Persing JA. Genetics of nonsyndromic craniosynostosis. *Plast Reconstr Surg*. 2018;141:1508-1516.
6. Persing JA, Jane JA, Shaffrey M. Virchow and the pathogenesis of craniosynostosis: a translation of his original work. *Plast Reconstr Surg*. 1989;83(4):738-742.
7. Fearon JA, Singh DJ, Beals SP, Yu JC. The diagnosis and treatment of single-sutural synostoses: Are computed tomographic scans necessary? *Plast Reconstr Surg*. 2007;120:1327-1331.
8. Renier D, Marchac D. Craniofacial surgery for craniosynostosis: functional and morphological results. *Ann Acad Med Singap*. 1988;17(3):415-426.
9. Kljajič M, Maltese G, Tarnow P, Sand P, Kölby L. The cognitive profile of children with nonsyndromic craniosynostosis. *Plast Reconstr Surg*. 2019;143(5):1037e-1052e.
10. Shipster C, Hearst D, Somerville A, et al. Speech, language, and cognitive development in children with isolated sagittal synostosis. *Dev Med Child Neurol*. 2003;45(1):34-43.
11. Utria AF, Lopez J, Cho RS, et al. Timing of cranial vault remodeling in nonsyndromic craniosynostosis: a single-institution 30-year experience. *J Neurosurg Pediatr*. 2016;18:629-634.
12. Fearon JA. Evidence-based medicine. *Plast Reconstr Surg*. 2014;133:1261-1275.
13. Seruya M, Borsuk DE, Khalifian S, Carson BS, Dalesio NM,

Dorafshar AH. Computer-aided design and manufacturing in craniosynostosis surgery. *J Craniofac Surg*. 2013;24:1100-1105.
14. Chim H, Wetjen N, Mardini S. Virtual surgical planning in craniofacial surgery. *Semin Plast Surg*. 2014;28:150-158.
15. Fisher M, Medina M III, Bojovic B, Ahn E, Dorafshar AH. Indications for computer-aided design and manufacturing in congenital craniofacial reconstruction. *Craniomaxillofac Trauma Reconstr*. 2016;9:235-241.
16. Cho RS, Lopez J, Musavi L, et al. Computer-assisted design and manufacturing assists less experienced surgeons in achieving equivalent outcomes in cranial vault reconstruction. *J Craniofac Surg*. 2019;30:2034-2038.
17. Macmillan A, Lopez J, Mundinger GS, Major M, Medina MA, Dorafshar AH. Virtual surgical planning for correction of delayed presentation scaphocephaly using a modified melbourne technique. *J Craniofac Surg*. 2018;29:914-919.
18. Fearon JA, Ditthakasem K, Garcia JC, Herbert M. Abandoning the supraorbital bandeau in anterior craniosynostosis repairs, for a single-segment reconstruction. *Plast Reconstr Surg*. 2018;142:334e-341e.
19. Fearon JA, Ditthaksem K, Chan WNJ, Herbet M. Long-term growth following trigonocephaly repairs: are overcorrections necessary? *Plast Reconstr Surg*. 2020;145:583e-590e.
20. Greensmith AL, Holmes AD, Lo P, Maxiner W, Heggie AA, Meara JG. Complete correction of severe scaphocephaly: the Melbourne method of total vault remodeling. *Plast Reconstr Surg*. 2008;121:1300-1310.

Chapter | 14 |

# Computer-assisted surgical planning congenital differences and anomalies: Treacher Collins syndrome

Richard A. Hopper, Mark Egbert, Hitesh Kapadia, Srinivas M. Susarla

CHAPTER OUTLINE



## Introduction

Although classically described as "mandibulofacial dysostosis," contemporary understanding of the three-dimensional (3D) skeletal dysmorphology in patients with Treacher Collins syndrome (TCS) extends to include midface hypoplasia involving the zygoma and maxilla.[1-6] The hallmark of severe deficiency is orbitozygomatic hypoplasia with a clockwise rotation deformity of the maxillomandibular complex related to severe mandibular ramus-condyle unit deficiency (Fig. 14.1).[1-6] This constellation of findings frequently results in critical narrowing of the upper airway and tracheostomy dependence.[7-10] As the deformity is nonprogressive, sequential interventions over time have proven effective at addressing the dysmorphology. In the most severe cases, the sequence of interventions includes costochondral graft placement to establish a mandible-skull base articulation followed by coordinated maxillomandibular distraction with advancement and counterclockwise rotation, zygomatic

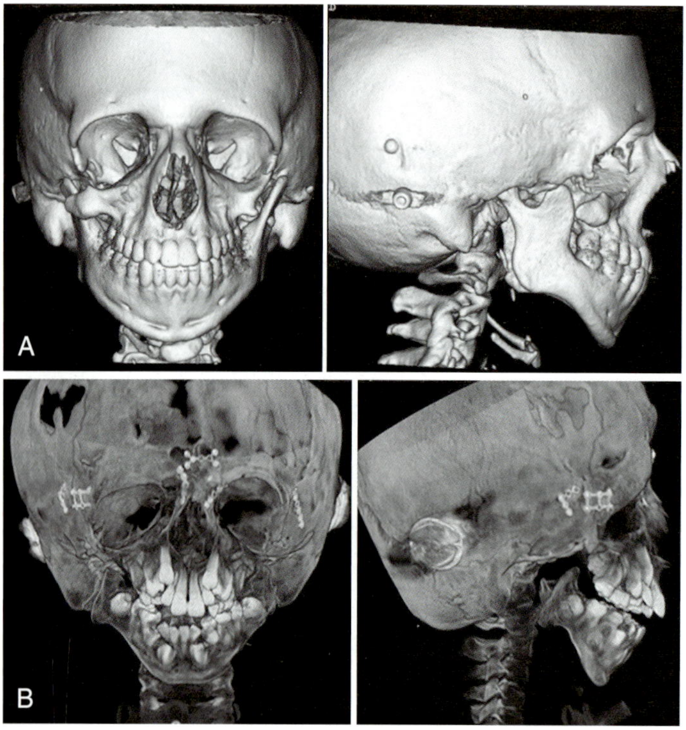


**Fig. 14.1** Phenotypic variation in Treacher Collins syndrome (TCS). There is a wide degree of variability in presentations of TCS. In mild cases, the skeletal dysmorphology is characterized by structures that are functional, but small (A). In severe cases, there is aplasia of the involved skeletal structures (B). A common feature of TCS, regardless of the degree of skeletal hypoplasia, is clockwise rotation of the maxillomandibular complex, with a long anterior face height, short posterior face height, and steep mandibular and palatal plane angles. Reconstructive planning should aim to establish a stable cranio-mandibular articulation, normalize the facial plane angles and facial height ratios, address malar deficiency, and improve the sagittal positioning of the maxillomandibular complex in conjunction with establishing a functional occlusion.

construction with calvarial bone graft, and orthognathic surgery at skeletal maturity to address residual airway disease and establish appropriate dentoskeletal relationships. Computer-assisted surgical planning (CaSP) has greatly enhanced the craniomaxillofacial surgeon's ability to precisely create the appropriate anatomic relationships at each step along this care pathway, ensuring a predictable plan of care.[11-13]

## Clinical considerations

### Ramus-condyle unit construction with costochondral grafts

Originally developed to describe the mandibular deficiency in craniofacial microsomia, the Pruzansky-Kaban classification has been applied to TCS.[14,15] The severity of the mandibular deficiency is related to the articulation between the ramus-condyle unit and glenoid fossa (Table 14.1). In the most severe cases (Pruzansky-Kaban type III), there is no articulation between the mandible and the skull base. In these patients, precise reconstitution of the anatomy is essential to establish a centric relationship between the mandible and temporal skull base and set the stage for subsequent interventions, which will rely on this articulation to correct the sagittal and vertical discrepancies of the maxillomandibular complex.

### Counterclockwise craniofacial distraction osteogenesis[16,17]

Once a stable centric relationship has been established, coordinated maxillomandibular rotation-advancement can be used to address the clockwise rotation deformity. In this stage of reconstruction, a Le Fort II osteotomy (or Le Fort III osteotomy in patients with developed zygomas) is performed in combination with bilateral mandibular inverted-L osteotomies. The osteotomized midface-mandibular complex is then advanced and counterclockwise

**Table 14.1** Pruzansky-Kaban classification of mandibular deformity

| Classification | Phenotype |
|---|---|
| Type 0 | Normal mandible |
| Type 1 | Hypoplastic mandible with all structures normal in shape and position |
| Type 2 | Small and abnormally shaped mandibular ramus with hypoplastic temporomandibular joint (TMJ) |
| Type 2A | With acceptable TMJ function |
| Type 2B | TMJ is anteriorly, medially, and inferiorly displaced and nonfunctional |
| Type 3 | Complete absence of ramus-condyle unit and TMJ |

rotated around the nasofrontal junction in a coordinated fashion utilizing distraction osteogenesis.

## Orbitozygomatic construction with full thickness calvarial bone grafts

Following appropriate reconstitution of the midface and mandibular anatomy with coordinated subcranial-mandibular distraction, many patients with TCS will be able to be decannulated. The stable skeletal framework for the central midface and craniomandibular articulation sets the stage for coordinated orthodontic-surgical management of the dentoskeletal relationships at skeletal maturity. For patients with zygomatic hypoplasia, reconstruction of the orbitozygomatic complexes can be undertaken as the next step in staged management. Since the rotation surgery is performed after 7 years of age, the subsequent malar reconstruction can be sized to anticipate the desired morphology at skeletal maturity.

Construction of the orbitozygomatic complexes is most reliably accomplished using full-thickness calvarial bone grafts. Partial-thickness grafts or grafts from other donor sites (iliac crest, rib) have unpredictable rates of incorporation/resorption. Our preference is to use parietal bone grafts, based upon the concordance between the curvature of the skull in this region and the contour necessary to create appropriate zygomatic projection.

## Workflow for computer-assisted design and computer-assisted manufacturing

The workflow for computer-assisted design and computer-assisted manufacturing (CAD/CAM) is shown in Fig. 14.2.

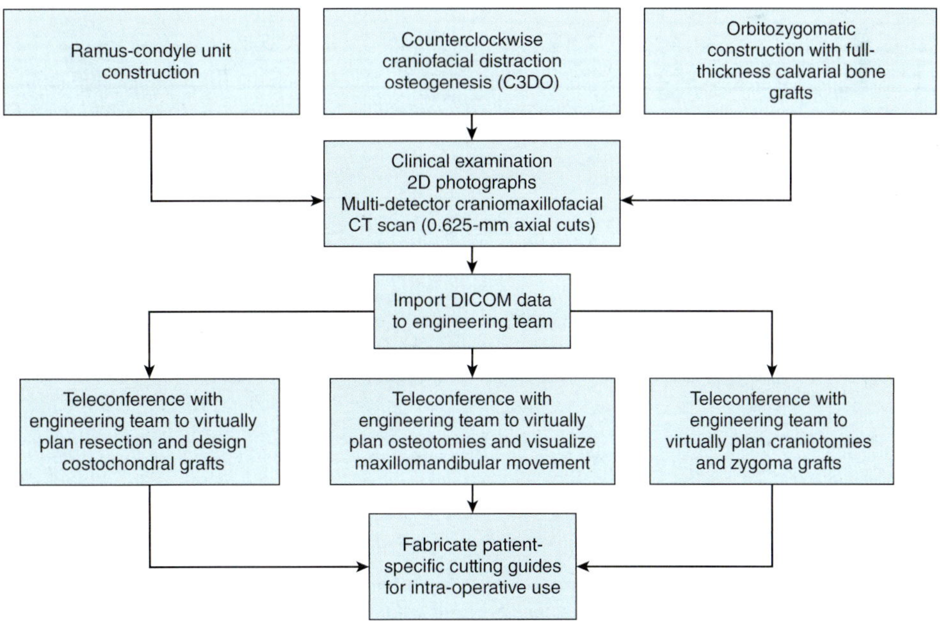


**Fig. 14.2** The workflow for computer-assisted design/computer-assisted manufacturing.

## Computer-assisted design

### Ramus-condyle unit construction with costochondral grafts

In patients with aplasia of the ramus-condyle units (Pruzansky-Kaban Type III, Fig. 14.1), first-stage reconstruction, ideally in the late primary dentition, involves the use of autologous rib grafts to establish a stable craniomandibular articulation, in anticipation of coordinated maxillomandibular distraction in the mixed dentition. In this regard, CaSP is a critical adjunct. The 3D anatomy of the dysmorphic mandible can be carefully mapped and customized cutting and positioning guides can be designed to harvest costochondral grafts of the exact size needed to create the mandible-glenoid fossa relationship (Fig. 14.3). CaSP in the 3D environment will also allow the surgeon to establish appropriate points for fixation, avoiding the inferior alveolar nerve and developing tooth buds.

### Counterclockwise craniofacial distraction osteogenesis

CaSP for this stage of reconstruction relies on the use of customized guides for the mandibular ramus osteotomies (Fig. 14.4). Surgical planning for inverted-L mandibular osteotomies in the computer-assisted environment has improved the safety and efficacy of the technique. The CaSP ensures safe osteotomy placement relative to the inferior alveolar nerve and developing succedaneous teeth, while also allowing adequate bone stock for hardware placement. A critical component of the coordinated distraction is offloading of the condylar (proximal) segments. This is accomplished using trans-pharyngeal pin placement within the proximal mandibular segments, which are frequently comprised of integrated costochondral grafts (as described above). Due to the paucity of bone stock in this region, positioning guides should include pilot holes for trans-pharyngeal and trans-facial pin placement, ensuring safe and accurate placement of the devices across the oropharynx and submental region.

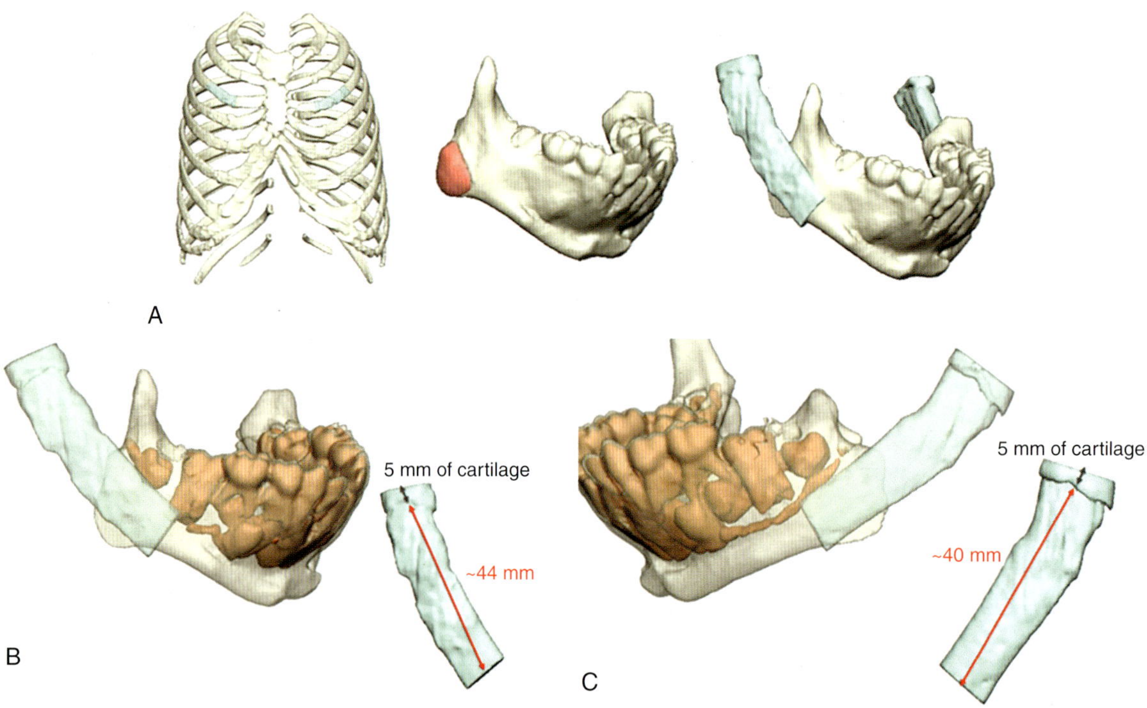


**Fig. 14.3** Ramus-condyle unit construction. (A) Rib harvest, mandible resection, mandible reconstruction. (B) Right mandible rib reconstruction uses cohort third left rib. (C) Left mandible rib reconstruction uses cohort third right rib.

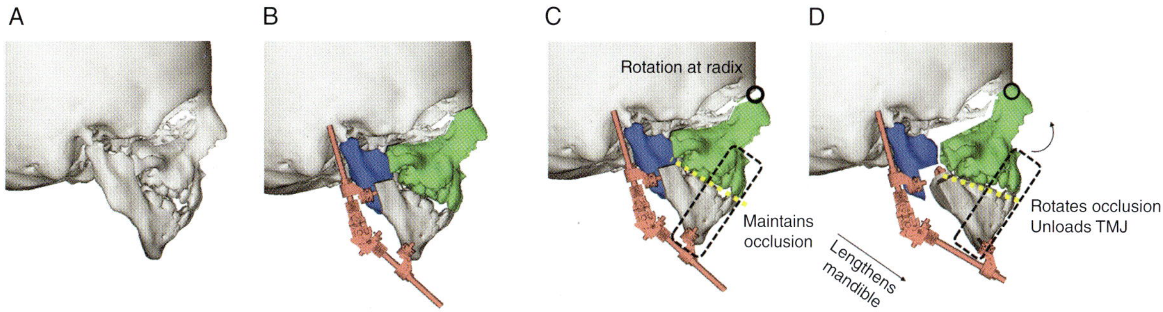


**Fig. 14.4** Counterclockwise craniofacial distraction osteogenesis (C3DO). Once a stable craniomandibular articulation has been established (ideally in the late primary dentition), coordinated maxillomandibular distraction is used to "derotate" the face (A). This intervention utilizes Le Fort II osteotomy and bilateral mandibular inverted-L osteotomies to isolate the anterior maxillomandibular complex, which is placed into intermaxillary fixation (B). External devices are then utilized to advance and counterclockwise rotate the midface and mandible in a coordinated fashion. Critical to the design and implementation of this operation is recognition of the forces transmitted to the proximal mandibular segment and temporomandibular joints. Stabilization of the proximal segments is accomplished with trans-pharyngeal pins; the fulcrum of rotation of the maxillomandibular complex is located at the nasofrontal junction (C). With the aid of an occlusal splint, the maxillomandibular complex is distracted anteriorly and superiorly, offloading the temporomandibular joints (D). (Modified with permission from Hopper RA, Kapadia H, Susarla SM. Surgical-orthodontic considerations in subcranial and frontofacial distraction. *Oral Maxillofac Surg Clin North Am*. 2020;32(2):309–20.)

The computer-assisted planning environment for this stage of reconstruction also allows the surgeon to anticipate the 3D changes that should occur at the distraction end point. Objective measurements from the computer-assisted plan can help the surgeon track progress during active distraction and make "mid-course" corrections in the vector of the midface device as needed.

### Orbitozygomatic construction with full thickness calvarial bone grafts

After establishing a stable craniomandibular articulation and appropriate maxillomandibular positioning, some patients may benefit from zygomatic construction, to improve lateral midface projection and afford support for the globes and periorbital soft tissues. Zygoma constructs are developed along the 3D computed tomography (CT) scan in the computer-assisted environment (Fig. 14.5). Full-thickness calvarial bone graft is ideally suited for this purpose. Within the computer-assisted environment, the surgeon can design templates that yield constructed zygomas with shape and projection that reestablishes a normal contour between the lateral midface and nasal radix, with the constructed infraorbital rim positioned approximately 7 to 10 mm anterior to the native supraorbital rim. These constructs are then mapped to the parietal skull, identifying the regions where the curvature of the exocortex most closely matches that of the zygoma.

## Computer-assisted manufacturing

### Ramus-condyle unit construction with costochondral grafts

In our practice, CAM is a useful adjunct for ramus-condyle unit construction in the context of customized guides that can assist with selective bony resection and ensuring the appropriate positioning of harvested grafts. The guide designs are adapted to the native mandibular anatomy, with guide holes for screw placement and fitted contours to help "dock" the graft and ensure appropriate angulation toward the skull base both anteroposteriorly as well as mediolaterally. This is critical to ensure that the constructed ramus-condyle unit creates the stable craniomandibular articulation necessary to support subsequent craniofacial distraction and orthognathic surgery at skeletal maturity (Fig. 14.6).

### Counterclockwise craniofacial distraction osteogenesis

Similar to planning for ramus-condyle unit construction using autologous rib grafts and 3D visualization of the mandible affords the surgeon the opportunity to identify the locations of developing teeth and inferior alveolar nerve. Precise osteotomy designs, developed in the computer-assisted environment, are translated into

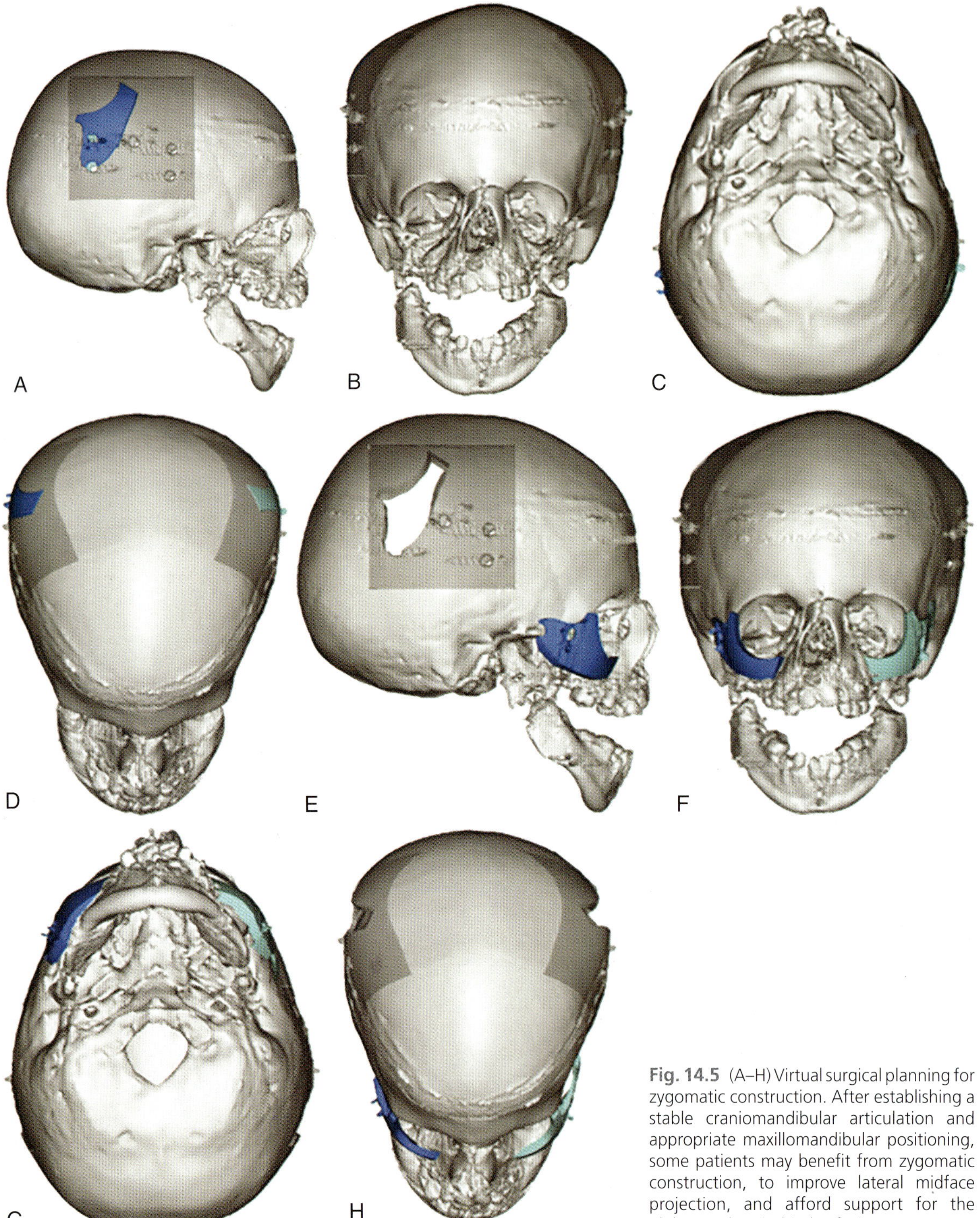


**Fig. 14.5** (A–H) Virtual surgical planning for zygomatic construction. After establishing a stable craniomandibular articulation and appropriate maxillomandibular positioning, some patients may benefit from zygomatic construction, to improve lateral midface projection, and afford support for the globes and periorbital soft tissues.

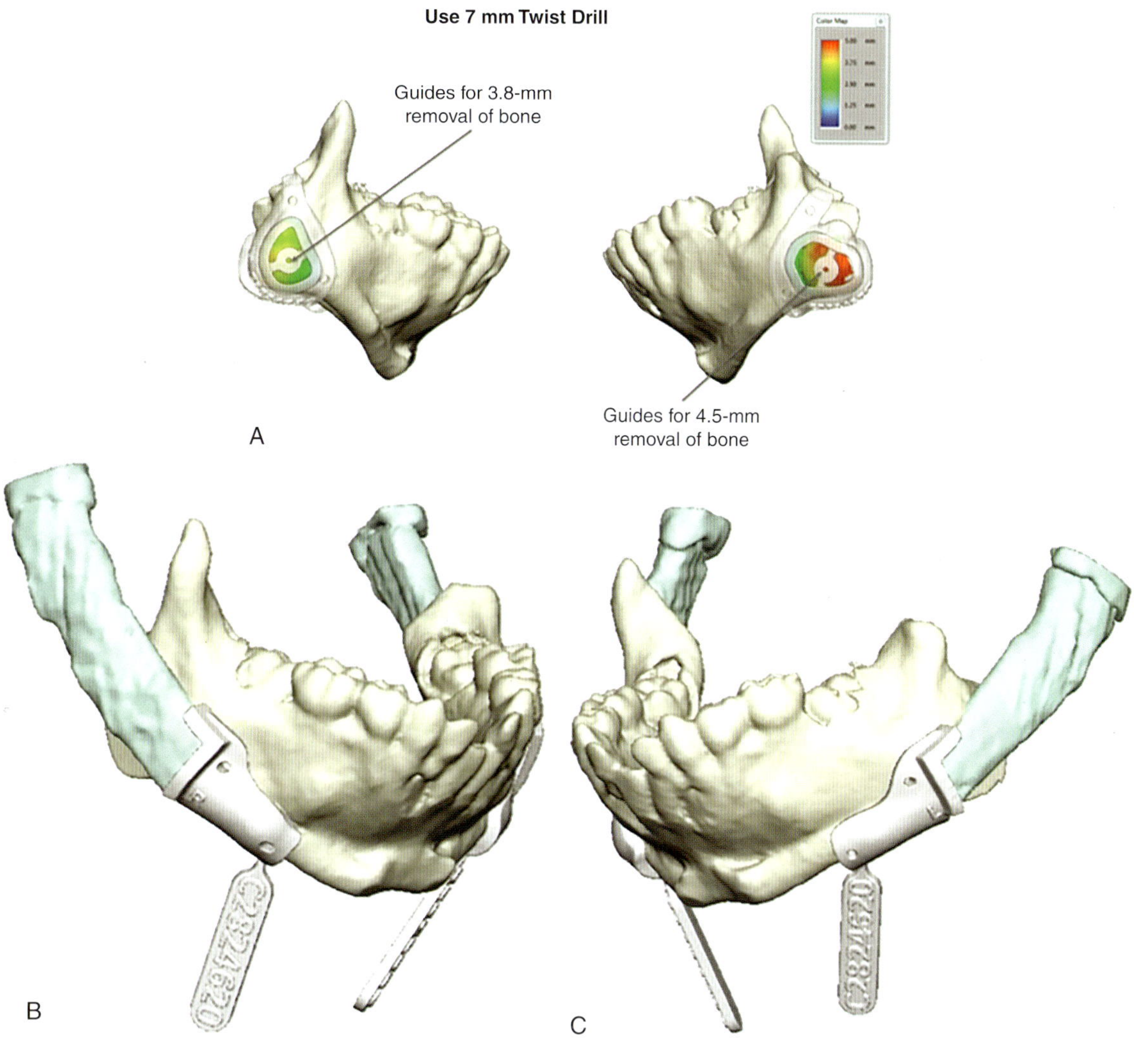


**Fig. 14.6** (A–C) Computer-assisted manufacturing for ramus-condyle unit construction.

customized guides used intraoperatively for the inverted-L osteotomy and trans-pharyngeal pin placement. The angulation between the plane of the posterior (trans-pharyngeal) and anterior (trans-facial) is precisely established by the positioning guide (Fig. 14.7).

## Orbitozygomatic construction with full-thickness calvarial bone grafts

Once the appropriate region for full-thickness calvarial bone graft harvest has been identified, customized cutting guides are fabricated for the craniotomy, with inset cutting templates for the constructed zygomas. Following full-thickness harvest, the constructed zygomas can be precisely cut from the parietal graft. The zygomatic constructs are then inset and affixed. The remnant parietal pieces are replaced in situ, with partial-thickness calvarial graft used to repair the cranial defects. We have found this presurgical computer-assisted planning saves considerable time in the operating room since the exact shape of graft needed for optimal bone contact has already been established (Fig. 14.8).

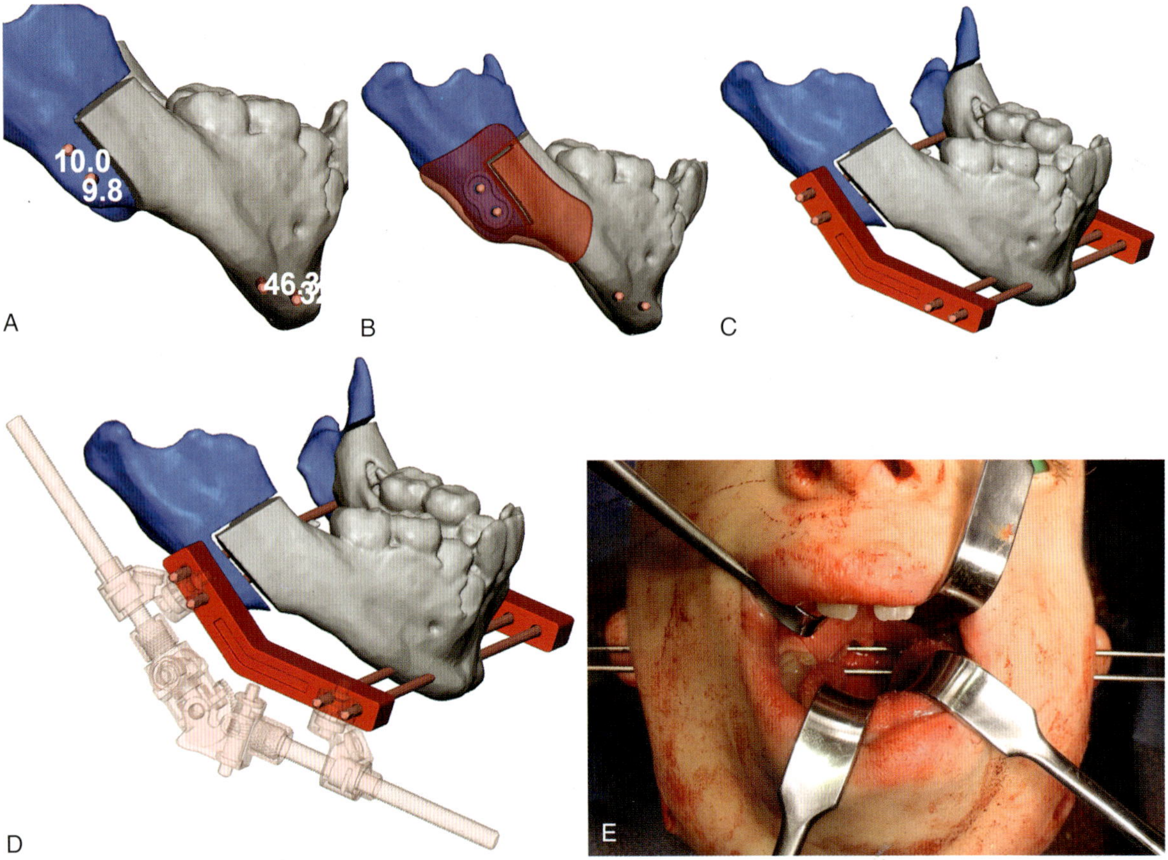


**Fig. 14.7** Computerized-surgical planning for counterclockwise craniofacial distraction osteogenesis mandible osteotomy. Surgical planning for inverted-L mandibular osteotomies in the virtual environment has improved the safety and efficacy of the technique. Similar to planning for ramus-condyle unit construction using autologous rib grafts, three-dimensional visualization of the mandible affords the surgeon the opportunity to identify the locations of developing teeth and inferior alveolar nerve (A). Precise osteotomy designs can then be developed, with customized guides used intraoperatively for the inverted-L osteotomy (B) and transpharyngeal pin placement (C–D). The angulation (E) between the plane of the posterior (transpharyngeal) and anterior (trans-facial) is precisely established by the positioning guide. (Modified with permission from Hopper RA, Kapadia H, Susarla SM. Surgical-orthodontic considerations in subcranial and frontofacial distraction. *Oral Maxillofac Surg Clin North Am*. 2020;32(2):309–20.)

## Operative technique

### Ramus-condyle unit construction with costochondral grafts

Ramus-condyle unit construction is performed through a transcervical (Risdon) approach. In some cases, this is preceded (at least 9 months prior) by enucleation of tooth follicles and corticocancellous iliac crest bone grafting to develop a platform for subsequent rib graft fixation.

Costochondral graft reconstruction is undertaken through Risdon incisions. The inferior border of the hypoplastic mandible is exposed, with care taken during the dissection to monitor for the marginal branch of the facial nerve and avoid iatrogenic injury. Once the mandible is exposed, prefabricated cutting guides are used to contour the proximal bone edge to allow passive adaptation of the rib graft to the native mandible. The guides are then used to identify the appropriate angulation for the rib graft placement; the path of the graft is then bluntly dissected within the infratemporal fossa until the skull base is reached (lateral to the lateral ptyergoid plates). The path of insertion is confirmed with stereotactic navigation. A costochondral graft with a 5-mm cartilaginous cap and intact perichondrial-periosteal junction is harvested from the third or fourth rib. An occlusal splint is used to establish the desired maxillomandibular relationship – the anterior open bite

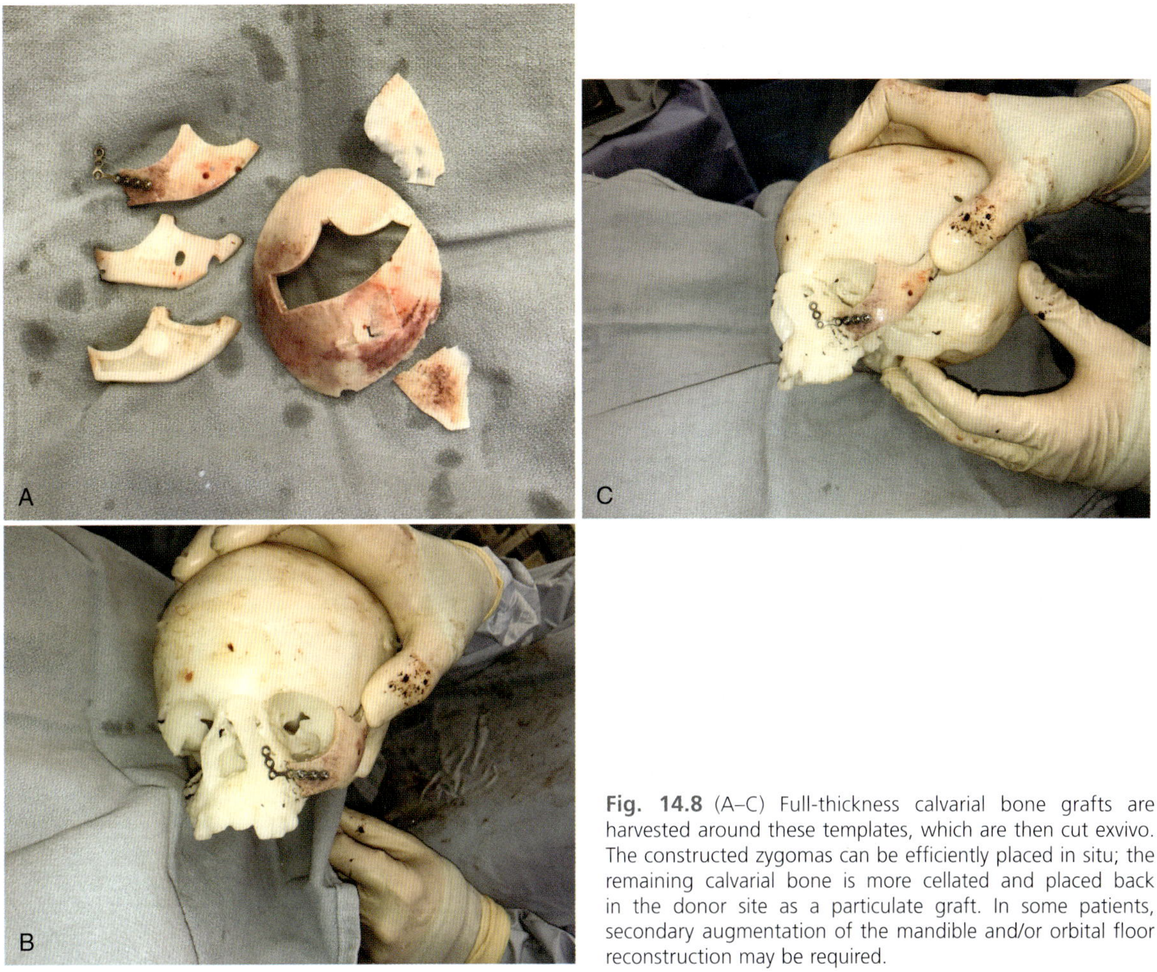


Fig. 14.8 (A–C) Full-thickness calvarial bone grafts are harvested around these templates, which are then cut exvivo. The constructed zygomas can be efficiently placed in situ; the remaining calvarial bone is more cellated and placed back in the donor site as a particulate graft. In some patients, secondary augmentation of the mandible and/or orbital floor reconstruction may be required.

malocclusion is not typically addressed at this time. The rib graft is then positioned and affixed using titanium miniplates and bicortical screws with the aid of the prefabricated guide. Stereotactic navigation can be used to verify the appropriate positioning relative to the skull base. The positioning guide is then removed and the incisions are closed in layers. Orthodontic bone anchors are placed between the central incisors to assist with elastic traction in the early postoperative period. The patient is maintained on a soft, non-chew diet for 4 weeks. The next stage of reconstruction (counterclockwise craniofacial distraction osteogenesis [C3DO]) is performed approximately 9 months later.

## Counterclockwise craniofacial distraction

The operation begins with a Le Fort II osteotomy (or Le Fort III osteotomy in patients with developed zygomas). A coronal incision is used, with subgaleal dissection. The anterior origin of the temporalis is released, but manipulation of the body of the muscle is minimized to prevent atrophy. Subperiosteal exposure begins approximately 2 cm above the supraorbital rims, skeletonizing the nasofrontal region, anterior portion of the zygomatic arch (if present), medial and lateral orbital walls, and orbital floor. Once this exposure is completed, the nasofrontal osteotomy is performed with a piezoelectric saw with a 5-mm wedge of bone removed to allow hinge rotation of the maxillomandibular complex. The osteotomy is then continued using the piezoelectric saw along the medial orbital wall, posterior to the medial canthal insertions. A thin osteotome is then used to connect the medial wall osteotomy to the orbital floor. Once this is accomplished, the lateral orbital wall is osteotomized at the junction of the frontozygomatic pillar with the zygomatic body and, if present, the zygomatic arch is osteotomized. A thin osteotome is then placed into the inferior orbital fissure and directed medially across the orbital floor to connect with the medial wall osteotomy. A curved osteotome placed into the inferior orbital fissure and directed inferiorly, anteriorly, and medially and then used to perform the pterygomaxillary disjunction. Finally, the septum is separated from the anterior skull base using a double ball nasal osteotome, with the tips directed inferior toward the posterior nasal spine.

Once this sequence of osteotomies is completed, the midface is gently downfractured with manual pressure and mobilized using Rowe-Kiley disimpaction forceps. Pilot holes are then drilled across the nasofrontal osteotomy site. A hinge is subsequently created by placing 28-gauge stainless steel wires or 3-0 polydioxanone sutures across the osteotomy site. The coronal incision is then closed.

After closure of the coronal incision, the Risdon incisions previously used for ramus-condyle unit construction are used to access the ramus. Customized cutting guides are then adapted to the mandibular ramus and secured in place using monocortical screws. Predictive holes in the guides are drilled to facilitate transfacial pin placement and the inverted-L mandibular osteotomies are marked and completed using a piezoelectric saw, stopping just shy of the inferior border. With the inferior border still intact, 2 pairs of 0.078" transfacial pins are passed via the predrilled holes on one side and transition across the pharynx posterior to the tonsillar pillars. A Frazier tip suction is then placed into the contralateral ramus pilot hole to guide the pins through the contralateral ramus. The inferior border osteotomies are then completed and the patient is placed into a customized acrylic occlusal splint, which is secured using piriform and lateral maxillary buttress wires. With the splint secured, maxillomandibular fixation is achieved using suspension wires from the midface to the mandible. External, multivector mandibular distraction devices are then attached to the transfacial pins, and an external midface distraction device (halo) is attached using cranial pins. With this framework established, activation posts are secured with 24-gauge wires to the splint via traction posts. The initial distraction vector is set with a 45-degree upward incline.

The patient is maintained under sedation in the intensive care unit for 2 days after surgery. Activation is initiated on postoperative day 5 via the midface distraction pins until visible tension is apparent on the splint wires. This ensures condylar offloading during active distraction. Distraction then commences at a rate of 1 mm/day at both the midface and mandibular sites, with the complex hinging on the nasofrontal junction. Distraction progress is monitored with serial lateral cephalograms. Once the appropriate distraction endpoint is reached, the consolidation period begins. After 5 to 7 days of initial consolidation, the maxillomandibular fixation is released to allow independent jaw movement. The maxillomandibular relationship is maintained using anterior elastics supported by bone anchors for the remainder of the consolidation period (12 weeks).

## Orbitozygomatic construction

Following successful consolidation, orbitozygomatic construction, if indicated, is undertaken at the time of distractor removal. The coronal incision is reopened, and full-thickness parietal bone grafts are harvested with the assistance of prefabricated cutting guides. The zygomatic bodies are then affixed using titanium miniplates. The remaining parietal bone is then used to fill the donor site calvarial defects.

## Case study

This patient underwent coordinated Le Fort II-mandible distraction C3DO followed by zygoma construction with full-thickness calvarial bone grafts. Prior to surgery, she has a classic deformity characterized by zygomatic aplasia and clockwise rotation of the maxillomandibular complex. Following C3DO and zygoma reconstruction, the facial proportions are improved (Fig. 14.9). The patient's airway expansion following distraction was sufficient to allow tracheostomy decannulation.

# Fidelity/verification

Verification of the appropriate anatomical relationships is done clinically and radiographically. Intraoperatively, following reconstruction of the ramus-condyle units, the mandible can be ranged to ensure a stable and consistent arc of mandibular motion. Postoperative imaging confirms the location of the rib grafts and fixation, though the use of positioning guides practically ensures high-fidelity placement. Following mandibular and midface osteotomies for C3DO, immediate postoperative imaging is used to verify the pin positioning and osteotomy trajectories. Serial lateral cephalometric films are taken during active distraction to ensure correct vector orientation and make "midcourse" corrections, as needed. The initial distraction vector is 45 degrees upward—once pogonion is in line with nasion, the midface distraction arm angle is increased to be as vertical as possible. This maximizes the rotational movement at end-distraction. A successful distraction endpoint is a normalized palatal plane, which typically requires a rotation of around 25 degrees.

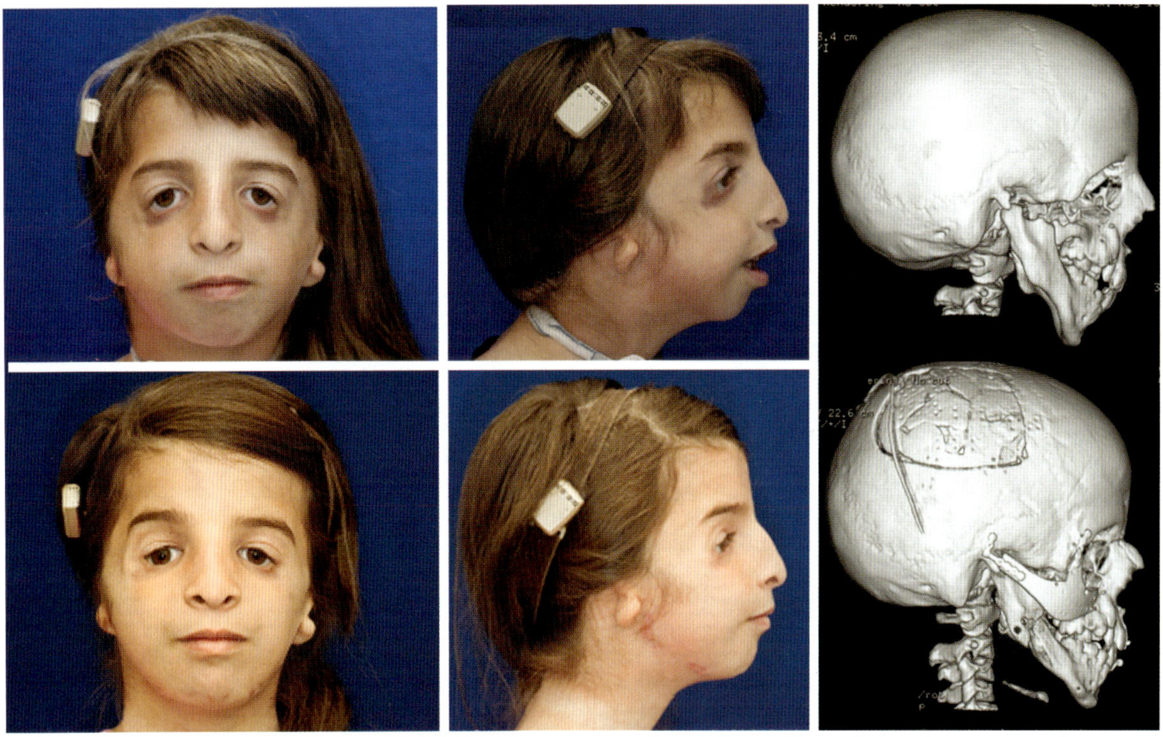

**Fig. 14.9** This patient underwent coordinated Le Fort II-mandible distraction with counterclockwise rotation (C3DO) followed by zygoma construction with full-thickness calvarial bone grafts. Prior to surgery, she has a classic deformity characterized by zygomatic aplasia and clockwise rotation of the maxillomandibular complex. Following C3DO and zygoma reconstruction, the facial proportions are improved. The patient's airway expansion following distraction was sufficient to allow tracheostomy decannulation. (From Susarla SM, Egbert MA, Kapadia H, Hopper RA. Management of the mandibular deformity in growing patients with Treacher Collins syndrome. In: Markiewicz MR, Yates D, ed. *Hemifacial Microsomia and Treacher-Collins Syndrome: Comprehensive Treatment of Associated Facial Deformities,* 1st ed. Springer Nature, US. 2021:379–92.)

Finally, in orbitozygomatic construction, the appropriate projection of the midface soft tissues is often evident immediately after positioning of the grafts and is subsequently confirmed by 3D CT imaging.

## Pearls/Pitfalls

- The surgeon should be keenly aware of the patient-specific anatomy that needs to be accounted for in osteotomy design. In particular, the position of the anterior skull base relative to the nasofrontal junction, the location and orientation of unerupted succedaneous teeth, and the position of the infraorbital and inferior alveolar nerves.
- Vector orientation with counterclockwise craniofacial distraction relies on a hinge point placed at the nasofrontal junction. Simulation of the counterclockwise rotational movement in the computer-assisted environment can help evaluate the progress during active distraction and allow for "midcourse" corrections, if needed.
- When performing orbitozygomatic reconstruction in this population, full-thickness calvarial bone grafts should be used. This source of graft allows for the most predictable recreation of the zygomatic projection and predictable healing.

## Outcomes/Complications

Construction of a stable craniomandibular articulation, followed by coordinated subcranial-mandibular distraction and subsequent zygoma construction complete the initial reconstructive course for patients with TCS. At the end of this sequence of care, the facial skeletal morphology should be characterized by improved maxillary and mandibular position, appropriate orbitozygomatic projection, and improved airway dynamics (frequently to the extent that tracheostomy is not required). For many patients, the goal should be to achieve this point of care by the late mixed dentition.

Once this skeletal foundation has been established, coordinated orthodontic-surgical care is undertaken, with the goal of addressing residual maxillomandibular discrepancy, malocclusion, and any residual airway obstruction at skeletal maturity. The prototypical dentofacial difference at this stage is a less severe recapitulation of the initial deformity. Some of the gains established in the first sequence of treatment may be lost due to partial relapse of the counterclockwise rotation, though this does not appear to create recurrent severe airway obstruction and repeat tracheostomy is rarely needed.[11,12,16,17] As such, the end-stage dentofacial difference is defined by shortened posterior face heights with steep mandibular plane angles, long anterior face heights, anterior open bites, and class II skeletal patterns with microgenia. This constellation of clinical findings is effectively treated with midface advancement at the Le Fort I level, bilateral mandibular ramus osteotomies, and genioplasty. Orthognathic surgery can be largely similar to that in patients with primary dentofacial deformities, as described elsewhere in the text.

## Conclusion

The facial morphology in TCS is a congenital, nonprogressive facial difference that is phenotypically variable. Mild cases present with minimal hypoplasia of the first branchial arch structures requiring little or no surgical intervention. In the most severe cases, however, patients with TCS will present with aplasia of the zygomatic bones, mandibular ramus-condyle units and glenoid fossae, along with the external and internal structures of the ear which requires careful coordination and planning of staged operative interventions. All patients with TCS will exhibit some degree of maxillomandibular discrepancy characterized by bimaxillary retrusion and microgenia with clockwise rotation of the palatal, occlusal, and mandibular planes. This typically results in a long anterior face height and short posterior face height, anterior open bite malocclusion, and physiologically consequential airway narrowing. CaSP has helped streamline the treatment for this complex constellation of problems, allowing precise construction of the appropriate condyle-skull base articulation, coordinated maxillomandibular counterclockwise distraction movements, customized zygomatic reconstruction, and efficient planning for bimaxillary orthognathic surgery.

## Take-home points

- CAD/CAM technology is highly useful in the management of the facial dysmorphology seen in patients with TCS.
- CaSP allows for the surgeon to develop precise osteotomies, avoiding critical structures such as the globes, skull base, developing dentition, and branches of the trigeminal nerve.
- CAD/CAM customized cutting guides and fixation devices can help the surgeon recreate the precise anatomic relationships for orbitozygomatic reconstruction.

## References

1. Marszalek B, Wojcicki P, Kobus K, Trzeciak WH. Clinical features, treatment and genetic background of Treacher Collins syndrome. *J Appl Genet*. 2002;43:223-233.
2. Plomp RG, van Lieshout MJ, Joosten KF, et al. Treacher Collins syndrome: a systematic review of evidence-based treatment and recommendations. *Plast Reconstr Surg*. 2016;137:191-204.
3. Posnick JC. Treacher Collins syndrome: evaluation and treatment. In: Posnick JC, ed. *Orthognathic Surgery: Principles and Practice*. London, UK: Elsevier; 2014:1059-1194.
4. Thompson JT, Anderson PJ, David DJ. Treacher Collins syndrome: protocol management from birth to maturity. *J Craniofac Surg*. 2009; 20:2028-2035.
5. Chong DK, Murray DJ, Britto JA, Tompson B, Forrest CR, Phillips JHA. Cephalometric analysis of maxillary and mandibular parameters in Treacher Collins syndrome. *Plast Reconstr Surg*. 2008;121:77e-84e.
6. Peterson-Falzone SJ, Figueroa AA. Longitudinal changes in cranial base angulation in mandibulofacial dysostosis. *Cleft Palate J*. 1989;26:31-35.
7. Akre H, Overland B, Asten P, Skogedal N, Heimdal K. Obstructive sleep apnea in Treacher Collins syndrome. *Eur Arch Otorhinolaryngol*. 2012;269: 331-337.
8. Plomp RG, Bredero-Boelhouwer HH, Joosten KF, et al. Obstructive sleep apnoea in Treacher Collins syndrome: prevalence, severity and cause. *Int J Oral Maxillofac Surg*. 2012;41:696-701.

9. Ma X, Forte AJ, Persing JA, Alonso N, Berlin NL, Steinbacher DM. Reduced three-dimensional airway volume is a function of skeletal dysmorphology in Treacher Collins syndrome. *Plast Reconstr Surg*. 2015;135: 382e-392e.
10. Ma X, Forte AJ, Berlin NL, Alonso N, Persing JA, Steinbacher DM. Reduced three-dimensional nasal airway volume in Treacher Collins syndrome and its association with craniofacial morphology. *Plast Reconstr Surg*. 2015;135:885e-894e.
11. Hopper RA, Wang HD, Mercan E, Kapadia H. Counterclockwise craniofacial distraction osteogenesis. *Clin Plast Surg*. 2021;48(3):445-454.
12. Hopper RA, Kapadia H, Susarla SM. Surgical-orthodontic considerations in subcranial and frontofacial distraction. *Oral Maxillofac Surg Clin North Am*. 2020;32(2):309-320.
13. Guo Y, Lopez J, Yang R, Macmillan A, Dorafshar AH. The use of virtual surgical planning in total facial skeletal reconstruction of Treacher Collins syndrome: a case report. *Craniomaxillofac Trauma Reconstr*. 2018;11(3):230-237.
14. Kaban LB, Mulliken JB, Murray JE. Three-dimensional approach to analysis and treatment of hemifacial microsomia. *Cleft Palate J*. 1981;18(2):90-99.
15. Figueroa AA, Pruzansky S. The external ear, mandible and other components of hemifacial microsomia. *J Maxillofac Surg*. 1982;10(4):200-211.
16. Susarla SM, Egbert MA, Kapadia H, Hopper RA. Management of the mandibular deformity in growing patients with Treacher Collins syndrome. In: Markiewicz MR, Yates D, ed. *Hemifacial Microsomia and Treacher-Collins Syndrome: Comprehensive Treatment of Associated Facial Deformities*. 1st ed. Springer Nature, US; 2021:379-392.
17. Hopper RA, Kapadia H, Susarla S, Bly R, Johnson K. Counterclockwise craniofacial distraction osteogenesis for tracheostomy-dependent children with Treacher Collins syndrome. *Plast Reconstr Surg*. 2018;142(2):447-457.

Chapter 15

# Computer-assisted surgical planning for craniofacial microsomia

*Roberto L. Flores, Paul A. Mittermiller, Pradip R. Shetye*

CHAPTER OUTLINE



## Introduction

Craniofacial microsomia is a congenital anomaly that results in the underdevelopment of one half or both sides of the face. It occurs in approximately 1:3000 to 1:5000 live births.[1] Treatment of this condition can involve multiple operations to augment the hard and soft tissue and improve facial symmetry. Two common procedures used for the correction of the skeletal differences in craniofacial microsomia are distraction osteogenesis of the mandible and orthognathic surgery. Other treatment options include bone grafting to the mandible or osseous free flap reconstruction of the mandible.

Computer-assisted surgical planning (CaSP) can be helpful during these complex operations. During distraction osteogenesis, CaSP can be helpful to plan the location of the osteotomies to avoid injury to critical structures and to determine and set the optimal distraction vectors preoperatively.[2,3]

CaSP is often used during orthognathic surgery for patients without craniofacial microsomia and has similar benefits for patients with craniofacial microsomia. These include the fabrication of custom cutting guides, custom plates, and printed dental splints.[4,5]

CaSP can also be used for the creation of custom implants that can help to camouflage asymmetries in the patient with craniofacial microsomia.

If free flap reconstruction of the mandible is performed, CaSP can facilitate and streamline the accurate completion of a complex three-dimensional (3D) reconstruction. These techniques will be covered in separate chapters of this book.

## Clinical considerations

### Distraction osteogenesis

The location of the osteotomies is critical when planning for distraction osteogenesis. It is critical to assess the quality of the bone and determine the location of the inferior alveolar nerve. Ideally, the osteotomy is designed superior to the foramen where the inferior alveolar nerve enters the mandible. The orientation of the cut should be perpendicular to the direction of distraction. There should be enough bone on either side of the osteotomy to hold screws and to distract the mandible in the appropriate orientation. The goal may be to lengthen the mandible in an anterior-posterior orientation, superior-inferior orientation, or both. Once the ideal location and orientation of the osteotomies is determined, cutting guides can be manufactured that have a higher degree of interaction with the mandible, allowing precise placement of the osteotomy on the patient's mandible. This sometimes requires wider periosteal undermining than would normally be done during the procedure. Sterile models of the mandible can also be produced on which the cutting guide can be placed to determine the adequacy of the fit and assist with locating the guide on the patient.

The thickness of the bone as well as avoidance of teeth and nerves are also critical factors that can be determined when planning the operation virtually and can inform screw placement and the location/orientation of osteotomy.

Virtually planning the placement of the osteotomies and distractors allows the advance determination of the vector and distance of activation.

## Orthognathic surgery

CaSP for orthognathic surgery in patients with hemifacial microsomia has similar advantages to its use with distraction osteogenesis. Osteotomies on the maxilla can be designed to avoid tooth roots and locate screw placement in robust and stable bone.

The movement of the Le Fort segment can be completely controlled by custom plates. The use of predictive screw holes withing the cutting guides, combined with custom plates, dictates translation and rotation in all three planes and axis. This computer- and hardware-controlled accuracy facilitates accurate intraoperative placement of the maxilla, which in turn, usually determines mandible placement. Although the plates determine the final location of the maxilla, dental splints can be used to confirm appropriate movement of the segment.

Mandibular osteotomies can also be designed to avoid injury to the inferior alveolar nerve. This is more relevant depending on which osteotomies, other than a sagittal split, are used, such as an inverted L osteotomy. Custom cutting guides can be used and custom plates manufactured that secure the predetermined movement.

With traditional orthognathic surgery, movement of the genioplasty is determined using two-dimensional cephalograms. This is usually insufficient in patients with hemifacial microsomia in 3D rotation and translation is required. CaSP can facilitate the planning and accurate execution of these complex movements and determine areas where bone may need to be contoured to optimize the facial framework.

Finally, bone grafts to the maxilla, mandible, and chin can all be designed by use of custom guides and shaping templates to improve stability and streamline the construction of accurately shaped bone grafts.

## Custom implants

Patients who have continued asymmetry after orthognathic surgery movements may benefit from custom implants. These can be used on the maxilla, mandible, or chin. If there is a deficiency of bone or soft tissue in those regions, custom implants can be designed virtually preoperatively and augment regions of the face in a patient-specific manner.

## Workflow for computer-assisted design/computer-assisted manufacturing

See Fig. 15.1.

## Computer-assisted design

Design planning:
- Key points in the design
- Video
- Anatomical design

A current thin cut computed tomography as well as a dental scan or high quality dental impressions are sent to the engineering team prior to planning

Planning should be done during a time that is free from distractions. It should not be done in the middle of office hours or an OR day.

Identification of midline and the horizontal plane of the patient is sometimes difficult and a best fit is can be required.

Whenever possible ensure that there is a components of bone to bone contact in the LeFort I segment to help with bony stability

Over correct the cant by about 2 degrees

Modify osteotomy of the mandibular segment as needed in cases of thin bone or poor bone stock

Ensure that the bony movements, the cutting guides and the plates are make sense from the standpoint of surgical exposure and soft tissue forces on the bone

(See Figs. 15.2–15.8, Table 15.1.)

## Computer-assisted manufacturing

- Stereolithographic models
- Video
- Guides (e.g., cutting guides, positioning guides)

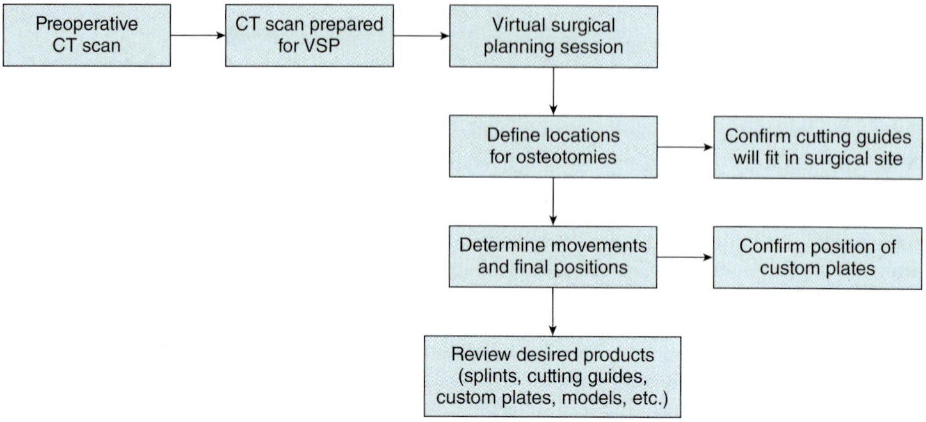


**Fig. 15.1** The process of computer-assisted surgical planning (CaSP) starts by obtaining imaging of the patient, usually in the form of a high-resolution computed tomography (CT) scan of the face (at least 1-mm cuts). The CT scan is then provided to the company assisting with CaSP. A planning session is arranged that includes an engineer, the surgeon, and potentially the craniofacial orthodontist. Depending on the procedure planned (distraction osteogenesis or orthognathic surgery), the location of the osteotomies are determined. With this osteotomy location, custom cutting guides can be created to ensure the osteotomies are placed in the positions that are planned preoperatively. The final position of the segments are then determined. For distraction osteogenesis, the angle of the distractors is decided. The custom cutting guides are made with predictive holes so that the distractors can be placed in the predetermined positions after the osteotomies are performed. If orthognathic surgery is planned, the custom plates can be manufactured that contain the information for the proposed movements. After the planning session, a plan is sent to the surgeon for review. If the plan is determined to be appropriate, the products are created and sent to the surgeon for the planned operation.

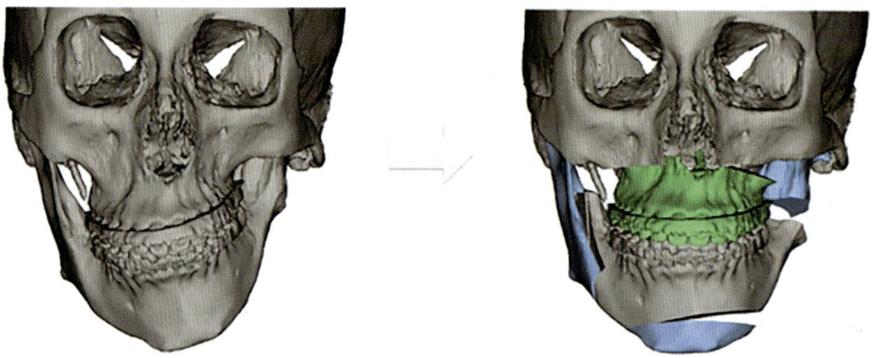

**Fig. 15.2** Computer-assisted surgical planning was performed on this patient with craniofacial microsomia who was to undergo orthognathic surgery with a Le Fort I osteotomy, a right-sided mandibular sagittal split osteotomy, a left-sided ramus osteotomy, and a genioplasty. The process will be described in detail in the following figures. She was noted to have a significant occlusal cant. Her dental relationships were corrected preoperatively. The plan was to correct the patient's cant and chin point deviation.

Stereolithographic models can be a useful but not required adjunct to reconstruction. They may serve as a means of understanding the fit of the cutting guides and plates. They can also be use to bend plates in the event that customiced plates are not used.

The cutting guides can be titanium based or polymer based. The titanium are more ridged but are more difficult to handle. The polymer based cutting guides are easier to handle but can be easily transected with a saw or drill.

It is important to inspect the size of the guide and implants. The proportions should be taken into consideration with the operative exposure for the case. The implants and guides may be segmented and assembled within the patient if the size is a challenge

Communications with the manufacturer is important to ensure that adequate time is given to production and manufacturing as to avoid cancelation of delay of surgery.

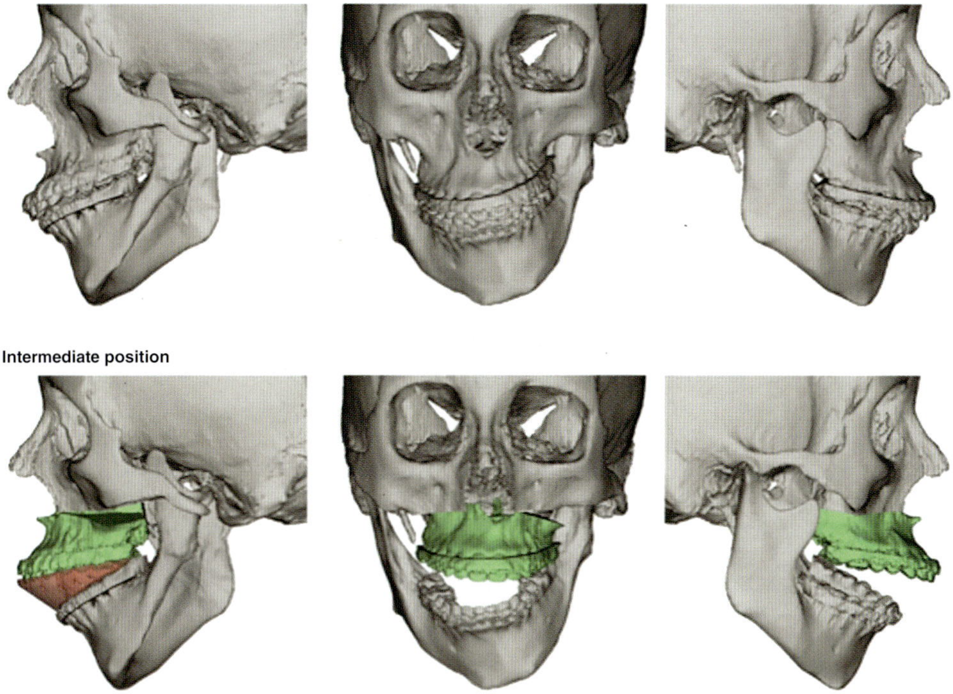


**Fig. 15.3** The first stage of the operation is similar to standard double jaw orthognathic surgery operations. This case was performed using a maxilla-first approach. A Le Fort I osteotomy was performed and the correct position for the maxilla was decided. Neither custom cutting guides nor custom plates were used for this operation; however, they could have been used. The position of the maxilla was built into the splint and the degree of vertical movement on the affected and unaffected sides were adjusted intraoperatively by measuring the distance from the nasal radix to the archwire on each side of the maxilla (affected and unaffected sides).

Carefully inspect all final plans before approval.
(See Figs. 15.9–15.11.)

## Operative technique

- Steps of the procedure
- Video
- Clinical cases
- Photos before and after
- Radiographs before and after and "fit" to plan

Orthognathic surgery using Computer-assistend surgical planning follows a similar progression to traditional orthognathic surgery. The surgical plan with the cutting guide and implant design should all be inspected prior to the start of surgery. All implants should also be inspected and confirmed to be present and sterile prior to the start of surgery. When performing the operative exposure, care should be taken to ensure that a meticulous subperiosteal plane is maintained throughout the areas of the jaws in which the guides and implants will interface. This careful dissection of all soft tissue from the bone is especially important around the edges of the bone where the footplates of the guides and implants will interact. Even a minor soft tissue interposition between the implant and bone can compromisre the surgical accuracy. When creating the registration holes, ensure that the holes are not overdrilled as this will compromised rigid fixation. Ensure that the appropriate cutting plane is maintained throughout all osteotomies. After the osteotomy is complete, carefully remove any bone that will prevent reduction of the jaw segment. This would be determined at the time of surgical planning. If the cutting guides were used properly, the custom plates should fit perfectly to the registration holes. The intermediate splint is an additional layer of assessment ensure that the maxilla is in an appropriate position (assuming a maxilla first surgery). However if the manufactured plate easily and anatomically fits the maxilla after rigid fixation is applied, the intermediate splint is not needed. As manufactured plates tend to be a higher profile and larger size, appropriate soft tissue closure is critical at the end of the procedure.

(See Figs. 15.12–15.15.)

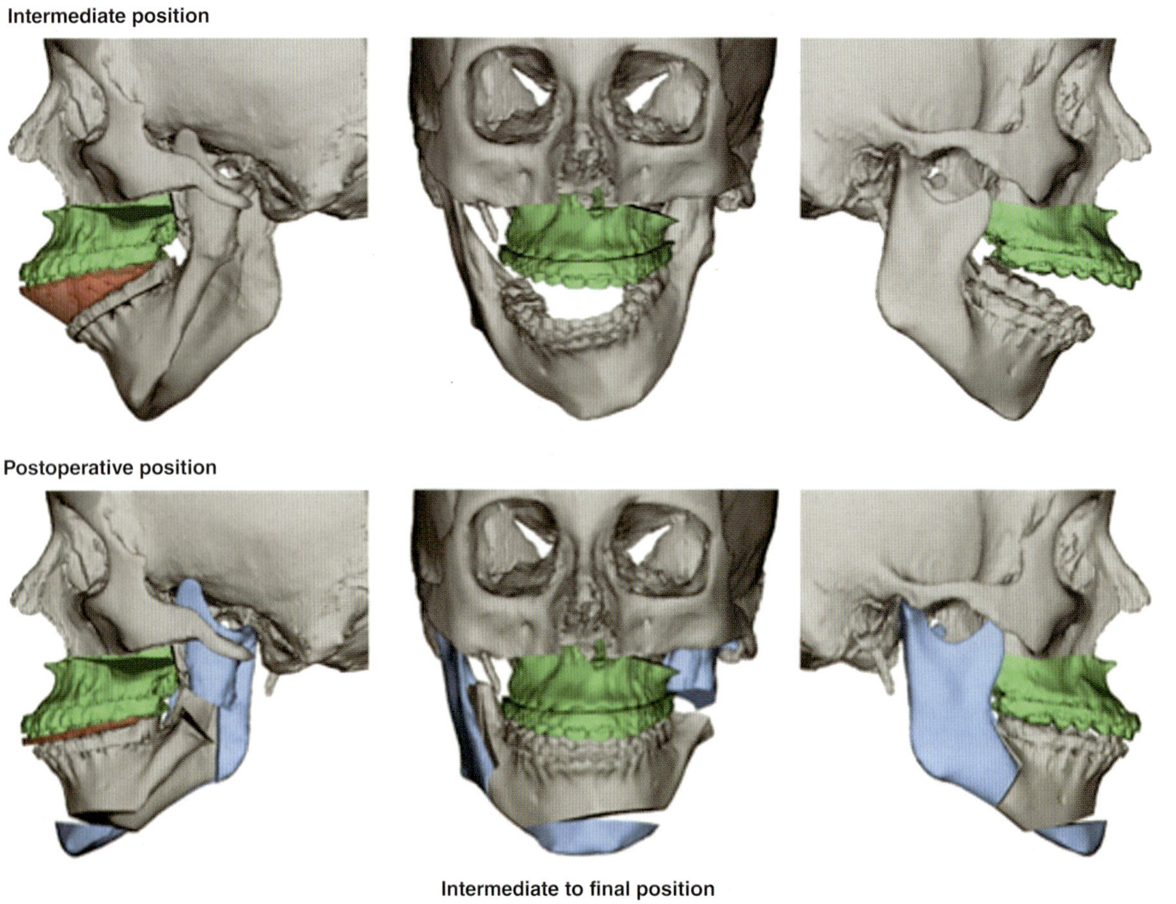


**Fig. 15.4** The second stage was then determined to be a sagittal split osteotomy and a bicortical osteotomy on the left, hypoplastic mandible. An asymmetric genioplasty was also performed. A final splint had been printed to set the tooth-bearing segment of the mandible to the Le Fort I segment.

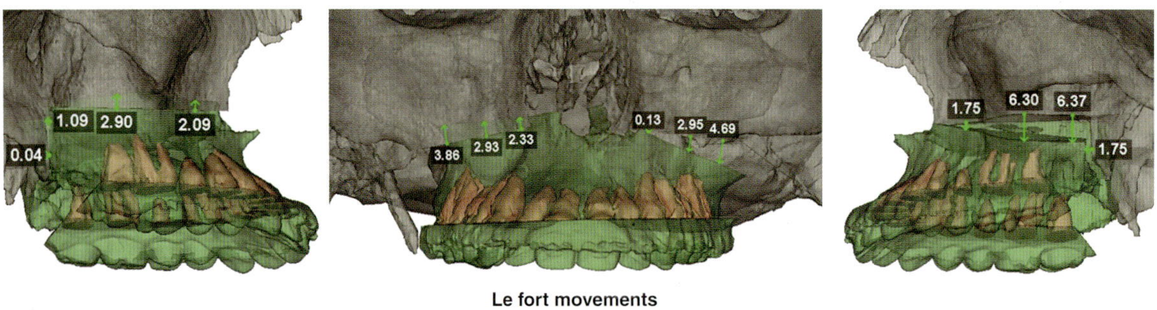


**Fig. 15.5** These images demonstrate the precise movements as seen on a virtual model. The right side of the Le Fort segment is being impacted while the left side is being disimpacted, with more movement occurring posteriorly.

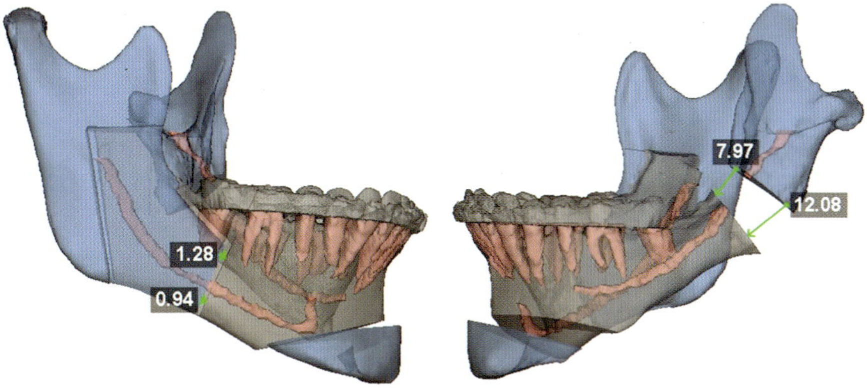


**Fig. 15.6** These images demonstrate the precise movements of the mandible as seen on a virtual model. The left side is being advanced to a significantly greater degree than the right side. Due to the high position of the mandibular foramen on the left, the osteotomy came across the mandibular canal.

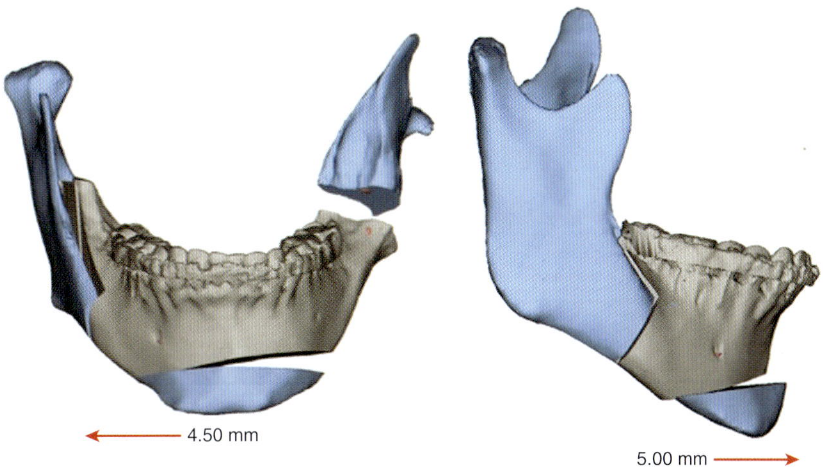


**Fig. 15.7** The genioplasty was designed to advance the chin, rotate toward the right, and translate toward the right.

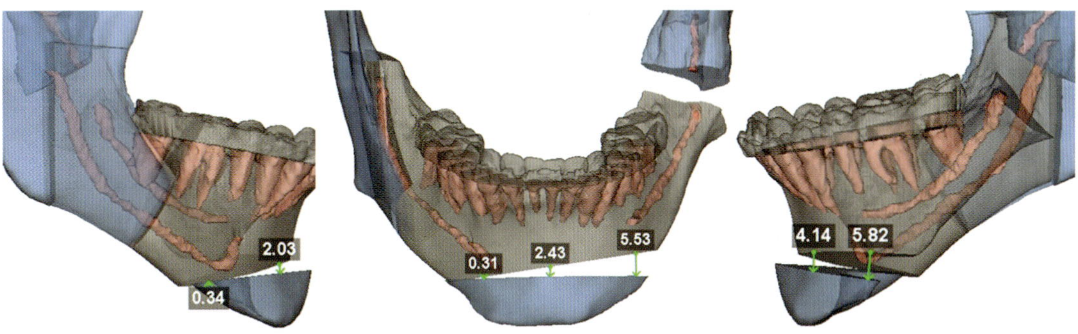


**Fig. 15.8** The genioplasty was tilted forward while being advanced and brought down asymmetrically to correct the patient's chin asymmetry.

**Table 15.1 Summary of movements**

The precise movements used during this case are included for review. The degree of the asymmetry in the movements can be seen in the measurements.

| Point | Name | Anterior/Posterior | Left/Right | Up/Down |
|---|---|---|---|---|
| ANS | Anterior nasal spine | 0.05 mm posterior | 4.21 mm left | 3.61 mm up |
| A | A point | 0.70 mm anterior | 3.07 mm left | 2.95 mm up |
| ISU1 | Midline of upper incisor | 3.50 mm anterior | 1.00 mm right | 4.00 mm up |
| U3L | Upper left canine | 2.93 mm anterior | 0.38 mm right | 0.45 mm down |
| U6L | Upper left anterior molar (mesiobuccal cusp) | 2.04 mm anterior | 0.73 mm left | 4.44 mm down |
| U3R | Upper right canine | 3.48 mm anterior | 0.86 mm right | 6.13 mm up |
| U6R | Upper right anterior molar (mesiobuccal cusp) | 2.92 mm anterior | 0.10mm right | 4.97 mm up |
| ISL1 | Midline of lower incisor | 5.47 mm anterior | 0.97 mm left | 3.47 mm up |
| L6L | Lower left anterior molar (mesiobuccal cusp) | 3.37 mm anterior | 1.00 mm left | 3.36 mm down |
| L6R | Lower right anterior molar (mesiobuccal cusp) | 6.18 mm anterior | 0.25 mm left | 3.97 mm up |
| B | B point | 7.48 mm anterior | 2.29 mm right | 1.74 mm up |
| Pog. | Pogonion | 14.10 mm anterior | 9.11 mm right | 1.07 mm down |

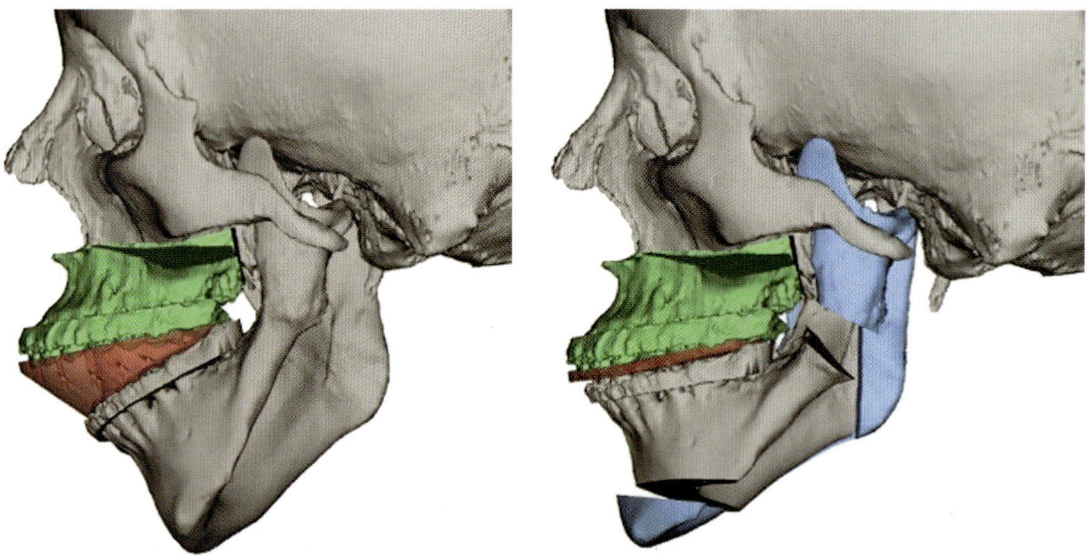


**Fig. 15.9** Custom splints were printed to allow for appropriate positioning of the Le Fort I and mandibular segments.

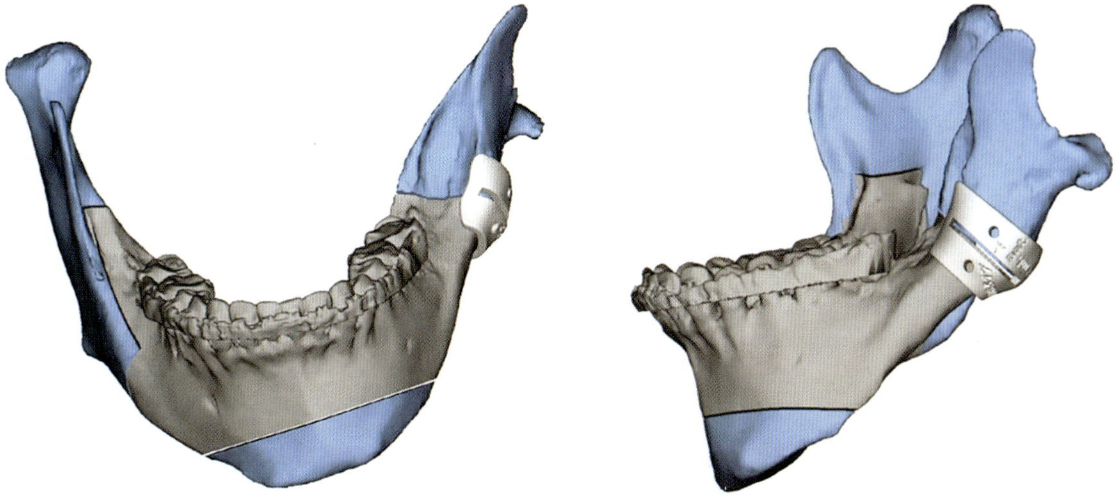

**Custom cutting guide to confirm osteotomy location**

**Fig. 15.10** A custom cutting guide was manufactured to accurately perform the mandibular osteotomy on the left side.

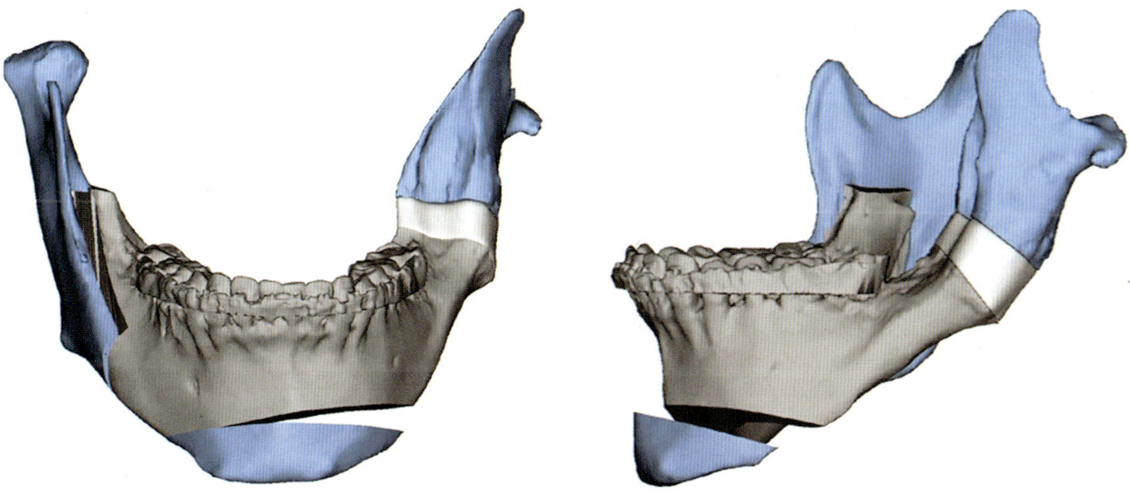

**Bone graft template**

**Fig. 15.11** A template was printed to mimic the bone graft that would be placed within the gap of the left mandible at the site of the osteotomy. This allowed for ex-vivo cutting of the bone graft to the planned dimensions.

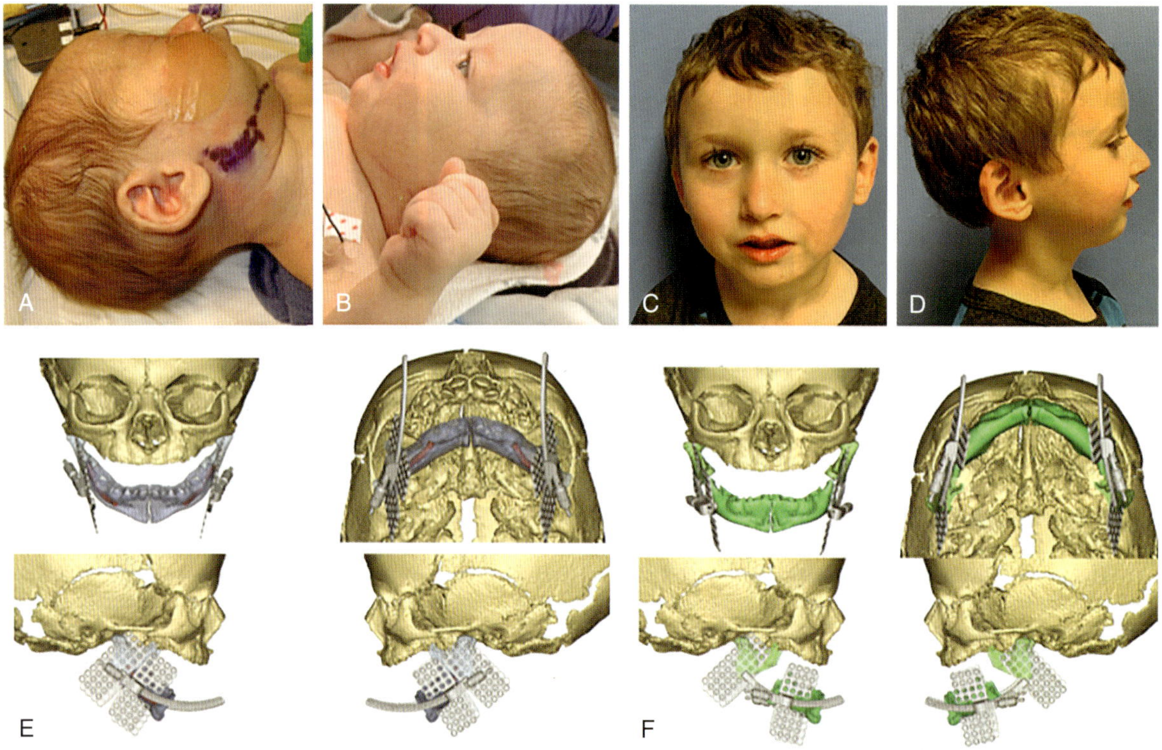


Fig. 16.3 Clinical example of a child with Pierre Robin sequence undergoing mandibular distraction osteogenesis. (A) Patient with preoperative image with operative markings. (B) Patient after completing consolidation phase at time of distractor removal. (C, D) Four years postoperative anteroposterior and lateral views. (E) Preoperative virtual surgical planning for mandibular osteotomies and distractor placement. (F) Anticipated computer-assisted surgical planning predicted advancement of the mandible to achieve occlusion.

scan if the surgeon so chooses. In a 2018 study by Li et al., the fidelity of the CAM/CAM surgical template for mandibular distraction in children treated for hemifacial microsomia was assessed by comparing the virtually planned and postoperative linear and angular differences for the distractor.[18] The largest linear deviation between the planned and the postoperative distractors was only 0.93 mm in the anteroposterior direction, and the largest in the horizontal plane was 4.64 degrees, even with the more restricted exposure of an intraoral incision. These differences were theorized to be because of the instability of the proximal ramus segment when the footplates of the distractor were being applied. Notably, of the 16 patients included in the study, there were no signs of permanent injury to the inferior alveolar nerve, dental roots, or tooth buds. In a study of six patients with hemifacial microsomia undergoing MDO, Sun et al. describe similar results with an overall difference in planned and actual ramus height of just 0.6 mm.[19]

Of course, one challenge of computer-assisted planning remains the inability to accurately simulate the effects of the overlying soft tissue or airway soft-tissue morphology. That said, conventional planning also has a similar disadvantage, although advances in 3D stereophotogrammetry and postoperative CT data may soon address this issue.[20] More critical than simulated airway morphology, however, is the challenge of predicting postoperative airway mechanics even with an expanded retroglossal space, which is influenced by a variety of factors, including airway tonicity, coordination, fluid dynamics and nonlaminar airflow, as well as anatomy.[21]

## Pearls/pitfalls

- CaSP allows the surgeon to determine optimal vector of distraction. Based on the patient's anatomical constraints, external or internal linear, multivector, or curvilinear devices may be selected for the patient's unique goals.

- Prior to proceeding with osteotomies, the bilateral subperiosteal dissection, cutting guide application, osteotomy marking, and predrilling of holes for the distractor footplates should be completed. Device implantation and fixation should always precede complete osteotomy. This ensures a more stable arch on which to secure the device footplates and safeguards an accurate vector of distraction.
- Our clinical practice favors the use of a piezoelectric saw for osteotomies in order to minimize trauma to nearby critical structures.

Although mortality from mandibular distraction is very low, early complications from MDO in the infant population range from infection and scarring,[22] to permanent dental injury, alveolar and marginal mandibular nerve damage,[23] device malposition, and bony nonunion and malunion.[24] Long-term complications include malocclusion and temporomandibular joint dysfunction.[25,26] For infants with Pierre Robin sequence who may be born premature, underweight, or more medically complex, surgical efficiency and decreased operative times are key to both surgical and medical success.[27] Furthermore, the diminutive size of the infant mandible necessitates precise osteotomies and hardware placement, as the margin for error is much narrower.[28] While CAD/CAM technology has its own disadvantages such as increased cost and time allotted for preoperative planning and custom device fabrication,[29] the efficiency and flexibility afforded by computer-assisted planning facilitates safer operations, shorter general anesthesia time, decreased blood loss, and more effective placement of hardware to avoid critical structures such as nascent tooth buds or nerves.[30]

## Conclusion

CAD/CAM technology allows the surgeon to use a single platform not just for device or cutting guide fabrication, but also for assessment of dysmorphology, quantitative and diagnostic confirmation, vector selection, and treatment planning.[31] Within the scope of neonatal and pediatric mandibular distraction osteogenesis, CaSP and the use of custom 3D templates allows for efficient, safe, and effective surgery while minimizing complications. Future directions for CAD/CAM technology and computer-assisted planning are to improve simulation of soft tissue expansion and airway morphometrics.

## Take-home points

- CaSP in TBAO or PRS patients aids in the precision and efficiency of the mandibular distraction process through target endpoint establishment, device and vector selection and the creation of key 3D printed deliverables (e.g., cutting and position guides) used in MDO surgery.
- CaSP can be integrated in multidisciplinary protocol design, informing the timing of real-time assessment tools (e.g., bedside PSG) that accurately evaluate clinical success of OSA resolution.
- Undersold features of CaSP (e.g., airway simulation) can be leveraged to optimize quality control via comparison of simulated and postoperative states.

## References


1. Paes EC, Mink van der Molen AB, Muradin MS, et al. A systematic review on the outcome of mandibular distraction osteogenesis in infants suffering robin sequence. *Clin Oral Investig*. 2013;17(8):1807-1820.
2. Mackay DR. Controversies in the diagnosis and management of the Robin sequence. *J Craniofac Surg*. 2011;22(2): 415-420.
3. Zhang RS, Hoppe IC, Taylor JA, Bartlett SP. Surgical management and outcomes of Pierre Robin sequence: a comparison of mandibular distraction osteogenesis and tongue-lip adhesion. *Plast Reconstr Surg*. 2018;142(2):480-509.
4. Van den Elzen AP, Semmekrot BA, Bongers EM, et al. Diagnosis and treatment of the Pierre Robin sequence: results of a retrospective clinical study and review of the literature. *Eur J Pediatr*. 2001;160(1):47-53.
5. Cacher M, Sautermeister J, Urschitz MS, Buchenau W, Arand J, Poets CF. An oral appliance with velar extension for treatment of obstructive sleep apnea in infants with Pierre Robin sequence. *Cleft Palate Craniofac J*. 2011;48(3):331-336.
6. Suri S, Ross RB, Tompson BD. Mandibular morphology and growth with and without hypodontia in subjects with Pierre Robin sequence. *Am J Orthod Dentofacial Orthop*. 2006;130(1):37-46.
7. Suri S, Ross RB, Tompson BD. Craniofacial morphology and adolescent facial growth in Pierre Robin sequence. *Am J Orthod Dentofacial Orthop*. 2010;137(6):763-774.
8. Figueroa AA, Glupker TJ, Fitz MG, BeGole EA. Mandible, tongue, and airway in Pierre Robin sequence: a longitudinal cephalometric study. *Cleft Palate Craniofac J*. 1991;28(4): 425-434.

9. Humphries LS, Reid RR, Ross CF, et al. Biomechanical and morphological analysis of Pierre Robin sequence mandible: finite element and morphometric study. *Anat Rec (Hoboken)*. 2021; 304(7):1375-1388.
10. Zellner, EG, Reid RR, Steinbacher DM. The Pierre Robin mandible is hypoplastic and morphologically abnormal. *J Craniofac Surg*. 2017; 28(8):1946-1949.
11. Lee JC, Bradley JP. Surgical considerations in Pierre Robin sequence. *Clin Plast Surg*. 2014; 41(2):211-217.
12. Oktay H, Baydaş B, Ersöz M. Using a modified nutrition plate for early intervention in a newborn infant with Pierre Robin sequence: a case report. *Cleft Palate Craniofac J*. 2006;43(3): 370-373.
13. Scott AR, Tibesar RJ, Sidman JD. Pierre Robin sequence: evaluation, management, indications for surgery, and pitfalls. *Otolaryngol Clin North Am*. 2012;45(3): 695-710.
14. Pfaff MJ, Steinbacher DM. Plastic Surgery applications using three-dimensional planning and computer-assisted design and manufacturing. *Plast Reconstr Surg*. 2016;137(3):603e-616e.
15. Resnick CM. Precise osteotomies for mandibular distraction in infants with Robin sequence using virtual surgical planning. *Int J Oral Maxillofac Surg*. 2018;47(1): 35-43.
16. Prescher H, Mokhlesi B, Mhlaba JM, et al. Polysomnography in the early consolidation phase of mandibular distraction as a tool to identify residual tongue-based airway obstruction and need for further distraction: a follow up study. *FACE*. 2021;2(1):71-77. doi:https://doi.org/10.1177/2732501621992463.
17. Humphries LS, Yates EK, Mhlaba JM, Collins JM, Baroody FM, Reid RR. Airway volume simulation in virtual mandibular distraction: a cohort study. *Plast Reconstr Surg*. 2018;141(4):1003-1009.
18. Li B, Sun H, Zeng F, Zhang T, Wang X. Accuracy of a CAD/CAM surgical template for mandibular distraction: a preliminary study. *Br J Oral Maxillofac Surg*. 2018;56(9):814-819.
19. Sun H, Li B, Zhao Z, Zhang L, Shen SG, Wang X. Error analysis of a CAD/CAM method for unidirectional mandibular distraction osteogenesis in the treatment of hemifacial microsomia. *Br J Oral Maxillofac Surg*. 2013;51(8):892-897.
20. Doscher ME, Garfein ES, Bent J, Tepper OM. Neonatal mandibular distraction osteogenesis: converting virtual surgical planning into an operative reality. *Int J Pediatr Otorhinolaryngol*. 2014;78(2):381-384.
21. Humphries LS, Roy T, Huang A, Collins J, Baroody FM, Reid RR. Airway morphological changes in Pierre Robin sequence: a retrospective study. *Cleft Palate Craniofac J*. 2020;57(7):828-839.
22. Scott AR, Tibesar RJ, Sidman JD. Pierre Robin sequence: evaluation, management, indications for surgery, and pitfalls. *Otolaryngol Clin North Am*. 2012;45(3): 695-710.
23. Mofid MM, Manson PN, Robertson BC, Tufaro AP, Elias JJ, Vander Kolk CA. Craniofacial distraction osteogenesis: a review of 3278 cases. *Plast Reconstr Surg*. 2001;108(5):1103-1107.
24. Master DL, Hanson PR, Gosain AK. Complications of mandibular distraction osteogenesis. *J Craniofac Surg*. 2010;21(5):1565-1570.
25. Reina-Romo E, Gómez-Benito MJ, Sampietro-Fuentes A, Domínguez J, García-Aznar JM. Three-dimensional simulation of mandibular distraction osteogenesis: mechanobiological analysis. *Ann Biomed Eng*. 2010; 39(1):35-43.
26. Zimmerman CE, Humphries LS, Roy T, Reid RR. Mandibular distraction for micrognathia in neonates. *NeoReviews*. 2018;19: 1-16.
27. Flores RL, Greathouse ST, Costa M, Tahiri Y, Soleimani T, Tholpady SS. Defining failure and its predictors in mandibular distraction for Robin sequence. *J Craniomaxillofac Surg*. 2015;43(8):1614-1619.
28. Mao Z, Zhang N, Cui Y. Three-dimensional printing of surgical guides for mandibular distraction osteogenesis in infancy. *Medicine (Baltimore)*. 2019;98(10):e14754.
29. Hanasono MM, Skoracki RJ. Computer-assisted design and rapid prototype modeling in microvascular mandible reconstruction. *Laryngoscope*. 2013;123(3):597-604.
30. Pfaff MJ, Steinbacher DM. Plastic surgery applications using three-dimensional planning and computer-assisted design and manufacturing. *Plast Reconstr Surg*. 2017;137(3):603e-616e.
31. Steinbacher DM. *Chapter 4: 3D Analysis, Planning and Model Surgery in Aesthetic Orthognathic Surgery and Rhinoplasty*. Hoboken, NJ: Wiley Blackwell; 2019:53-75.

Chapter 17

# Computer-assisted planning congenital differences and anomalies: craniopagus twin separation

*Andrew Timberlake, Andre Alcon, Mickey Gideon, Eldad Silbertstein, Noor ul Owase Jeelani, David A. Staffenberg*

CHAPTER OUTLINE



## Introduction

Craniofacial surgery commonly involves carefully orchestrated surgery between plastic surgeons, neurosurgeons and other specialists. In some cases, the neurosurgeons provide a craniotomy for access to the midface. For example, correction of orbital hypertelorism or monobloc frontofacial advancement. In other cases, neurosurgeons are performing craniectomies that the plastic surgeons will remodel and reassemble. Commonly, plastic surgeons and neurosurgeons will work side by side to repair fractures involving the skull base, frontal sinus, and the orbital roof. A common theme is that one team leads and the other follows. It is always important for each discipline to keep in mind that the way that they proceed will have an impact on the other discipline. This requires advanced experience and exemplifies what we call interdisciplinary care as opposed the multidisciplinary care, or simply working together. This is particularly important when we discuss the care of craniopagus twins.

Amongst the congenital craniofacial disorders that are faced by such a team, craniopagus twins are remarkably rare. The risks are doubled because two children are being operated on at once and interventions on one are likely to impact the other until they are effectively separated. It is crucial to recognize that in such conjoined twinning the anatomy is quite variable, beyond the anomalies of other more common craniofacial disorders.

Textbooks, surgical atlases, and anatomical dissection, whether on cadavers or done virtually, are necessary to teach surgeons at every stage of their training and career. Imaging the craniofacial skeleton has allowed planning since radiographs were first available. Advances in imaging have allowed surgeons to understand the pertinent anatomy of their specific patients in greater detail over the years. In the early days two-dimensional (2D) radiographs allowed diagnosis and surgical planning that enabled our mentors and those before to achieve remarkable success, although this seems rather primitive today. Imaging technology was translated to the operating room indirectly. In other words, the images were transferred to the patient through the additional knowledge, experience, and imagination of the surgeon. This continued to be the case with the age of computer tomography. With the further development of software that was able to reconstruct a three-dimensional (3D) image from the computed tomography (CT) scan, teaching, diagnosis, and treatment were elevated to a new level. Although the quality of imaging was clear enough for a layperson to appreciate, the transfer of this information was still a leap to the surgical field.

Historically, the information provided in radiographic imaging provide the surgical team information about the normal and abnormal anatomy of the craniopagus. This allowed the team to assess the feasibility of separation. The individual steps required to actually separate them remained in the surgeon's imagination. The advent of virtual planning revolutionized the way in which the anatomy could be visualized, manipulated and communicated. This can be seen in many ways throughout the chapters of this textbook. This allows the key decisions to be made before going to the operating room. This provides the team the luxury of time to assess options without wasting time under anesthesia. Additionally, the virtual planning provides the family images that can be reviewed with the surgical team prior to surgery. This valuable addition to informed consent is readily apparent. After being purely visual, imaging became tangible when it was possible to manufacture stereolithographic models through 3D printing. This allowed surgeons and their students to perform osteotomies on the stereolithographic models, a step up from practicing these procedures on models of a normal craniofacial skeleton. The capability for a surgeon to hold the anomalous anatomy in their hands is very powerful indeed. A 3D model is indispensable when demonstrating complex surgery to patients and other surgical team members. These stereolithographic models can be "printed" from different materials, including those that can be drawn on with pencils. This allows skin flaps and osteotomies to be planned while sitting at a desk, at any time, while options are considered, demonstrated, and discussed with other team members. Planning for complex cases, such as craniopagus separation surgery, may take several weeks or months.

As well as being used to create stereolithographic models, 3D information can also be transferred to a workstation in the operating room. Sterilized wands can be used in the operative field showing the surgeon immediately where the tip of the wand is in the CT and/or magnetic resonance imaging (MRI), and most powerfully, what adjacent structures lie close in the patient's anatomy but are not yet visible to the naked, even magnified eye.

Additional benefits include hardware, such as plates and mesh, that can be contoured directly on the model and then sterilized for surgery. This saves time during surgery and may also confirm correct placement according to the fit of the contoured hardware. Ultimately this technology allows custom implants and hardware to be produced with precision, also saving time in surgery. Note that despite this, training, skill, and judgment are still required for the safe planning and conduct of these operations. Implant materials continue to be developed and refined, and their compatibility and durability must be taken into account. Experience, training, and skill remain quintessentially important.

## Classification System

Craniopagus twinning presents a unique challenge because complex anatomy required for survival and quality of life is shared between the twins, and successful separation depends on correctly partitioning these structures, making surgical planning critical in such cases. Craniopagus twins are classified into a four-category system that assesses the twins for a vertical or angular configuration, and the presence or absence of significantly shared dural venous sinuses.[1] In the angular subtype, the cerebral hemispheres are arranged horizontally within a shared cranium, whereas in the vertical subtype, a longitudinal arrangement with one continuous cranium housing the cerebral hemispheres is present. The surgical approach to separation of each type will be slightly different; however, this framework allows for prioritization and planning of early surgical procedures that will occur prior to final separation (see Figs. 17.1 and 17.2).

## Craniofacial Surgery

Detailed planning is exceptionally important in such cases because: (1) Rarity of the deformity inevitably reduces teams' personal experience with treatment; (2) There is variability in anatomy; (3) The large number of team members involved in surgery requires complicated coordination; and (4) The surgical procedure itself is multistaged. Thus computer-assisted simulation may have a significant impact on coordinating such a complex task with many participants.

## Background

As with many rare challenges, the separation of craniopagus twins may be seen as either too complex to achieve. Surprisingly, on the other hand, such a separation may be interpreted as a straightforward matter of dividing the shared tissue along the conjoined plane, taking whatever amount of time is needed. Of course, separation is never simple when the craniopagus twins share any or all of the following: Dural sinus, cerebral vasculature, brain, and of course bone and scalp. Surprisingly, one does not need to go back too far into surgical history to see examples of this overly simple interpretation of the clinical problem. The complexity is readily apparent when we see that the approach of the neurosurgeons will impact the success or failure of the plastic surgeons and vice versa. Like the conjoined twins, the success of the two surgical teams is inextricably linked. The plastic surgical team must plan for the appropriate amount of scalp to reconstruct the separated heads while providing adequate exposure for the neurosurgeons. The incisions must be designed in order to minimize the risk of brain exposure, or exposure of dura grafts

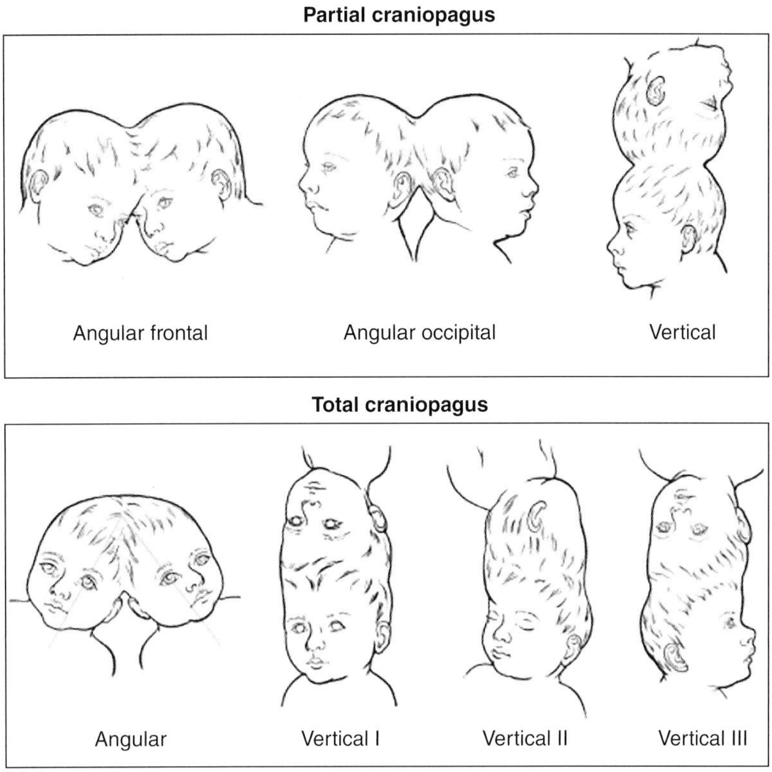


**Fig. 17.1** Classification of craniopagus. "Partial" and "Total" forms of the craniopagus malformation. (From Stone JL, Goodrich JT. The craniopagus malformation: classification and implications for surgical separation. *Brain*. 2006;129(5):1084–95.)

if dehiscence occurs. On the other hand, if the neurosurgeons interrupt too much shared veins between the twins brains, venous engorgement, and potentially venous stasis will result. This may impact the outcome due to increased bleeding and venous infarcts, but will also result in increased brain swelling that cannot be covered with the expanded scalp. Preparation and planning is key. Planning virtually allows easier collaboration between the teams and allows the surgeons to arrive in the operating room with the advantage of preparation. Similar to many reconstructive problems this paradigm mandates that the neurosurgical team performs the separation with the plastic surgeons providing closure at the end of the separation. As with the separation of many other types of conjoined twins, these approaches have historically included the use of tissue expansion prior to separation followed by separation surgery.[2-5] In the most capable hands, at the best medical centers, the mortality reported in the literature over the past 50 years is greater than 50%. Craniofacial surgery frequently demands a coordinated effort between plastic surgery and neurosurgery and many other specialties, and separating craniopagus twins takes this coordination to a stratospheric level. It is, however, this coordination that is of paramount importance. Success clearly requires an understanding of the complex interrelationship between the "separation" and the "reconstruction", and that decisions made for one aspect of the surgery will have a profound impact on another aspect of the surgery. The impact can be disastrous, or if planned well, can be advantageous.

The separation of craniopagus conjoined twins is a very rare and complex challenge requiring exquisite coordination between the neurosurgeon and plastic surgeon. Success lies, in part, in the recognition that a successful outcome demands that each recognizes that their component parts of the surgery have an impact on the other's parts. In other words, a superb result by one may be marred by poor planning by the other. It should be clear, for instance, that poorly planned or executed flaps will likely lead to cerebrospinal (CSF) fluid leak, meningitis, and possibly brain exposure and death. For the plastic surgeon, it soon becomes clear that unexpected cerebral edema will undo the best planned flaps. Herein lies the strength of the staged technique, as well as the importance in recognizing the nuances of planning.

As already stated, when too many bridging veins from the sagittal sinus are interrupted acutely, the alternate

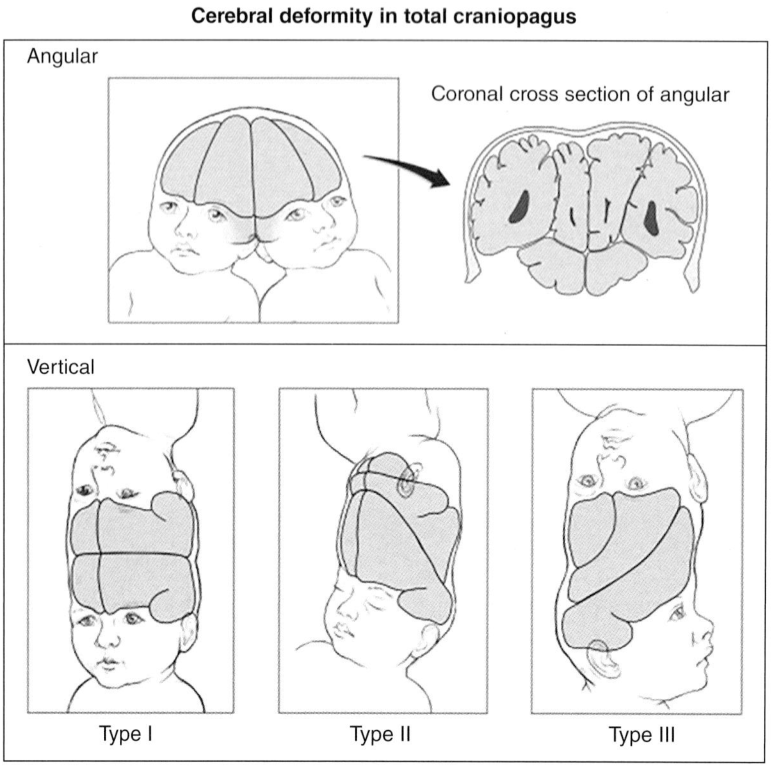


Fig. 17.2 Cerebral deformity in total craniopagus. (From Stone JL, Goodrich JT. The craniopagus malformation: classification and implications for surgical separation. *Brain*. 2006;129(5):1084–95.)

venous pathways (venous collaterals) are overwhelmed and cerebral edema occurs, possibly even leading to venous infarcts. Once cerebral edema ensues, successful scalp coverage becomes much more challenging. Using a staged approach, the bridging veins are able to gradually dilate and carry the increased demands. Our experience is that at the time of final separation, there is very little cerebral edema. This increases the success rate of closure, allowing the vascularized flaps to heal without CSF leak or other consequent problems.

Given that the first incision of the first stage will be a part of the final flap design, planning is crucial. A variety of flap designs may be considered. It must be remembered that vascularized free tissue transfer in an infant is far less useful than in an adult because the relative surface area of an infant's scalp is twice that of an adult, and vascularized free flaps (e.g., the latissimus dorsi and rectus abdominis muscles) are comparatively smaller than in adults. Tissue expansion should be used as well to maximize the amount of available vascularized tissue.

There are many options for dura replacement. We have considered expanded tensor fascia lata from the twins' thighs, but the fascia lata has a grain and will frequently leak. Despite our usual commitment to autologous tissues, we have chosen Durasys (Cook, USA) because of its watertight properties. Another option is to use the pericranium for dura replacement as a graft or as a pedicled flap. This flap can then receive bone or skin grafts.

The planning of the scalp flaps may be counterintuitive. The senior author (DAS) recommends a 3D model, such as a RapidView Model (Medical Modeling, LLC, Golden, CO, USA) of the skin surface from neck to neck and including the ears, be produced which the plastic surgeon can use to design and modify the plans well ahead of the first stage of surgery. A #2 pencil can be used on this surface like 3D paper, measured, erased and modified. These designs must be reviewed with other team members, so all understand the implications of the design, coverage and protection. Proper flap design will avoid suture lines at the vertex since this is, by definition, the most distal part of the flap and therefore the part of the flap most likely to suffer necrosis and the part most difficult to replace. Furthermore, the vertex is likely to have a dura graft, which will require time to develop its own vascular supply. If the dura graft (autologous, heterotopic, or alloplastic) is not yet well-healed, it will not support an overlying skin graft. Corners and angles should be avoided to keep the best blood supply and avoid the need for trimming. The flaps should include reliable blood supply. The most suitable design is a sinusoidal pattern, which allows one flap to turn over across the vertex of one twin, while the other does the same to cover the other twin. This approach was designed for the separation of vertical type I craniopagus from the Philippines in 2004.[3,6]

## Steps in Design

1. Consider first the region and area of congruence and extrapolate for head convexity in order to estimate the two expected defects.
2. Consider the interaxial angulation of the twins: As the angle decreases from 180 degrees, flaps of varying lengths may be designed. The next step will determine where the long flap should be designed. The flaps are planned and marked carefully on the twins in the first stage and opened as needed. Previously healed parts of the incision will need to be reopened at the final stage (Figs. 17.3 and 17.4).

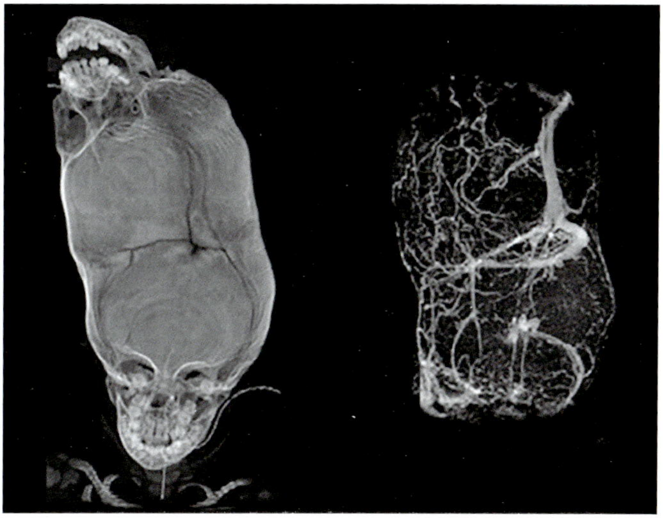

**Fig. 17.3** A sinusoidal pattern.

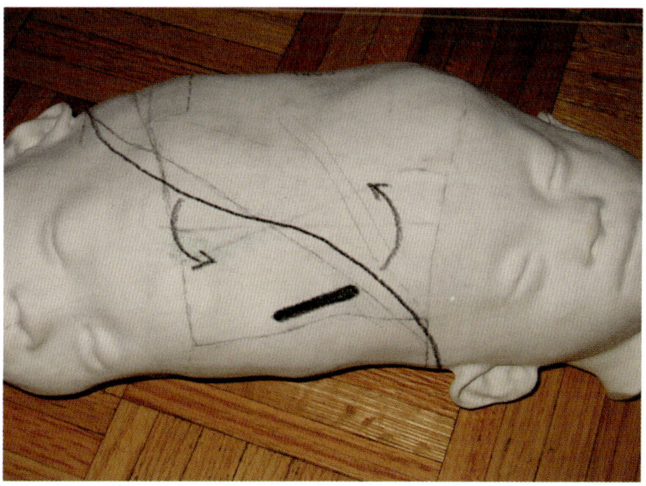

**Fig. 17.4** The flaps are planned and marked carefully on the twins in the first stage and opened as needed.

3. Consider the final recipient of the sinus lake: How the shared sinus is divided or distributed dictates how much of the shared dura each twin gets. This is crucial, and the twin that gets less native dura should be provided with the larger scalp flap. This larger vascularized scalp flap will be necessary to cover the dura graft or substitute used to close the defect of the dura. A skin graft, if needed, will only heal on native vascularized dura. Having emphasized this, the twin who will receive the sinus lake will ultimately need more volume. This may lead the shortsighted surgeon to design the longer flap for this twin. The twin receiving the lake will require a smaller dura graft, and therefore the flap must cover that small graft, but any shortfall can be closed with a skin graft or acellular dermal graft (e.g., AlloDerm, LifeCell, NJ, USA). The twin who does not receive the lake will have a smaller volume or surface area to cover, but will need a larger dura graft. This larger dura graft must be covered successfully with a healthy vascularized scalp flap at the time of separation. It is this twin, therefore, who should receive the larger (or longer) flap. If an acellular dermis graft is used on the native dura initially, it can be grafted later with a thin split thickness skin graft once healthy granulation tissue is noted. It is important to recognize that there is often dura intervening between the two brains with a variable size defect within it.
4. Consider hairline and pattern of hair growth: When examining the flaps, the direction of hair growth is an important detail in design and execution. The sinusoidal flaps allow transfer of hair from one twin to the other (like a "Yin Yang") so a cowlick, or hair growing against the grain, is avoided.
5. Consider tissue expansion: Tissue expansion allows the team to increase the amount of available vascularized scalp. It is more challenging than usual in a staged procedure because of the existing scars, which increases the risk of exposure and infection. It is important to note that the expansion must be available at the time of final separation, so we recommend placing them in a separate procedure 7 weeks before separation. The expanders are allowed to heal for 3 weeks after which 10% of their final volume is instilled sterilely every 3 days. If the expanders are removed at the beginning of the separation surgery, the expanded scalp may shrink, and the advantage is lost. Therefore, we recommend placing the expanders through small incisions away from the base of the flaps. By placing the expanders away from the plane of conjoining, the expanders can be left in place during the final neurosurgical separation. They are only removed at the time of final closure.
6. Resect enough native skull to avoid impinging on the blood supply of the flaps from below.
7. Consider bony fixation: Resorbable fixation is unnecessary. Use suture or titanium hardware to secure each craniotomy so that they can be easily opened at the time of separation.
8. Consider autologous bone grafting at the time of separation. Remember that the addition of non-vascularized bone, on top of non-vascularized dura may increase the risk of infection. Bone grafting will not be possible in areas where the scalp flap does not fully cover. When in doubt, do not bone graft primarily, although grafting at a later stage may be an additional challenge.

Computer-assisted 3D-models after every stage significantly assists planning of the next stage modifying previous plan if needed and facilitate communication between team members.

## References


1. Stone JL, Goodrich JT. The craniopagus malformation: classification and implications for surgical separation. *Brain*. 2006;129:1084-1095.
2. Heuer GG, Madsen PJ, Flanders TM, et al. Separation of craniopagus twins by a multidisciplinary team. *N Engl J Med*. 2019;380:358-364.
3. Staffenberg DA, Goodrich JT. Separation of craniopagus conjoined twins with a staged approach. *J Craniofac Surg*. 2012;23:2004-2010.
4. Wood BC, Sher SR, Mitchell BJ, et al. Conjoined twin separation: integration of three-dimensional modeling for optimization of surgical planning. *J Craniofac Surg*. 2017;28:4-10.
5. Eley KA, Rossi-Espagnet MC, Schievano S, et al. Multiparametric imaging for presurgical planning of craniopagus twins: The experience of two tertiary pediatric hospitals with six sets of twins. *Radiology*. 2021;298:18-27.
6. Goodrich JT, Staffenberg DA. Craniopagus twins: clinical and surgical management. *Childs Nerv Syst*. 2004;20:618-624.

## Suggested Reading


Bassi M, Antonelli V, Tomassini A, et al. Synchronized "one-step" resection and cranio-orbital reconstruction for spheno-orbital lesions with custom made implant. *J Craniofac Surg*. 2021;32: 1870-1873.

Bucholz RD, Yoon KW, Shively RE. Temporoparietal craniopagus. Case report and review of the literature. *J Neurosurg*. 1987;66:72-79.

Chang EI, Jenkins MP, Patel SA, Topham NS. Long-term operative outcomes of preoperative computed tomography-guided virtual surgical planning for osteocutaneous free flap mandible reconstruction. *Plast Reconstr Surg*. 2016;137:619-623.

Chen Z, Mo S, Fan X, You Y, Ye G, Zhou N. A Meta-analysis and systematic review comparing the effectiveness of traditional and virtual surgical planning for orthognathic surgery: based on randomized clinical trials. *J Oral Maxillofac Surg*. 2021;79:471. e1-471.e19.

Gaist G, Piazza G, Galassi E, Cavina C, Salvioli GP. Craniopagus twins. An unsuccessful separation and a clinical review of the entity. *Childs Nerv Syst*. 1987;3:327-333.

Goh KY. Separation surgery for total vertical craniopagus twins. *Childs Nerv Syst*. 2004;20:567-575.

Grossman HJ, Sugar O, Greeley PW, Sadove MS. Surgical separation in craniopagus. *J Am Med Assoc*. 1953;153:201-207.

Gupta D, Kedia S, Rath GP, et al. A century with craniopagus twin separation surgeries: nihilism to optimism. *Neurosurgery*. 2022;91:27-42.

Hammoudeh JA, Howell LK, Boutros S, Scott MA, Urata MM. Current status of surgical planning for orthognathic surgery: traditional methods versus 3D surgical planning. *Plast Reconstr Surg Glob Open*. 2015;3:e307.

Hsu SS, Geteno J, Bryan Bell R, et al. Accuracy of a computer-aided surgical simulation protocol for orthognathic surgery: a prospective multicenter study. *J Oral Maxillofac Surg*. 2013;71:128-142.

Jansen O, Mehrabi VA, Sartor K. Neuroradiological findings in adult cranially conjoined twins. Case report. *J Neurosurg*. 1998;89:635-639.

Marras CE, Caria A, Benedictis ADE, et al. Successful staged separation of total angular craniopagus. *J Neurosurg Sci*. 2022. [Epub ahead of print]

O'Connell JE. Craniopagus twins: surgical anatomy and embryology and their implications. *J Neurol Neurosurg Psychiatry*. 1976;39:1-22.

Roser SM, Ramachandra S, Blair H, et al. The accuracy of virtual surgical planning in free fibula mandibular reconstruction: comparison of planned and final results. *J Oral Maxillofac Surg*. 2010;68: 2824-2832.

Todorov AB, Cohen KL, Spilotro V, Landau E. Craniopagus twins. *J Neurol Neurosurg Psychiatry*. 1974;37:1291-1298.

van Ouwerkerk WJ, van den Berg R, Allison CE, et al. Craniopagus: the Suriname-Amsterdam conjunction. *Childs Nerv Syst*. 2004;20:625-634.

Walker M, Browd SR. Craniopagus twins: embryology, classification, surgical anatomy, and separation. *Childs Nerv Syst*. 2004;20:554-566.

Winston KR, Rockoff MA, Mulliken JB, Strand RD, Murray JE. Surgical division of craniopagi. *Neurosurgery*. 1987;21:782-791.

Winston KR. Craniopagi: anatomical characteristics and classification. *Neurosurgery*. 1987;21:769-781.

Zhang N, Liu S, Hu Z, et al. Accuracy of virtual surgical planning in two-jaw orthognathic surgery: comparison of planned and actual results. *Oral Surg Oral Med Oral Pathol Oral Radiol*. 2016;122: 143-151.

Zinser MJ, Sailer HF, Ritter L, et al. A paradigm shift in orthognathic surgery? A comparison of navigation, computer-aided designed/computer-aided manufactured splints, and "classic" intermaxillary splints to surgical transfer of virtual orthognathic planning. *J Oral Maxillofac Surg*. 2013;71:2151.e1-2151.e21.

Chapter 18

# Computer-assisted planning in craniomaxillofacial trauma: orbital fractures

*Pasha Shakoori, Idean Roohani, Joseph Lopez*

CHAPTER OUTLINE



## Introduction

Several indications necessitate posttraumatic orbital reconstruction. For example, restrictive diplopia secondary to entrapment of extraocular muscles can lead to irreversible muscle ischemia and necrosis within hours, thus requiring emergent surgery. In particular, pediatric patients are especially susceptible to extraocular muscle entrapment due to the increased bone elasticity in their orbital floor—resulting in self-reduction as opposed to a fracture.[1] Enophthalmos secondary to orbital herniation or implant displacement can lead to globe malposition and increased orbital volume due to loss of structural support, ultimately necessitating surgery as well. Given the reconstructive complexity of orbital floor repair and the high risk of patient dissatisfaction, there is an essential need for improved accuracy and precision.

Over the past two decades, radiographic advances have allowed not only the introduction of computer-assisted surgical planning (CaSP) but have also created headway for the creation of custom patient-specific implants to cover the orbital defect. This revolutionary technology has improved the accuracy, efficiency, and safety in the surgical management of orbital fractures. Aside from enhanced operative efficacy, these innovations have significantly improved patient outcomes and satisfaction.[2]

Ocular injuries are frequently seen in orbital floor fractures. As such, prompt ophthalmologic consultation is imperative in all suspected cases of orbital fracture to evaluate for ocular trauma. However, when the consultor is initially evaluating the patient, they must be mindful of the relative contraindications that may delay orbital reconstruction, such as hyphema, retinal tear, or lens displacement. Inversely, there are no known absolute contraindications to CaSP.

In this chapter, the authors present their preferred computer-assisted design/computer-assisted manufacturing (CAD/CAM) workflow to perform posttraumatic orbital reconstruction. This methodology has been validated by the senior author (J.L) and thus the chapter will focus on the nuances of this approach and provide information to surgeons who hope to utilize CAD/CAM-based orbital reconstruction.

## Clinical considerations

The first step of assessment for a patient presenting with suspected orbital fracture secondary to trauma is to perform a thorough trauma survey, ensuring the patient's airway, breathing, and circulation is not compromised. Afterward, the clinical examination should begin with the inspection of the globe and orbit—pecifically examining the enophthalmos, dystopia, periorbital edema and ecchymosis, orbital rim step-off, and subconjunctival hemorrhage. Additionally, comprehensive neurologic and eye examinations are warranted in patients evaluated for post-traumatic orbital repair including assessment of extraocular movements and vision.

During the assessment of extraocular movements, the presence of strabismus can be further differentiated based on restrictive or neurogenic etiology. This is critical because orbital reconstruction is likely to improve restrictive strabismus but unlikely to improve paralytic strabismus. Thus, whenever evaluating an orbital injury a forced duction test must be conducted in order to determine if a patient's pathology is secondary to a restrictive etiology. Additionally, exophthalmometric measurement of the globe position relative to the lateral orbital rim should be performed to determine abnormally low orbital volume.

Beyond the physical exam, a thorough patient history should be taken. Determining the mechanism of injury, time of injury, ocular complaints, and prior facial trauma or procedures are vital pieces of information. Notably, facial implant utilization should be investigated for any patient with prior facial trauma. Patients who acutely present with an orbital fracture may report symptoms of diplopia, dystopia, periorbital pain, and paresthesia along the infraorbital dermatome. Therefore, understanding the events prior to the onset of these symptoms should be assessed to gain insight into the etiology, severity of damage, and to determine appropriate next steps.

Like most acute trauma evaluations, thin-cut (~1-mm) computed tomography (CT) scan is the first choice for diagnostic radiographic evaluation due to its thorough evaluation of the bony anatomy within the orbit. Magnetic resonance imaging (MRI) can be utilized if the patient has any contraindications to CT imaging. Not only is an up-to-date CT image essential for proper evaluation for orbital reconstruction, but it is also necessary for the manufacturing of patient-specific custom plates. Diagnostic imaging should focus on assessing the orbital volume of the affected eye compared to the uninjured side.

## Workflow for computer-aided design/computer-assisted manufacturing

The workflow for CAD/CAM-based orbital reconstruction is presented in ppt 18.1.

## Computer-assisted design

Using CAD has several benefits as it relates to orbital reconstruction. First, CAD offers the intersectionality of three data sources: clinical information, patient photos, and three-dimensional (3D) skeletal imaging. This provides a unique opportunity to see all three datasets work synchronously together and allows the radiographic imaging used in CAD to provide morphometric data, such as the anteroposterior (AP) orbital floor length (approximately 30 mm) and the orbital floor angle (~21 degrees).[3,4] Accordingly, it is essential to obtain adequate preoperative multiplanar-view CT images, consisting of axial, coronal, sagittal, and 3D reconstruction.

Secondly, CAD offers auto-segmentation of the unaffected orbit to visualize the preinjured globe. The contralateral segment is then mirrored and repositioned to ensure anatomically accurate repair of the defective side. In cases of bilateral orbital floor fractures, obtaining recent CT imaging would be the most ideal for patient-specific restoration. If unavailable, normative modeling utilizing pooled data as a reference model can generate a normative approximation. In all these cases, CAD ultimately facilitates the ability to customize patient-specific implants, facilitate 3D visualization intraoperatively, and provide real-time spatial measurements allowing the surgeon to understand their distance from critical anatomic landmarks—such as the posterior ledge of the orbit.

Postoperatively, CAD also has immense utility. It can quantify the magnitude of fracture reduction, plate position, and volume restoration. An overview of various CAD tools applicable to orbital floor reconstruction can be seen in ppt 18.2.

## Computer-assisted manufacturing

Computer-assisted surgical planning (CaSP), comprised of CAD and CAM, has been essential for accurate and sophisticated orbital reconstruction.[5] As previously mentioned, a recent preoperative orbital CT is needed to analyze the intricacy of orbital anatomy of the contralateral, uninjured side. From there, CAD can then be used to design and fabricate patient-specific implants. Not only are these implants tailored to the patient's unique anatomy, but these custom plates are also manufactured with drill guides and predrilled screw holes. These features of CAM-based implants have improved not only the accuracy of the procedure, but also significantly reduced the need for bony revision surgeries.[6] For these reasons and more, the

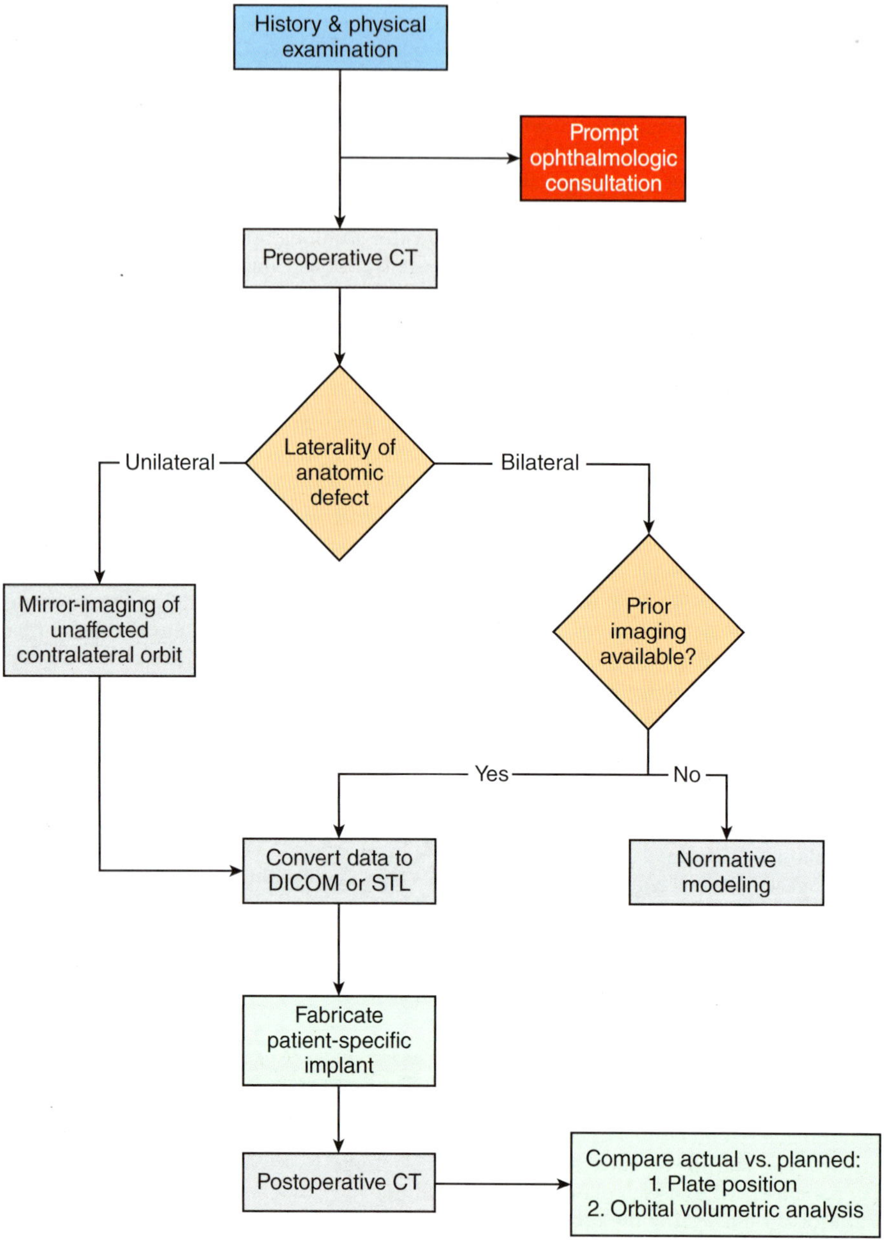


**ppt 18.1** Workflow for computer-assisted design/computer-assisted manufacturing-based orbital reconstruction.

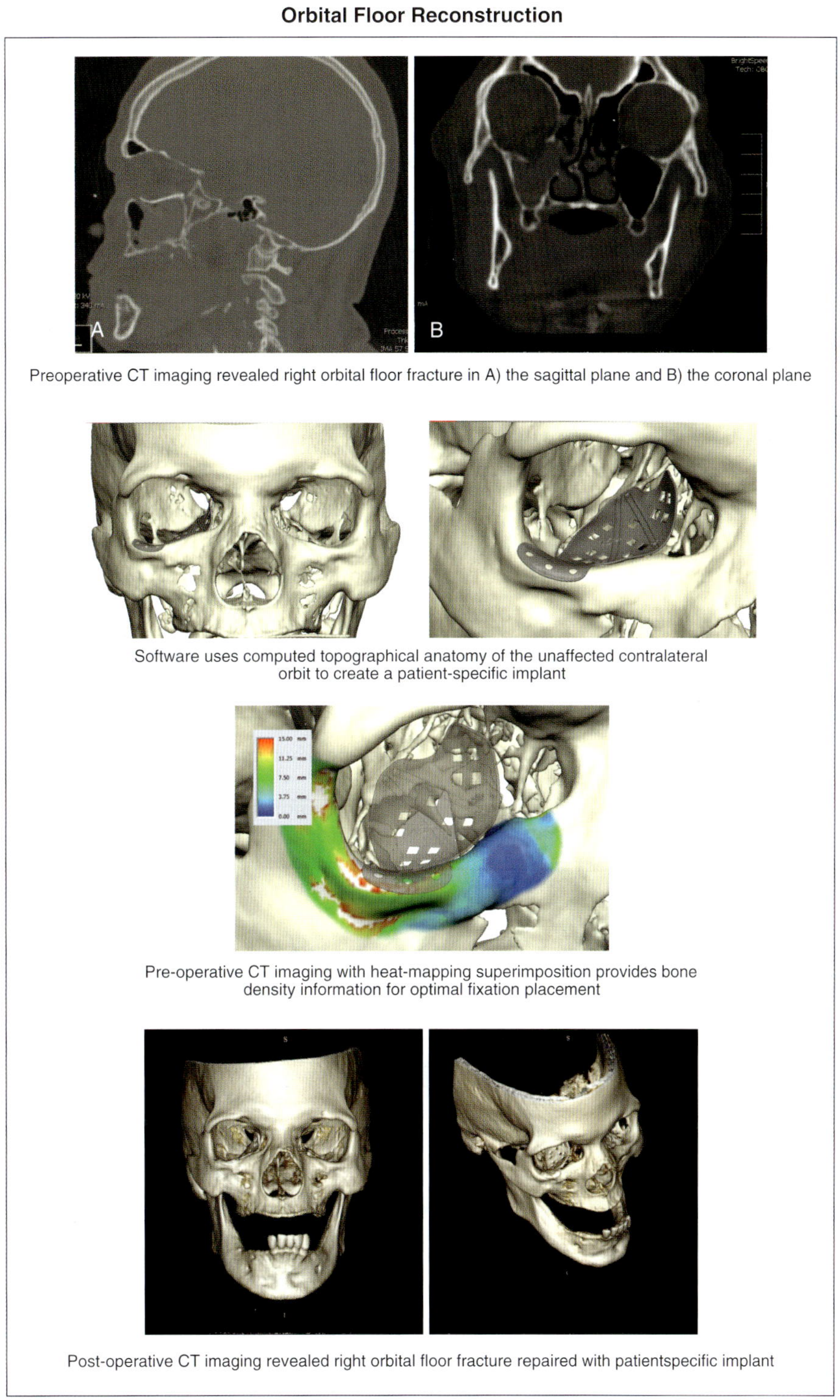


**ppt 18.2** An overview of various computer-assisted design tools applicable to orbital floor reconstruction.

all emerged from the innovation of CaSP. All of which have aided plastic and maxillofacial surgeons to improve outcomes in patients requiring complex orbital reconstruction.[8,9] However, despite these technological advancements, complications still arise. As with any surgical procedure, patients should be thoroughly counseled on the possibility of persistent symptoms.

Among the variety of incisional approaches, the subciliary incision is associated with the most complications, specifically, ectropion is seen in up to 14% of cases. And though the transconjunctival approach has the lowest complications rate, there is still a risk of developing entropion.[10] Despite these risks, previous studies have noted clinically significant improvement in enophthalmos and hypoglobus in 50% of patients following posttraumatic orbital reconstruction.[11] Of note, other studies have observed early intervention before 1 week did not yield improved outcomes due to significant periorbital edema. However, delayed intervention beyond 2 weeks increased the risk of persistent postoperative diplopia or enophthalmos. Thus, a consensus on operative timing 1 to 2 weeks following the incident was made to optimize edema control and minimize scar formation.[12] Though a consensus has been reached, future studies will need to provide evidence-based guidelines to evaluate the validity of this timing hypothesis. Collectively, there is a paucity in the literature assessing the efficacy of applying CaSP to orbital reconstruction and objectively evaluating patient outcomes. Future studies are needed to assess the efficacy of this new and exciting approach.

## Conclusion

The innovation of CAD/CAM technology has been an invaluable improvement in the planning, treatment, and patient outcomes in orbital floor reconstruction. Due to the intricacy of the internal orbit and its proximity to critical anatomic structures, CAD/CAM and real-time intraoperative navigation are ideal for this region. Through segmental mirror-imaging, patient-specific implants are able to be fabricated and used efficiently to achieve preinjurious orbital volume. With this technology, complex repairs become more simple, more predictable, and safer for patients.

## Take-home points

- Prompt ophthalmologic consultation is critical in all cases of orbital fractures.
- CAD integrates clinical data, patient photos, and 3D CT imaging into a single process.
- CAD utilizes the segmental mirror imaging of the contralateral uninjured orbit to restore the orbital volume of the affected side and approximate an appropriately sized plate.
- CAM offers the capability to 3D print customized plates that are based on a patient's unique anatomy.
- Ultimately, reconstruction of the orbital floor attempts to restore the orbital volume as it once was prior to the injury.

## References


1. Maloney K. Non-displaced pediatric orbital fracture with displacement of the inferior rectus muscle into the maxillary sinus: a case report and review of the literature. *Int J Oral Maxillofac Surg*. 2014;43(1):29-31.
2. Pelo S, Gasparini G, Garagiola U, et al. Surgery-first orthognathic approach vs traditional orthognathic approach: oral health-related quality of life assessed with 2 questionnaires. *Am J Orthod Dentofacial Orthop*. 2017;152(2):250-254.
3. Kang HS, Han JJ, Oh HK, Kook MS, Jung S, Park HJ. Anatomical studies of the orbital cavity using three-dimensional computed tomography. *J Craniofac Surg*. 2016;27(6):1583-1588.
4. Nikizad H, Schubert W. Role of plain radiographs in assessing appropriate placement of orbital implants for repair of floor fractures. *Craniomaxillofac Trauma Reconstr*. 2020;13(3):192-197.
5. Gellrich NC, Schramm A, Hammer B, et al. Computer-assisted secondary reconstruction of unilateral posttraumatic orbital deformity. *Plast Reconstr Surg*. 2002;110(6):1417-1429.
6. Lauer G, Pradel W, Schneider M, Eckelt U. Efficacy of computer-assisted surgery in secondary orbital reconstruction. *J Craniomaxillofac Surg*. 2006;34(5):299-305.
7. Bly RA, Chang SH, Cudejkova M, Liu JJ, Moe KS. Computer-guided orbital reconstruction to improve outcomes. *JAMA Facial Plast Surg*. 2013;15(2):113-120.
8. Jansen J, Schreurs R, Dubois L, Maal TJJ, Gooris PJJ, Becking AG. The advantages of advanced computer-assisted diagnostics and three-dimensional preoperative planning on implant position in orbital reconstruction. *J Craniomaxillofac Surg*. 2018;46(4):715-721.

9. Udhay P, Bhattacharjee K, Ananthnarayanan P, Sundar G. Computer-assisted navigation in orbitofacial surgery. *Indian J Ophthalmol*. 2019;67(7):995. doi:10.4103/ijo.ijo_807_18.
10. Ridgway EB, Chen C, Colakoglu S, Gautam S, Lee BT. The incidence of lower eyelid malposition after facial fracture repair: a retrospective study and meta-analysis comparing subtarsal, subciliary, and transconjunctival incisions. *Plast Reconstr Surg*. 2009;124(5):1578.
11. Freihofer HP. Effectiveness of secondary post-traumatic periorbital reconstruction. *J Craniomaxillofac Surg*. 1995;23(3):143-150.
12. Jazayeri HE, Khavanin N, Dorafshar AH. Does early repair of orbital fractures result in superior patient outcomes? A systematic review and meta-analysis. *J Oral Maxillofac Surg*. 2020;78(4):e15-e16.

Chapter | 19 |

# Computer-assisted planning in craniomaxillofacial trauma: mandibular fractures

*Jennifer N. Akin, George Kokosis, Amir H. Dorafshar*

CHAPTER OUTLINE



## Introduction

Repair of traumatic mandibular fractures is a complex process requiring assessment of the degree of comminution, extent of soft tissue injury and restoration of preinjury occlusion.[3] Traditionally, mandibular trauma is managed via intermaxillary fixation (IMF) and open reduction-internal fixation (ORIF) using titanium plates bent intraoperatively.[3] This process requires subjective determination of intraoperative occlusion and plate contouring is time consuming and may lack accuracy.[3] Additionally, the use of extraoral incisions to adequately visualize the reduction carries an increased risk of morbidity due to possible structural or nerve injury and can result in an aesthetically unpleasing scar.[1,2] Computer aided design and computer aided manufacturing (CAD/CAM) has revolutionized complex craniofacial and orthognathic surgery as it enables advanced preoperative planning along with fabrication of three-dimensional (3D) models, customized plates, osteotomy guides, and splints. Through the implementation of these technologies the focus of craniofacial surgeries is able to shift from a surgeon's subjective assessment to a more facile interface of preoperative planning and enhanced intraoperative execution. This shift has in turn led to improved precision, efficiency and patient outcomes. Although CAD/CAM is now a staple of many scheduled craniofacial surgeries, there is increasing literature on its application in patients undergoing traumatic craniofacial reconstruction.

The use of CAD/CAM in treatment of acute facial trauma has been mostly described in orbital and midface trauma. However, new studies are emerging describing CAD/CAM implementation in the management of acute mandibular trauma. Reconstruction of mandibular trauma can be difficult, depending on the extent of intraoral and extraoral soft tissue damage, the degree of comminution and the need to reestablish proper occlusion. It can be further complicated in edentulous patients, due to poor bone stock and absence of dentition to assist in fracture reduction. Frequently, acute mandibular fractures are managed with serial debridements and use of load-bearing plates to bridge any segmental bone loss.

The use of CAD/CAM application in this setting has been documented in only a handful of studies.[3] These emerging studies, however, describe a variety of ways CAD/CAM can be utilized to address the reconstructive challenges posed by acute mandibular trauma. One such method is to use CAD/CAM to assist in prebending plates. In this method the patient's admission computed tomography (CT) scan is uploaded into a CAD/CAM program which allows the mandibular segments to be virtually reduced and preinjury occlusion to be restored. The virtually reduced mandible can then be printed as a 3D model. The CAD/CAM and 3D printing can either be outsourced or, if resources are available, can be performed and printed in-house.[3] Standard plates can then be bent preoperatively to fit this model, thereby reducing OR time and ensuring proper fit. It is also possible to use CAD/CAM to virtually reduce a fractured mandible and then commission custom milled or laser sintered titanium plates. While the printing of custom plates can take several days and delay an operation, they eliminate the need for plate bending and provide a method of guiding and confirming the reduction. Titanium plates are also inherently stronger and lower profile making them less palpable.[1] Finally, for comminuted or edentulous mandibular fractures surgical splints can be fabricated using CAD/CAM technology. These splints can then assist in the anatomical reduction of bony segments and provide immobilization during maxillomandibular fixation (MMF) or ORIF application.

Therefore, advantages of using CAD/CAM in this setting include shorter OR time, less invasive repair through intraoral incision, use of stronger, anatomically configured, lower profile plates, and less subjectivity in reconstruction. However, CAD/CAM implementation does require coordination with bioengineers, longer lead time for custom models, plates, guides, and splints. Additionally, the cost of custom pieces can be substantial, and may not be fully offset by reduction in cost from reduced OR time.

## Clinical considerations

Virtual reduction using CAD/CAM software is done based on occlusion and condyle position.[3] The first step of virtual reduction is to ensure that mandibular condyles are appropriately seated within the mandibular fossa. Once this is completed the mandibular bone fragments can be aligned to create "virtual IMF" using wear facets and dental midlines as a guide. In the case of edentulous mandibular fractures, mandibular symmetry can be assessed using anatomic landmarks such as the midline of nasal bones, intercondylar distance, and the mental protuberance.[4] Virtual reduction with a team of experienced radiologists, oral/maxillofacial surgeons, or outside vendor bioengineers can be completed in approximately 20 minutes, however, this process is dependent on the user's familiarity with the software and anatomy.[3]

Based on resources, plates can be custom milled, 3D printed with laser sintering or prebent using a standard plate. Whether custom milled, laser sintered or prebent plates are being used, the process of fracture reduction and plating is very similar. First, the patient should be placed in intermaxillary fixation (IMF). This step can be challenging in patients with edentulous mandibular fractures where preexisting dentures or gunning splints are typically used to achieve IMF. However, fabrication of gunning splints in an acute trauma setting can be difficult to obtain since they require dental impressions and stone models. CAD/CAM technology can be used instead to design a maxillary mandibular splint based on the virtual reduction. This splint can then be used as a guide intraoperatively to guide fracture reduction and establish proper vertical dimension.

Once IMF is achieved the plate is then fixed to the largest fracture segment and each subsequent piece is reapproximated one at a time using bicortical screws. For more comminuted or complex injuries, monocortical simplification plates can be used first to bring smaller bone fragments together prior to placing larger plates. A minimum of three screws should ideally be used to hold the anterior and posterior pieces of the fracture with one screw in each of the larger comminuted pieces. Bone stock should be assessed preoperatively using the admission CT scan and screw position must be planned for areas of adequate bone stock. Ideally at least four screw holes should be available in major segments and at least two holes in comminuted segments thereby allowing for redundancy in the number of screw holes in case of unforeseen failure at one of the sites.[1] In severe cases of mandibular trauma the mental nerve may be severed; however, if the mental nerve is preserved it should be meticulously dissected and skeletonized in order to minimize risk of injury. The plate should then be placed inferior to the nerve.[1]

Once the plate is secured, appropriate anatomical occlusion should be confirmed by clinical assessment before the patient has left the OR. A postoperative CT scan in the early postoperative period can also be used to confirm appropriate skeletal occlusion.[1]

## Workflow for computer aided design/computer aided manufacturing

Please see Fig. 19.1.

## Computer aided design

Utilization of CAD/CAM for facial trauma typically involves a team of surgeons and biomedical engineers

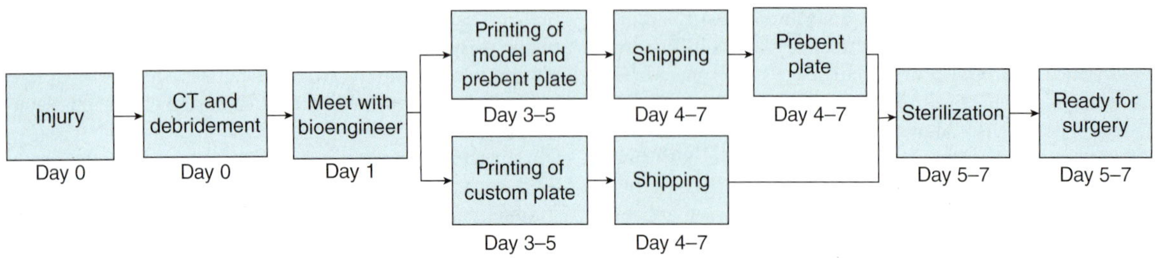


**Fig. 19.1** Timeline of day of injury to delivery of plate for use in the operating room.

from a modeling company. Alternatively, some institutions have in-house radiologists well versed in the software required to virtually reduce a mandible. After virtual reduction of the mandible is complete, files are exported to a 3D printing software as stereolithography (STL) files. In this format the file is aligned on the print bed and supports are generated prior to printing. Models are printed using a biocompatible resin and then washed with fresh isopropyl alcohol prior to curing.[3] After curing is complete standard titanium locking reconstruction plates can be prebent using the model as a guide. Once the plate is appropriately prebent it is then sterilized in preparation for surgery. Similarly, surgical splint design, including shape, thickness, and location of splint holes, is done using computer software during the planning meeting. The custom surgical splint is then 3D printed using a biocompatible resin.[6] When using custom printed titanium plates, the virtual reduction is completed and then plates are virtually superimposed on the computer model. The plate's position is then adjusted virtually to contour with the reduced mandible and so that screw holes are placed in areas of adequate bone density. Once appropriate contour positioning of the plate is achieved the file is once again exported to 3D printing software and the plate is constructed using milling or laser sintering technology. A milled plate is created through a process of "subtractive" printing. Through this process a block of titanium has layers gradually removed (milled) until the remaining titanium fits the computer model. Laser sintering, on the other hand, is a form of "additive" printing in which titanium particles are "welded" together using a laser until the plate is formed. This custom plate is then shipped to the hospital where it undergoes sterilization prior to the patient's surgery.[1]

## Computer aided manufacturing

Stereolithographic models (Fig. 19.2–19.5).

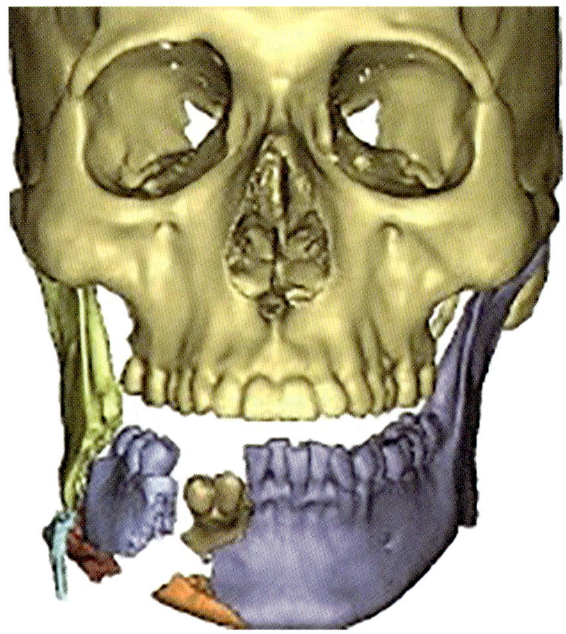

**Fig. 19.2** Three-dimensional rendition of mandibular fracture using admission computed tomography.

## Operative technique

### Steps of the procedure (Video 19.1)

1. Patient undergoes washout and repair of lacerations on the day of trauma.
2. Using admission CT scan and 3D reformats, the patient's fracture and occlusion is restored virtually.
   a. Occlusion is restored virtually using best fit of wear facets and maximal intercuspation.
   b. In edentulous fractures mandibular symmetry can be assessed using anatomic landmarks such as the

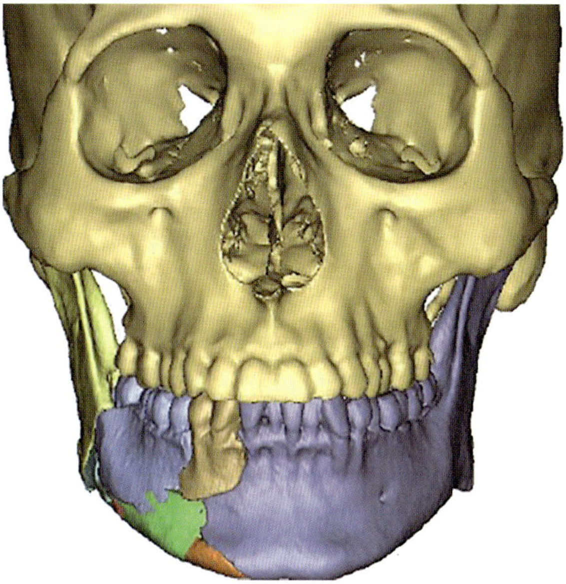

Fig. 19.3 Virtually reconstructed mandibular fracture using computer-assisted surgical planning.

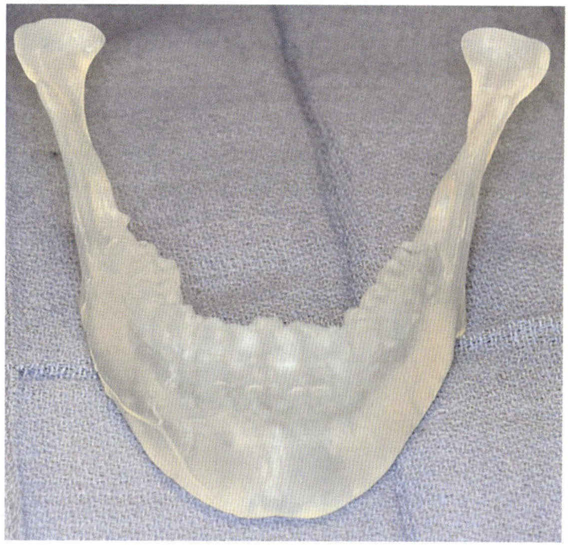

Fig. 19.5 3D printed model of reconstructed mandibular fracture.

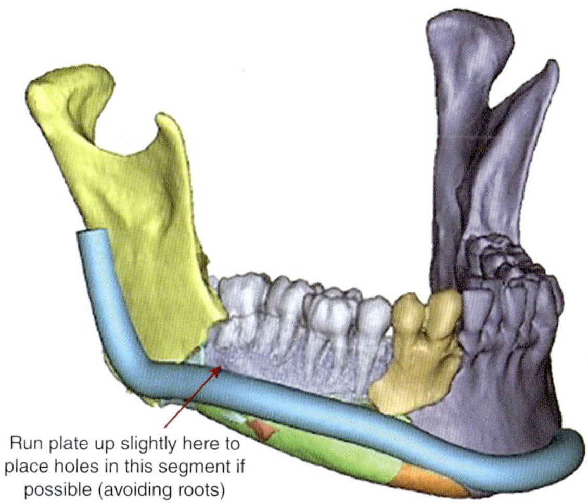


Fig. 19.4 Overlay of custom plate designed for fracture fixation.

midline of nasal bones, intercondylar distance, and the mental protuberance.[3]

3. Printing.
   a. Restored mandible model can be printed allowing plates to be prebent.
   b. Milled 2.0-mm plate or a laser sintered custom titanium plate can be commissioned to bridge the defect with the patient in occlusion.
   c. Gunning splints can then assist in the anatomical reduction of bony segments.
4. Surgery (Fig. 19.6).
   a. Plate is fixed to the largest fracture segment.
5. For more complex or comminuted injuries, first use monocortical simplification plates to bring smaller bone fragments together prior to placing larger plates.
   a. Each subsequent piece is reapproximated one at a time using bicortical screws.
   b. Intraoral incisions closed.
6. Confirmation (Fig. 19.7).
   a. Occlusion is confirmed via clinical assessment before the patient leaves the operating room.
   b. Postoperative CT scan is obtained in the early postoperative period in order to assess the results and confirm skeletal occlusion.
   c. The patient is then followed in clinic to confirm occlusion.[1]

## Fidelity/verification

Appropriate anatomic occlusion is confirmed via clinical assessment during surgery before the patient leaves the OR. Position of the reconstructive plate over the fragments without step offs and appropriate seating of the condyles during range of motion of the mandible at the end of the case can help confirm appropriate results. A postoperative CT scan is obtained in the early postoperative period in order to assess the results and confirm skeletal occlusion. The patient is then followed in clinic to confirm occlusion.[1]

## Pearls/pitfalls

- Working with an experienced team of industry professionals or in-house staff is vital for efficient and accurate virtual planning and CAD/CAM design in the setting of acute trauma.
- Condyle position must be a central focus during planning to achieve appropriate final occlusion and prevent condyle displacement.
- Virtual design should include redundancy in screw holes in case of stripping or unforeseen failure at one site.
- Anatomic occlusion should be confirmed throughout the operative and early postoperative period using

### Clinical cases

Photos before and after

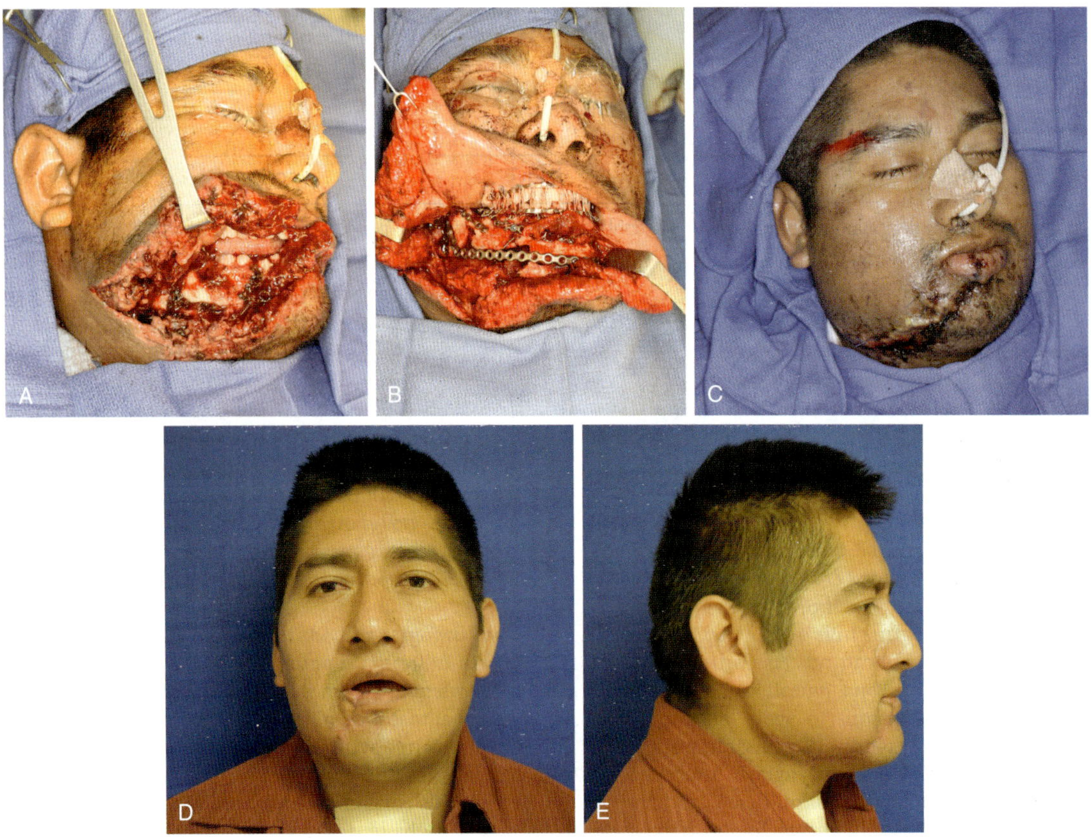


**Fig. 19.6** Intraoperative and postoperative photos of a patient that suffered a blast injury resulting in an open right hemi-mandibular fracture with significant soft tissue injury. (From Kokosis G, Davidson EH, Pedreira BS, Macmillan A, Dorafshar AH. The use of computer aided design and manufacturing in acute mandibular trauma reconstruction. *J Oral Maxillofac Surg*. 2018;76(5):1036–43.)

Radiographs before and after and "fit" to plan

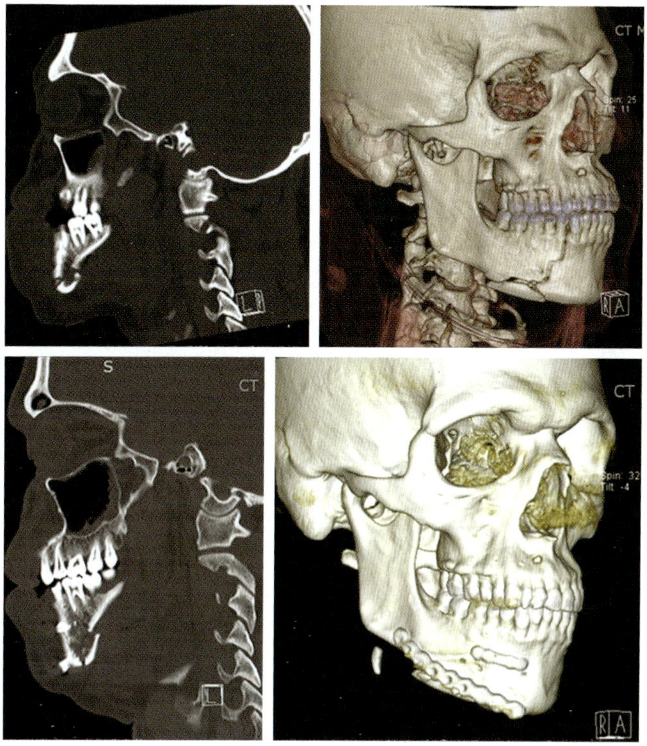


**Fig. 19.7** Preoperative *(upper left)* and postoperative *(lower left)* computed tomography scans and preoperative *(upper right)* and postoperative *(lower right)* three-dimensional scans of patient. (From Kokosis G, Davidson EH, Pedreira BS, Macmillan A, Dorafshar AH. The use of computer aided design and manufacturing in acute mandibular trauma reconstruction. *J Oral Maxillofac Surg.* 2018;76(5):1036–43.)

clinical assessment and CT imaging to ensure virtual occlusion is accurate.

- Virtually designed dental splints should be considered in order to reduce, fixate, and stabilize complex mandibular fractures.

## Outcomes/complications

There have been several studies addressing the use of CAD/CAM technologies in traumatic mandibular reconstruction. Kokosis et al. used CAD/CAM to virtually reduce fractures then used an intraoral incision to secure either a custom milled plate or a prebent standard plate. None of their patients developed any postoperative complications except for one patient that experienced minor dehiscence of the intraoral incision. This minor complication resolved with local wound care.[1] In this study, the implementation of CAD/CAM facilitated confident reduction through an intraoral approach, which reduces the risk of marginal mandibular nerve injury and orocutaneous fistula which can occur via an extraoral approach with concomitant intraoral traumatic laceration.[1] At the time of the study the average interval from injury to custom plate availability was 7 days. This protocol was then optimized and reduced to only 4 days, which could still be prohibitive in some settings.

For patients with edentulous or highly comminuted mandibular fractures Wang et al.[5] and Kongsong et al.[6] utilized CAD-CAM technologies to design and print dental splints. These authors reported no complications and demonstrated that the use of CAD/CAM to construct dental splints decreased operating time and improved fracture stability in complex cases.

## Conclusion

CAD/CAM in the setting of mandibular trauma gives surgical teams the ability to preplan complex comminuted fracture reductions and subsequently print 3D models, dental splints, and custom plates. Prebending standard plates using custom models or commission of custom milled plates or laser sintered plates can improve efficiency. Having a patient-specific plate also enables more confident reduction via an intraoral incision thus reducing subjectivity of repair and decreasing risk of morbidity. Although operative efficiency is improved, there can be longer lead time of 4 to 14 days for manufacturing and shipping of custom models and milled plates. More studies are currently needed to elucidate if the increased cost of custom models and plates is offset by the cost savings of reduced OR time. Overall, CAD/CAM technologies have become a mainstay in reconstructive surgeries, and these methods can be safely and effectively utilized in the setting of acute complex mandibular trauma.

## Take-home points

- CAD/CAM technologies can be used to assist in prebending standard plates or to produce custom milled plates or laser sintered for traumatic mandibular fractures,
- CAD/CAM technology can be used to produce dental splints to assist in mandibular reduction in edentulous mandibular fractures,
- CAD/CAM application in mandibular trauma reconstruction can increase efficiency by eliminating the need for in situ plate bending and serving as a method to guide and confirm the reduction,
- The use of prebent or custom printed plate can facilitate reduction and visualization through an intraoral incision,
- CAD/CAM can be a safe and useful adjunct for treating complex traumatic mandibular fractures.[1]

## References


1. Kokosis G, Davidson EH, Pedreira BS, Macmillan A, Dorafshar AH. The use of computer-aided design and manufacturing in acute mandibular trauma reconstruction. *J Oral Maxillofac Surg*. 2018;76(5):1036-1043.
2. Chrcanovic BR. Open versus closed reduction: comminuted mandibular fractures. *J Oral Maxillofac Surg*. 2013;17:95-104.
3. Marschall JS, Dutra V, Flint RL, et al. In-house digital workflow for the management of acute mandible fractures. *J Oral Maxillofac Surg*. 2019;77(10):2084.e1-2084.e9.
4. Wagner JD, Baack B, Brown GA, Kelly J. Rapid 3-dimensional prototyping for surgical repair of maxillofacial fractures: a technical note. *J Oral Maxillofac Surg*. 2004;62:898.
5. Wang HD, Frost C, Cusano A, Dorafshar AH. Management of bilateral edentulous mandible fractures through an intraoral approach using CAD/CAM technology: a case report. *J Oral Maxillofac Surg*. 2018;76(5):1056.e1-1056.e6.
6. Kongsong W, Somsak S. Utilization of virtual surgical planning for surgical splint-assisted comminuted maxillomandibular fracture reduction and/or fixation. *Craniomaxillofac Trauma Reconstr*. 2020;13(4):334-341.


## Suggested Reading


Elegbede A, Diaconu SC, McNichols CHL, et al. Office-based three-dimensional printing workflow for craniomaxillofacial fracture repair. *J Craniofac Surg*. 2018;29:e440,

King BJ, Park EP, Christensen BJ, Danrad R. On-site 3-dimensional printing and preoperative adaptation decrease operative time for mandibular fracture repair. *J Oral Maxillofac Surg*. 2018;76:1950.e1.

Mazzoni S, Bianchi A, Schiariti G, et al. Computer-aided design and computer-aided manufacturing cutting guides and customized titanium plates are useful in upper maxilla waferless repositioning. *J Oral Maxillofac Surg*. 2015;73:701.

Chapter 20

# Computer-assisted surgical planning in craniomaxillofacial trauma: zygomaticomaxillary complex fractures and secondary reconstruction

*Tulsi Roy, Joseph Lopez, Amir H. Dorafshar*

**CHAPTER OUTLINE**



## Introduction

Zygomaticomaxillary complex (ZMC) fractures are one of the most common facial fractures, second only to nasal bone fractures.[1,2] The ZMC plays a key functional and aesthetic role for the face—the zygomatic arch serves as the cranial insertion point for the masseter, and the zygomatic complex provides an anatomic separation between the maxillary sinus, orbit, and temporal fossa. Aesthetically, the ZMC provides a normal cheek contour and is principal to establishing an appropriate and symmetric facial width.[3]

As with most facial fractures, accurate reduction and expeditious surgical fixation of the ZMC is desirable because reestablishing pretraumatic facial contour is challenging after scarring and bony remodeling have transpired.[2,4] Given the ZMC's numerous bony attachments and at-times complex translational and rotational displacement, computer-assisted surgical planning (CaSP) and computer-assisted design and manufacturing (CAD/CAM) can be helpful in restoring premorbid facial morphology and orbital volume.[5,6] This chapter will discuss clinical management using CAD/CAM in treating ZMC fractures acutely as well as in the setting of secondary reconstruction.

## Clinical considerations

Depending on the vector, force, and mechanism of injury, damage to the ZMC can be highly variable, and for this reason, a litany of diagnostic classification systems exists to standardize surgical treatment and postoperative care of these fractures. These classifications typically distinguish categories based on the degree of displacement, comminution, and rotation of the bony segments.[7] A detailed discussion of each of these systems is outside the scope of this chapter, but, broadly speaking, the morphology, displacement, and degree of comminution of the fracture pattern (as well as the presence of other concomitant facial fractures) will ultimately guide the surgeon in their maneuvers for adequate reduction and internal fixation.

Clinically, disruption of the ZMC through blunt or penetrating trauma can result in asymmetry and malar flattening with facial widening, exophthalmos or enophthalmos, increased scleral show, or trismus. If significantly displaced, step-offs and crepitus along the zygomatic arch or orbital rim can also be appreciated on palpation. Because of the proximity of the infraorbital nerve, facial paresthesia may also be present and nerve decompression may be warranted at the time of fracture fixation.[8] As with all facial fractures, the gold standard for diagnosis and presurgical planning of the ZMC remains non-contrast computed tomography (CT) imaging of the craniofacial skeleton. Special consideration should also be taken to observe any areas of coronoid involvement as a possible cause of trismus due to impingement from a posteriorly displaced or rotated zygoma.

A special note should be made regarding ocular injury, which frequently accompanies ZMC and other midfacial fractures that disrupt the integrity of the orbital skeleton. Subconjunctival hemorrhage and corneal abrasion are the most frequently diagnosed ocular injuries in this context, but more serious complications such as hyphema, vitreous hemorrhage, retinal hemorrhage, extraocular muscle entrapment, canthal ligament detachment, and globe rupture may also be present.[9] For this reason, in the acute setting, a thorough ophthalmologic evaluation and an assessment of visual acuity is necessary to diagnose and treat any potentially blinding complications before fracture fixation can safely proceed. Operative fracture treatment in this context should be delayed until stabilization of the ocular injury and ophthalmology clearance has been elicited, and in certain cases, it may be desirable to delay treatment further until improvement in periorbital edema to aid intraoperative visualization of the zygomaticosphenoid suture and orbital floor.

Nondisplaced or incomplete ZMC fractures may be managed nonoperatively with sinus precautions and a soft diet. For displaced ZMC fractures, however, technical considerations range from one to four points of fixation in the literature with no clear consensus. In a recent meta-analysis examining the number of fixation points for ZMC fractures, the overall quality of current evidence for the number of points of exposure and fixation of ZMC fractures was poor.[10] That said, it is largely accepted that while some translation and rotational movement can be mitigated with the use of a single miniplate,[11] a second or third plate provides further stability, counteracting the strong displacing forces from the masseter muscle. When analyzing the few randomized controlled trials that compared two- and three-point fixation, three-point fixation of ZMC fractures was shown to improve fracture stability and yield less long-term vertical orbital dystopia. The surgeon should, however, weigh the potential gains in stability against the risks of additional exposure, periosteal stripping, ectropion, and soft tissue scarring.[12] Broadly speaking, in our experience, with most facial fractures, a greater degree of comminution and fracture complexity increases the need for more fixation points.

For those patients who have either missed their window for open reduction and internal fixation or for those whose fractures are inadequately reduced during prior fixation,[13] secondary reconstruction of ZMC fractures may be required. In most ZMC fractures, the zygoma is usually displaced laterally and inferiorly due to masseteric pull,[14] thereby increasing intraorbital volume, and development of enophthalmos.[15] In these instances, patients may present with residual post-traumatic deformity such as malar flattening, hypoglobus, trismus, and facial asymmetry. Once again, up-to-date CT imaging of the craniofacial skeleton is important for visualizing the topography of prior fractures, noting the presence of any previous radio-opaque hardware or foreign bodies, and observing any areas of impingement or bony interference. Depending on the severity of the deformity, correction of facial projection or orbital symmetry may require soft tissue resuspension or augmentation, malar implants, or zygomatic repositioning osteotomies.

## Workflow for computer-assisted design/computer-assisted manufacturing

Owing to the variability and complexity of injury patterns, CaSP can be useful in both the primary and secondary reconstructive setting.[16] In primary open reduction and internal fixation, CT data can be used to visualize or generate stereolithographic models of the facial skeleton and ZMC in three dimensions and better characterize any rotational component to its displacement, which can often prove challenging to represent in two-dimensional axial or sagittal images.[17] Using this information, the surgeon can better plan their movements to disimpact and derotate the zygoma during surgery. Secondly, not only can the surgery be simulated, but custom titanium plates can also be fabricated to assist in precise fracture reduction and subsequent fixation. The location and placement of these plates and their screw holes can be planned in areas of stable bone stock, which is particularly helpful when restoring contour in the face of significant comminution when precise fracture alignment is particularly challenging. Similarly, orbital volume can be evaluated, and the orbital floor can be reestablished with a custom implant model based on the floor contour of the intact contralateral orbit.[18] Thirdly, any functional interferences from other bony structures can be detected or simulated virtually, and coronoidectomy can be planned if deemed necessary.

Obtaining a baseline low-dose, high fidelity maxillofacial CT scan is the first step for any preoperative virtual surgical planning and is essential when utilizing CAD/CAM for generation of stereolithographic models or the manufacturing of any custom prefabricated plates or implants.[19] Scans are then uploaded to a third-party vendor for CaSP. Digital mobilization of fracture fragments can then be simulated, and subsequent realignment in the correct position can provide the basis for custom plate fabrication, a process that may take 1 to 2 weeks. Care should be taken to consider the number of fixation points, exposure access, incision length(s), and implant size in operative planning and implant design.

When using CaSP in the primary reconstructive setting, once the fractures have been digitally reduced, the zygomaticofrontal suture typically serves as the preferred reference for custom plate fabrication, owing to its strength, reliability, and ease of surgical access. In these instances, the plate can be designed with a "lip" or extension to hug the internal contour orbit and superiorly to lock into place. These extensions on the plate facilitate precise implant placement and decrease the likelihood of fracture rotation around the zygomaticosphenoid suture during the plating sequence. Theoretically, custom implants can also be designed for the zygomaticomaxillary and orbital fractures as well, but in the setting of impacted or heavily comminuted ZMC fractures, even with CaSP, it can be challenging to predict the extent of orbital floor defects or areas of adequate maxillary bone stock after disimpaction and the reduction of any other concomitant midface fractures.

In the case of secondary reconstruction for ZMC fractures, the use of CaSP has several distinct advantages: once the degree of skeletal deformity and of enophthalmos has been characterized, the decision can be made to perform custom onlay malar implant for recontouring versus repositioning zygomatic osteotomies.[14] An intact or uninjured contralateral side can be mirrored and used as a template for onlay creation or to plan cutting guides and implants to "recreate" the prior fracture and reposition the zygoma en-bloc. Prior hardware used for fixation can be easily visualized and, if removal is necessary, this can be simulated prior to any custom implant planning. Should malar implants be selected, they should be designed with at least two holes for screw fixation to prevent rotation of the implant.[20] If zygomatic repositioning is needed, then cutting guides with predictive holes can be designed for osteotomies along the maxilla and inferior and lateral orbital rims. After the ZMC is digitally repositioned, a custom prefabricated orbital plate can be designed to restore orbital volume with an extension or lip to fixate the osteotomy at the inferior orbital rim.

## Operative technique

The operative procedure begins with the induction of general anesthesia and orotracheal intubation. After infiltration of local anesthesia with epinephrine, extraoral incisions can be made to expose the fractures. If existing lacerations are present, these can always substitute for the approaches for reduction. If no lacerations are present, the zygomaticofrontal fracture can be approached through a lateral brow or upper blepharoplasty incision. The fracture along the zygomaticosphenoid suture should be visualized through the surgeon's preferred exposure of the orbital floor, either a transconjunctival, subciliary, or transcutaneous approach. The zygomaticomaxillary suture should be exposed intraorally through an upper vestibular approach. Generally, the zygomatic arch itself rarely requires fixation, but for severely displaced and comminuted arch fractures and those that are associated with multiple midfacial fractures that necessitate maximal exposure, a coronal incision should be planned to visualize and reconstruct the arch. After subperiosteal dissection of all fractures, the ZMC should then be mobilized and reduced. A Carroll-Girard screw may be deployed to assist in disimpaction, if necessary. Plating should be begin with the zygomaticofrontal suture, using the custom plate with extensions predetermined by the CaSP. Following confirmation of adequate reduction at the lateral orbit and zygomaticosphenoid suture, the zygomaticomaxillary buttress and the orbital rim can be plated, depending on the need for two- or three-point fixation.[10,21] Finally, an inventory of the orbital floor should be taken, and the floor should be repaired if a significant defect exists. Following plating, resuspension of the soft tissues of the malar eminence is recommended to minimize traction on the infraorbital tissue and limit the development of ectropion. The tissue can be secured to the orbital rim plate or directly to the bone with the use of a wire-passing drill, before cutaneous and intraoral incisions are closed.[2] A clinical example is provided in Fig. 20.1.

If zygomatic repositioning is necessary for secondary reconstruction, consideration should be given to the amount of exposure required for osteotomy creation. Lateral cantholysis and extended upper blepharoplasty or lateral brow incisions can provide the increased exposure of the periorbita necessary for additional instrumentation. After cutting guides with predictive holes are placed along the orbital rim, the maxillary osteotomy can be marked and created using a reciprocating or piezo-electric saw, before joining it intraorbitally to a second osteotomy carried through the zygomaticofrontal bone and lateral orbit. After the periorbital and maxillary osteotomies, a final osteotomy can be created intraorally through the zygomatic arch in

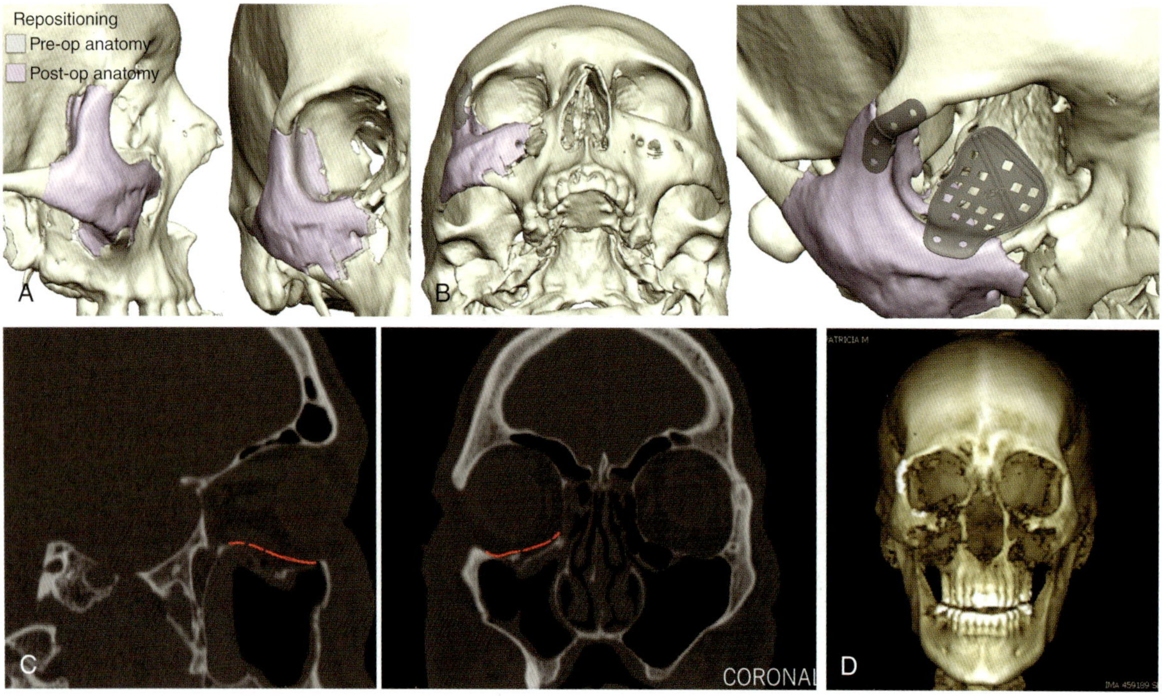


**Fig. 20.1** The use of computer-assisted design/computer-assisted manufacturing for primary zygomaticomaxillary complex fracture repair. (A) Lateral *(left)* and frontal *(right)* views of planned preoperative and postoperative zygoma position. (B) Basal view *(left)* and oblique view *(right)* of lateral orbital rim and orbital floor prefabricated plates. Note the extension or "lip" of the lateral orbital plate that extends medially to wrap around the rim. (C) Sagittal *(left)* and coronal *(right)* computed tomography (CT) scan views demonstrating planned orbital floor plate position. (D) Final postoperative CT scan demonstrating adequate fracture reduction with custom plates in place.

order to reposition the zygoma based on the movements delineated by the CaSP. Once osteotomy completion is confirmed, any areas of bony interference should be removed with a saw or burr before rotating and repositioning the zygoma into its final location. A small low-profile miniplate or wire can be placed along the lateral orbital rim in order to secure the zygoma while maintaining some flexibility to adjust the orbital floor plate and screw it into place along the inferior orbital rim and the ZM. Following zygoma fixation, malar projection should be assessed for symmetry before midface resuspension and incision closure. Clinical examples are provided in Figs. 20.2 and 20.3.

## Fidelity/verification

If institutional capabilities permit, intraoperative CT scan can be particularly helpful in assessing fracture reduction, bony interference, and malar eminence symmetry, and adjustments to the plate or bone can be made efficiently and avoid the need for a secondary revision procedure.[22,23] The accuracy of postoperative results following CaSP acute fracture fixation or zygomatic repositioning can also be evaluated with a postoperative CT scan, ideally with three-dimensional (3D) reconstruction. Whether an intraoperative or postoperative CT scan is obtained, malar projection and facial width can be measured and compared to a contralateral uninjured side. Similarly, such data can also be used to quantify and compare orbital volume. These precise measures prove particularly beneficial in the setting of soft tissue and periorbital edema, which can obscure assessment of facial symmetry or spatial relationships of the globe in the early postoperative period.

The soft tissue envelope is a key consideration in evaluating facial balance and malar projection. Ellis et al. reported that facial asymmetry that did not exceed 2 mm was difficult to perceive by experienced clinicians.[24] In a separate study evaluating facial asymmetry after ZMC fracture, Kim et al. found that patients often complain of soft tissue asymmetry when comparing with the contralateral

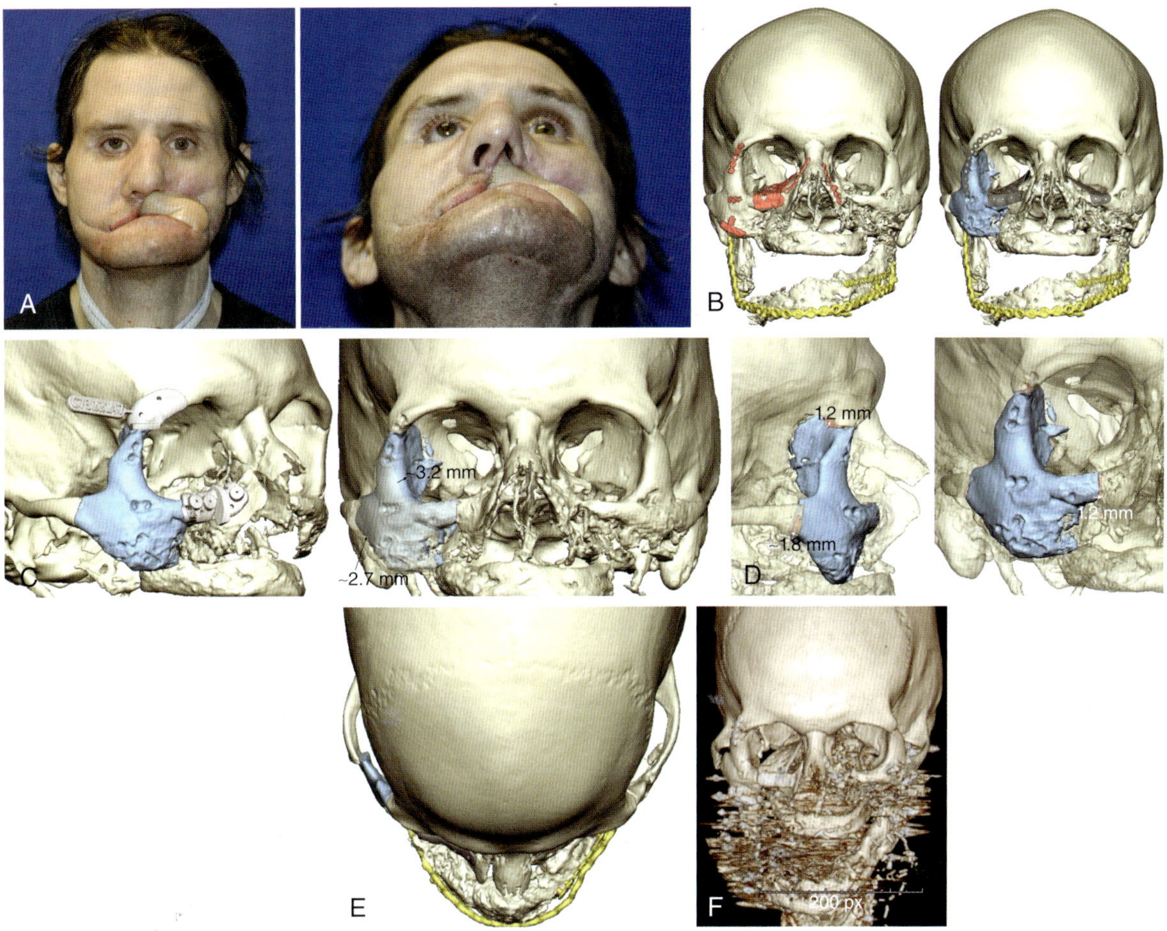


**Fig. 20.2** Secondary reconstruction of zygomaticomaxillary complex fracture with right zygomatic repositioning. (A) Preoperative frontal view *(left)* and basal view *(right)* photos of a patient with a posttraumatic deformity following primary repair. Note the right-sided malar flattening and widening, with significant enophthalmos and scleral show. (B) A three-dimensional (3D) preoperative *(left)* and postoperative *(right)* simulated zygoma position. *Red* indicates preexisting hardware. *Blue* indicates zygoma. (C) A 3D-simulated cutting guide placement for zygomatic osteotomies along the inferior and lateral orbital rim. (D) Lateral *(left)* and oblique *(right)* planned zygoma movement. Red indicates areas of bony interference/overlap fated for removal. (E) Bird's-eye view of the final simulated position of the zygoma. Note the step-off along the zygomatic arch. (F) A 3D-reconstructed computed tomography scan of the patient demonstrating a newly medially and superiorly positioned right zygoma fixated along the zygomaticofrontal suture and the inferior orbital rim with a custom orbital floor plate. Patient has extensive radiologic artifact secondary to retained metal foreign bodies from prior ballistic injury.

side of the face even when bone fragments were accurately reduced.[25] Unfortunately, the ZMC fracture pattern is diverse and soft tissue change after reduction surgery is difficult to predict.[26] Blunt and penetrating trauma to the soft tissues can lead to scarring, atrophy, and contour irregularities. If facial asymmetry persists despite adequate bony reduction and fixation, the craniofacial surgeon can be reassured that the skeletal framework is no longer deficient and therefore plan to address the facial soft tissue envelope separately with soft tissue augmentation through local tissue rearrangement or fat grafting. Regardless of whether the surgeon is performing zygomatic repositioning or malar implant placement, the bulk of surgical judgment should be done in the preoperative planning stage, as relying solely on intraoperative assessment of the overlying soft tissue is prone to distortion secondary to edema, surgical access, patient positioning, and the presence of the endotracheal tube.

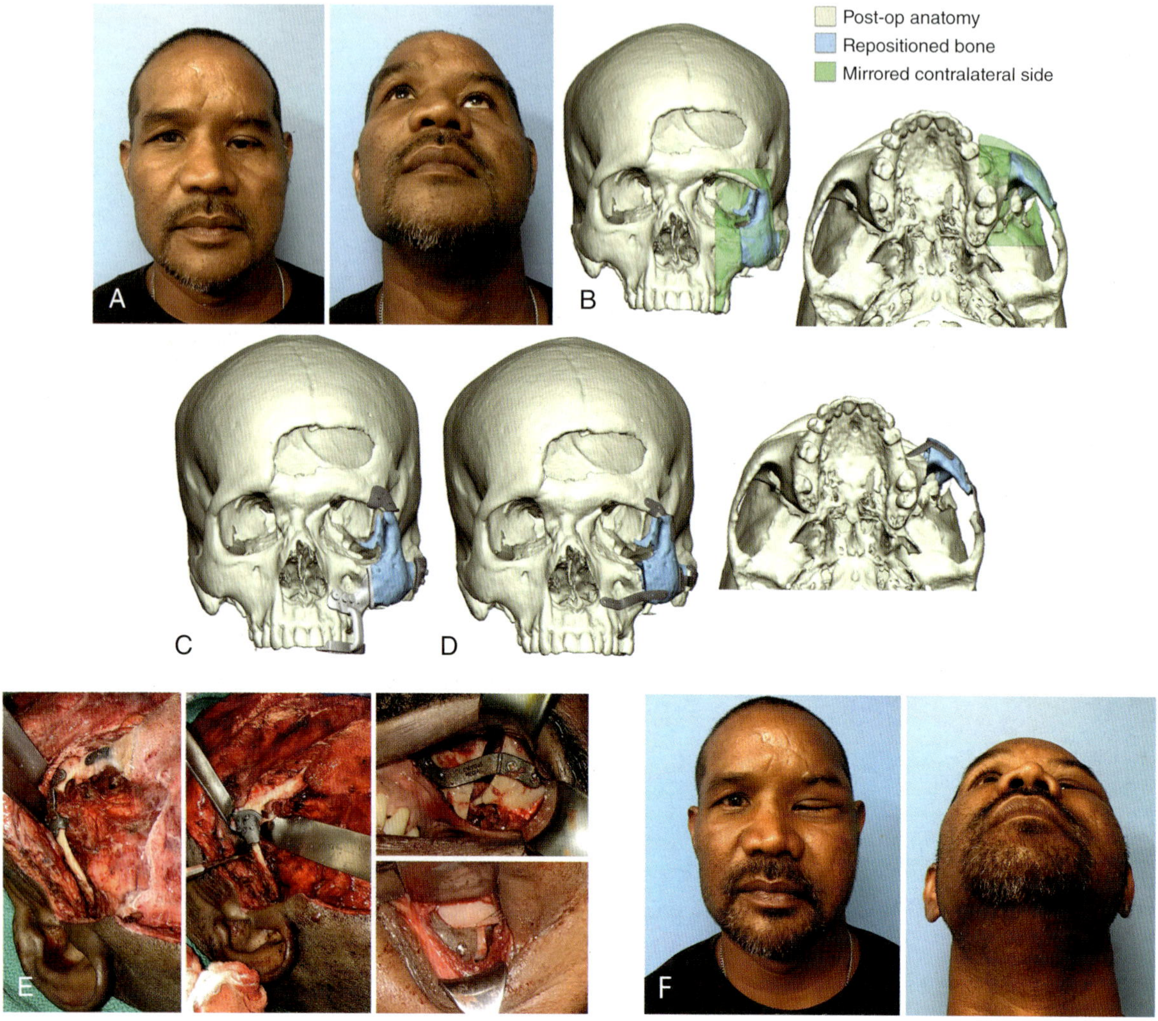


**Fig. 20.3** Secondary reconstruction of left zygomaticomaxillary complex (ZMC) fracture with left zygomatic repositioning. (A) Preoperative frontal view *(left)* and basal view *(right)* photos of a patient with a posttraumatic malar flattening, orbital malposition, and enophthalmos. (B) A three-dimensional (3D) simulated zygoma with mirrored contralateral zygoma *(green)* and repositioned zygoma *(blue)*. (C) A 3D-simulated cutting guide placement for zygomatic osteotomies. (D) Simulated repositioned zygoma with custom plates along all four bony articulations of the ZMC. (E) Intraoperative photographs demonstrating prefabricated hardware securing osteotomies at the levels of the lateral orbit, zygomatic arch, zygomaticomaxillary buttress, and inferior orbital rim. (F) Two-week postoperative photographs of the patient. Despite residual expected edema, frontal view *(left)* and basal view *(right)* demonstrate improvement in malar projection and globe position.

## Pearls/pitfalls

- The process of acquiring prefabricated plates typically requires at least 1 week. For this reason, the authors recommend reserving CAD/CAM for secondary reconstruction and in select acute trauma patients with significantly comminuted and displaced fractures, particularly those in which fracture reduction is anticipated to be challenging.
- In the primary trauma reconstructive setting, the length and shape of prefabricated orbital floor plates may be challenging to predict prior to surgical disimpaction of the ZMC. For this reason, the zygomaticofrontal suture provides a more reliable template for custom plate

fabrication. Compared to a single flexible miniplate used in traditional fracture reduction, a custom plate designed with an extension to wrap medially around the lateral orbital rim can minimize rotational forces on the zygoma to facilitate precise fracture reduction at the other articulations of the ZMC.

- Custom plates around the orbit should be designed to be as low-profile as reasonably possible to avoid contour irregularities and minimize palpability.
- Postoperatively, patients should avoid pressure to the malar region and adhere to a soft diet to limit the displacing forces on the reduced or newly repositioned zygoma.

## Complications

Possible complications from internal fixation of ZMC fractures and zygomatic repositioning include bleeding, infection, bony malunion, and nonunion. Retrobulbar hematoma and damage to the orbital contents, including the globe and extraocular muscles, is also a potential risk incurred during subperiosteal dissection or osteotomy. While 3D planning and CAD/CAM require additional upfront logistics and cost, CaSP and CAD/CAM provide additional surgical efficiency and confidence and eliminate the need for aesthetic "guesswork" with implant or bony repositioning.[19] Unlike traditional methods, which require repeated attempts at intraoperative implant contouring and placement, by decreasing intraoperative time and curtailing multiple attempts at implant repositioning, trauma and edema of the periorbital tissues can be minimized. Although the use of CaSP in orbital reconstruction is the topic of another chapter, it should also be stated here that the use of prefabricated orbital plates not only accurately restores the continuity of the orbital floor, but it also decreases the risk of incarceration of orbital contents and impingement of vital orbital structures.

## Conclusions

- CAS allows the surgeon to assess spatial relationships, calculate orbital volume, and determine optimal vector for fracture reduction or zygomatic repositioning.
- By reliably reestablishing a symmetric skeletal foundation with 3D planning and CAD/CAM, the soft tissue envelope can then be restored separately without needing to compensate for an inadequate bony framework.
- Minor secondary deformities from zygoma malposition with adequate intraorbital volume can be managed by onlay grafting. CAD/CAM facilitates the creation of precise onlay malar implants mirrored on the normal contralateral side.
- CAS can enable more precise zygoma repositioning in three dimensions—with a degree of reliability and reproducibility that is challenging to achieve with traditional methods.

## References


1. Strong EB, Gary C. Management of zygomaticomaxillary complex fractures. *Facial Plast Surg Clin North Am*. 2017;25(4):547-562.
2. Herford AM, Miller M, Cantu D. Orbitozygomaticomaxillary complex fractures. In: Dorafshar A, Rodriguez ED, Manson P, eds. *Facial Trauma Surgery: From Primary Repair to Reconstruction*. Edinburgh; London; New York; Oxford: Elsevier. 2020:137-146.
3. Ho JPTF, Schreurs R, Aydi S, et al. Natural variation of the zygomaticomaxillary complex symmetry in normal individuals. *J Craniomaxillofac Surg*. 2017:45(12):1927-1933.
4. Sharaf BA, Morris JM, Kuruoglu D. EPPOCRATIS: A point-of-care utilization of virtual surgical planning and three-dimensional printing for the management of acute craniomaxillofacial trauma. *J Clin Med*. 2021:10(23):5640.
5. Gong X, He Y, An J, et al. Application of a computer-assisted navigation system (CANS) in the delayed treatment of zygomatic fractures: A randomized controlled trial. *J Oral Maxillofac Surg*. 2017;75(7):1450-1463.
6. Shaheen HA, Shaker S, Ibrahim WH, et al. Delayed complex fronto-zygomatico-orbital reconstruction using patient specific 3D printed implants: A report of three complex cases – A short communication. *J Plast Reconstr Aesthet Surg*. 2022;75(10):3877-3903.
7. Dreizin D, Nam AJ, Diaconu SC, et al. Multidetector CT of midfacial fractures: Classification systems, principles of reduction, and common complications. *Radiographics*. 2018;38(1):248-274.
8. Dubron K, Verbist M, Shaheen E, et al. Incidence, aetiology, and associated fracture patterns of infraorbital nerve injuries following zygomaticomaxillary complex fractures: A retrospective analysis of 272 patients. *Craniomaxillofac Trauma Reconstr*. 2022;15(2):139-146.

9. Malik AH, Shah AA, Ahmad I, Shah BA. Ocular injuries in patients of zygomatico-complex (ZMC) fractures. *J Maxillofac Oral Surg*. 2017;16(2):243-247.
10. Jazayeri HE, Khavanin N, Yu JW, et al. Fixation points in the treatment of traumatic zygomaticomaxillary complex fractures: A systematic review and meta-analysis. *J Oral Maxillofac Surg*. 2019;77(10):2064-2073.
11. Shokri T, Sokoya M, Cohn JE, Bahrami A, Inman J, Ducic Y. Single-point fixation for noncomminuted zygomaticomaxillary complex fractures: A 20-year experience. *J Oral Maxillofac Surg*. 2020; 78(5):778-781.
12. Rana M, Warraich R, Tahir S, et al. Surgical treatment of zygomatic bone fracture using two points fixation versus three point fixation: A randomised prospective clinical trial. *Trials*. 2012;13:36.
13. Watzinger F, Wanschitz F, Wagner A, et al. Computer-aided navigation in secondary reconstruction of post-traumatic deformities of the zygoma. *J Craniomaxillofac Surg*. 1997;25(4):198-202.
14. Aman HM, Alenezi A, Ducic Y, Reddy LV. Secondary reconstruction of the zygomaticomaxillary complex. *Semin Plast Surg*. 2020; 34(4):254-259.
15. Manson PN, Grivas A, Rosenbaum A, Vannier M, Zinreich J, Iliff N. Studies on enophthalmos: II. The measurement of orbital injuries and their treatment by quantitative computed tomography. *Plast Reconstr Surg*. 1986;77(2):203-214.
16. Day KM, Kelley PK, Harshbarger RJ, et al. Advanced three-dimensional technologies in craniofacial reconstruction. *Plast Reconstr Surg*. 2021;148(1):94e-108e.
17. Zhang X, Han CY, Dai MJ, et al. Application of computer-assisted surgery techniques in the management of zygomatic complex fractures. *Chin J Traumatol*. 2018;21(5):281-286.
18. Chepurnyi Y, Zhukovtseva O, Kopchak A, Kanura O. Clinical application of automated virtual orbital reconstruction for orbital fracture management with patient-specific implants: A prospective comparative study. *J Craniomaxillofac Surg*. 2022;50(9):686-691.
19. Reddy S, Macmillan A, Dorafshar A. Virtual surgical planning. In: Dorafshar A, Rodriguez E, Manson P, eds. *Facial Trauma Surgery: From Primary Repair to Reconstruction*. Edinburgh; London; New York; Oxford: Elsevier; 2020:483-492.
20. Steinbacher DM. Alloplastic facial augmentation. In: Steinbacher, ed. *Aesthetic Rhinoplasty and Orthognathic Surgery*. Hoboken: Wiley Blackwell; 2019:559-572.
21. Raghoebar II, Rozema FR, de Lange J, Dubois L. Surgical treatment of fractures of the zygomaticomaxillary complex: effect of fixation on repositioning and stability. A systematic review. *Br J Oral Maxillofac Surg*. 2022;60(4):397-411.
22. van Hout WM, Van Cann EM, Muradin MS, Frank MH, Koole R. Intraoperative imaging for the repair of zygomaticomaxillary complex fractures: a comprehensive review of the literature. *J Craniomaxillofac Surg*. 2014;42(8):1918-1923.
23. van Hout WM, de Kort WWB, Ten Harkel TC, Van Cann EM, Rosenberg AJWP. Zygomaticomaxillary complex fracture repair with intraoperative CBCT imaging. A prospective cohort study. *J Craniomaxillofac Surg*. 2022;50(1):54-60.
24. Ellis E III, el-Attar A, Moos KF. An analysis of 2,067 cases of zygomatico-orbital fracture. *J Oral Maxillofac Surg*. 1985;43(6):417-428.
25. Kim DH, Kim RH, Lee J, Chee YD, Kwon KH. Evaluation of soft tissue asymmetry using cone-beam computed tomography after open reduction and internal fixation of zygomaticomaxillary complex fracture. *J Korean Assoc Oral Maxillofac Surg*. 2014;40(3): 103-110.
26. Khaqani MS, Tavosi F, Gholami M, Eftekharian HR, Khojastepour L. Analysis of facial symmetry after zygomatic bone fracture management. *J Oral Maxillofac Surg*. 2018;76(3):595-604.

Chapter | 21 |

# Computer-assisted surgical planning and navigation in cranio-orbital tumor resection

*Julio Acero, Patricia de Leyva*

**CHAPTER OUTLINE**



## Introduction

The cranio-orbital region is a complex anatomical area that accommodates structures of great functional importance such as the brain, the internal carotid artery and the cavernous sinus, the optic nerves, and chiasm or the globe. This region can be affected by a variety of tumors that can originate primarily or spread through the anatomical pathways from neighboring structures. Treatment of tumors of the cranio-orbital region is a challenge for the surgeon. In fact, it remains the most complex and controversial aspect of head and neck surgery in terms of disease control and reconstruction.[1] Access and visualization in this area are usually limited and a complete exposure of the surgical site is often difficult to achieve.[2] Endoscopic approaches to the skull base have been introduced with success although open approaches are still necessary in many situations.[3,4] For these reasons, oncologic surgery of the cranio-orbital region and skull base must be carefully evaluated and planned, and the reconstructive approach must be thoroughly designed.[5] An optimal reconstruction of the resulting defect is essential to avoid severe complications, such as cerebrospinal fluid (CSF) leak and meningitis. Prior to the advent of computer-assisted design and computer-assisted manufacturing (CAD/CAM) surgery planning, outcomes after traditional surgical planning depended mostly on the surgeon's experience and were less predictable. Computer-assisted surgery constitutes a major breakthrough, being especially useful in the treatment of tumors affecting the craniofacial region.[4] Computer-assisted surgical planning (CaSP), design of the reconstruction and manufacturing of patient-specific implants (PSI) and cutting guides (CAD/CAM procedures) as well as surgical navigation, provide the possibility of an accurate three-dimensional (3D) preoperative planning of the oncological resection as well as performing complex reconstructions with highly predictable postoperative results. Navigation systems integrate the imaging with the surgical field, allowing the surgeon to visualize the actual position of a surgical pointer in real time on the monitor displaying the computed tomography (CT) and/or magnetic resonance imaging (MRI) data of the patient. It offers a more accurate approach to essential anatomical structures such as the optic nerve, the internal carotid artery, and the cavernous sinus, thus increasing safety of the procedure, which is a critical concept in cranio-orbital surgery. It is necessary to remark that although accurate 3D planning and computer-assisted surgery improve predictability and precision of the procedure, the technical complexity and additional cost could be a major drawback for many institutions.

## Clinical considerations

Management of cranio-orbital tumors requires a thorough knowledge of craniofacial anatomy. Careful presurgical planning including clinical examination, imaging techniques with CT scan and MRI, as well as angiography, if indicated, is mandatory. Radiological evaluation of the craniofacial skeleton should be performed with a submillimeter data set and reconstructed in the axial, coronal, and sagittal planes.[6,7]

The location, invasion, and tumor extension are determining factors in the selection of the surgical approach and resectability of the tumor itself and should be taken into account in preoperative planning. With the current software and tools, the margins of resection can be designed, and vital structures outlined preoperatively with great accuracy, in order to be intraoperatively navigated during tumor ablation, improving the precision of the resection, while minimizing damage to healthy tissue. Surgical planning allows for such resection to be performed with greater confidence when visual cues are absent. In addition, navigation helps reduce the risk of damaging surrounding vital structures. The coupling of real-time 3D-navigation and CaSP further enhances these advantages to provide real-time feedback.[8,9]

Furthermore, the incorporation of other imaging modalities, such as 3D-CT angiography, and MRI, into navigation surgery facilitates the comprehension of vital structures within the surgical field such as the internal carotid artery or the optic nerve. Important landmarks, such as the foramen ovale and foramen rotundum, can be outlined before surgery as well, to help anatomical orientation during the procedure.

As navigation at the skull base is not influenced by shifting of the brain or soft tissue, precision is greater than in other neurosurgical procedures. Once the system is calibrated, surgical navigation allows the enhancement of both surgical precision and accuracy owing to real-time confirmation of position, without the need to obtain additional intraoperative images that expose patients to additional radiation. The use of a navigation system also reduces the duration of surgery at radical resections, although it increases the preoperative preparation time.[10]

Regarding reconstruction, immediate repair of defects in the cranio-orbital region is needed to achieve an adequate aesthetic and functional result. Resections in the orbital region involving a lack of eye globe support need reconstruction of the orbital walls to ensure symmetry and function; in cases of orbital exenteration, filling of the defect is mandatory, in order to isolate the sinonasal cavity. Resections affecting the skull base also need isolation of the intracranial contents from the aerodigestive tract.

Depending on the size and location of the defect, local or regional flaps, such as galeal-pericranial or temporalis muscle flap, can be used. In cases of massive resections, microvascular flaps are usually preferred (either osteocutaneous or musculocutaneous free flaps).[11] In maxillary resections, fibular, scapular, and iliac crest flaps are the most suitable options.[10] In orbital exenterations, a temporalis flap can be chosen, or a bulkier flap such as an ALT or rectus abdominis flap. In cases of complex orbito-zygomatic craniectomies, PSIs provide better (and simpler, surgery-wise) aesthetic results. Computer-assisted surgery is a helpful tool in both the planning and designing of the reconstruction, and the intraoperative checking of the positioning of the flap according to the planning. Currently, high-resolution CT scan and magnetic resonance multiplanar imaging can be merged to visualize and virtually manipulate the tumor, which can be segmented and a preferred surgical margin outlined. A mirror image of the healthy side can be added, for example in cases of orbital exenterations or tumors requiring an orbitozygomatic craniectomy, to plan for a symmetrical reconstruction. A PSI can then be designed: titanium meshes for orbital wall reconstruction can be "drawn" as desired, or an STL (Standard Triangle Language) file can be imported, to fit a true-to-original reconstruction, or patient-specific titanium plates for the fibula segments. Even the cutting guides with drilling holes and screws with different lengths depending on the depth of the bone can be anticipated, providing the optimal angles for fibula flap osteotomies to easily match the desired 3D shape to achieve symmetry in the zygomatic area. Alternatively, a 3D-printing and rapid-prototyping technique can be used to prebend a standard titanium mesh on a stereolithographic model of the patient with the mirrored healthy orbit. This mesh is afterwards sterilized and ready to use, easily fitting into the orbital wall, thus minimizing intraoperative time. In the cranio-orbital region a similar procedure to produce a specific implant made of polyetheretherketone (PEEK) is very useful because of the intricate topography and characteristics of the region. Shape adaptability and biocompatibility make this material a great option to bear in mind when planning reconstruction of the orbital-maxillary-zygomatic and pterional/sphenoid wing area.[12,13] In reconstruction of the defect with microvascular bony flaps, CAS has been reported to significantly reduce time of flap ischemia as well as operative time, when compared with non-guided surgery.[10,14,15]

## Workflow for computer-assisted design/computer-assisted manufacturing

The workflow for CAD/CAM based cranio-facial oncologic resection is shown in Fig. 21.1.

## Computer-assisted design

Accurate planning of the resection and reconstruction is essential in order to obtain an adequate result in the surgical treatment of craniofacial tumors. Conventional surgical procedures are based mainly in the surgeon's experience and are often associated with imprecise oncologic and reconstructive results as well as certain intraoperative risks. A 3D preoperative plan provides accurate information on tumor location and relationship to critical anatomical structures such as the optic nerve, cavernous sinus, and so on as mentioned before in this chapter. Holographic models with mixed reality technology are being introduced in the computer-assisted planning workflow and will contribute to a better understanding of each case. Moreover, the design of safer resection margins at the workstation is possible with this technology as well as computer-assisted preoperative planning of the reconstruction in the craniofacial region with PSIs or bone flaps to repair the defect.

The following CAD planning sequence is based on a case of relapsing fibrous dysplasia with massive orbital involvement (Fig. 21.2A) (Video 21.1, Video 21.2).

## Computer-assisted manufacturing and intraoperative navigation

The surgical planning is transferred into the surgical field in order to reproduce the surgical project, thus performing an accurate excision of the tumor and the correct reconstruction of the bone resection. Osteotomy cutting guides are manufactured using 3D printing procedures in order to transfer the resection planning and the design of a bone flap, if indicated. Rapid prototyping models (Fig. 21.3) can be printed out to better understand the resection and to perform a preoperative modeling of fixation plates or titanium implants. Also, especially in complex cases, direct production of the PSI from the computer-assisted plan can be performed as a routine procedure, thus avoiding the necessity of printing an intermediate model. Although an accurate transferring of the resection planning can be performed by means of the cutting guides in cases of accessible surfaces, such as the external surface of the zygomatic bone and the frontotemporal region, in complex defects involving deep areas of the orbit and the

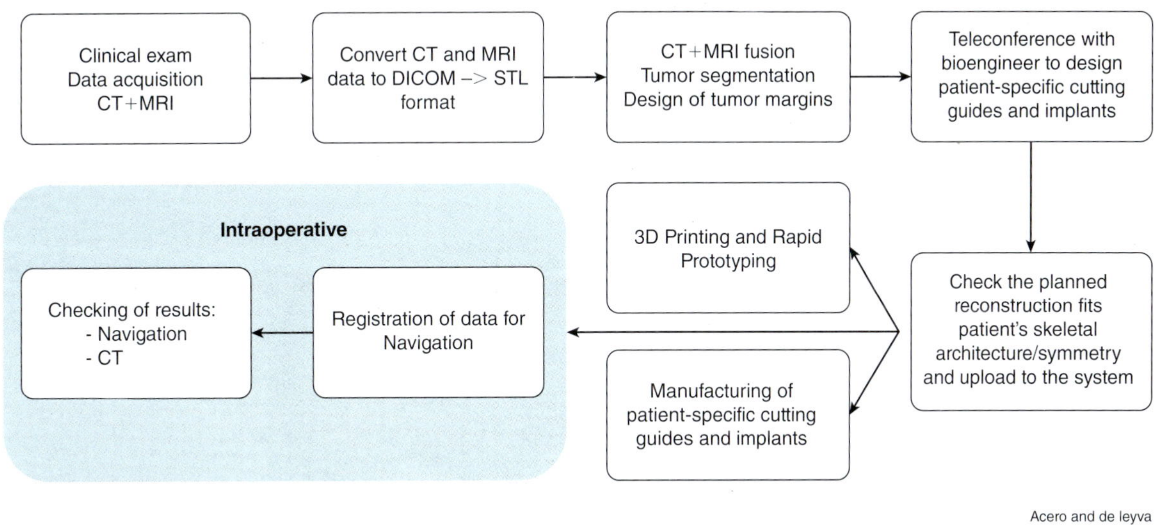


**Fig. 21.1** Workflow for computer-assisted design and computer-assisted manufacturing based cranio-facial oncologic resection.

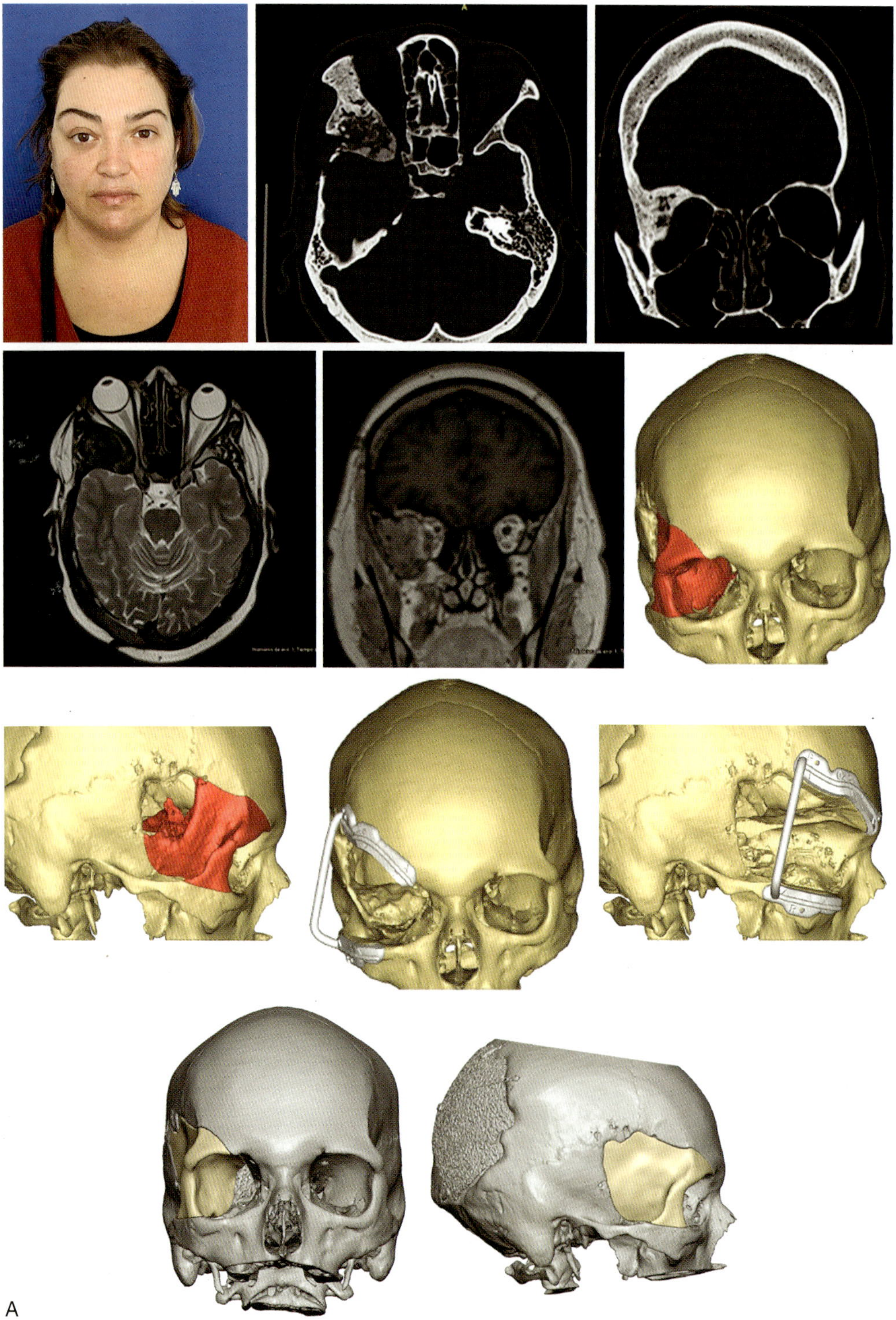

A

**Fig. 21.2** (A) Computer-assisted design planning sequence.

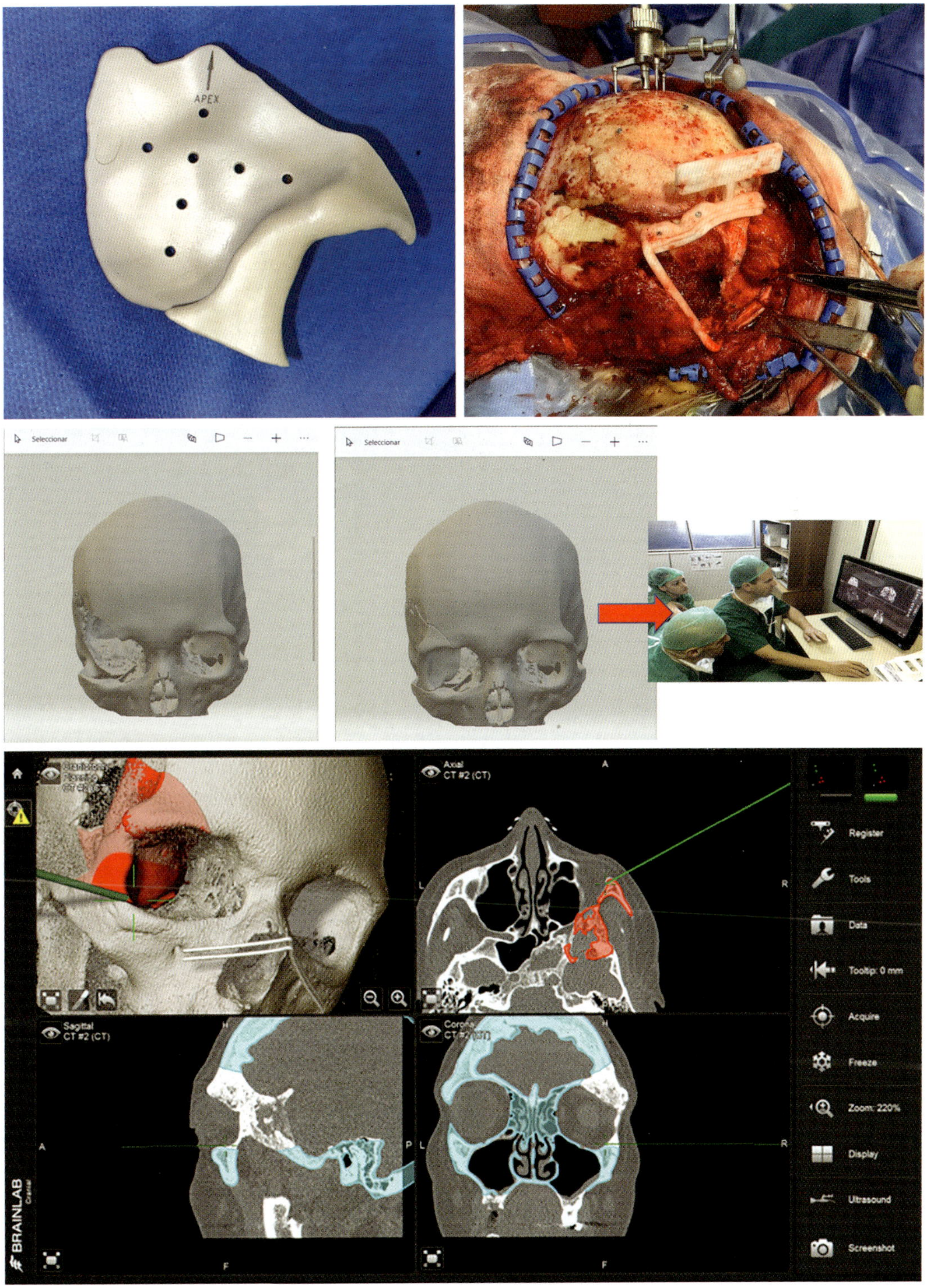


Fig. 21.2, cont'd (B) Computer-assisted manufacturing.

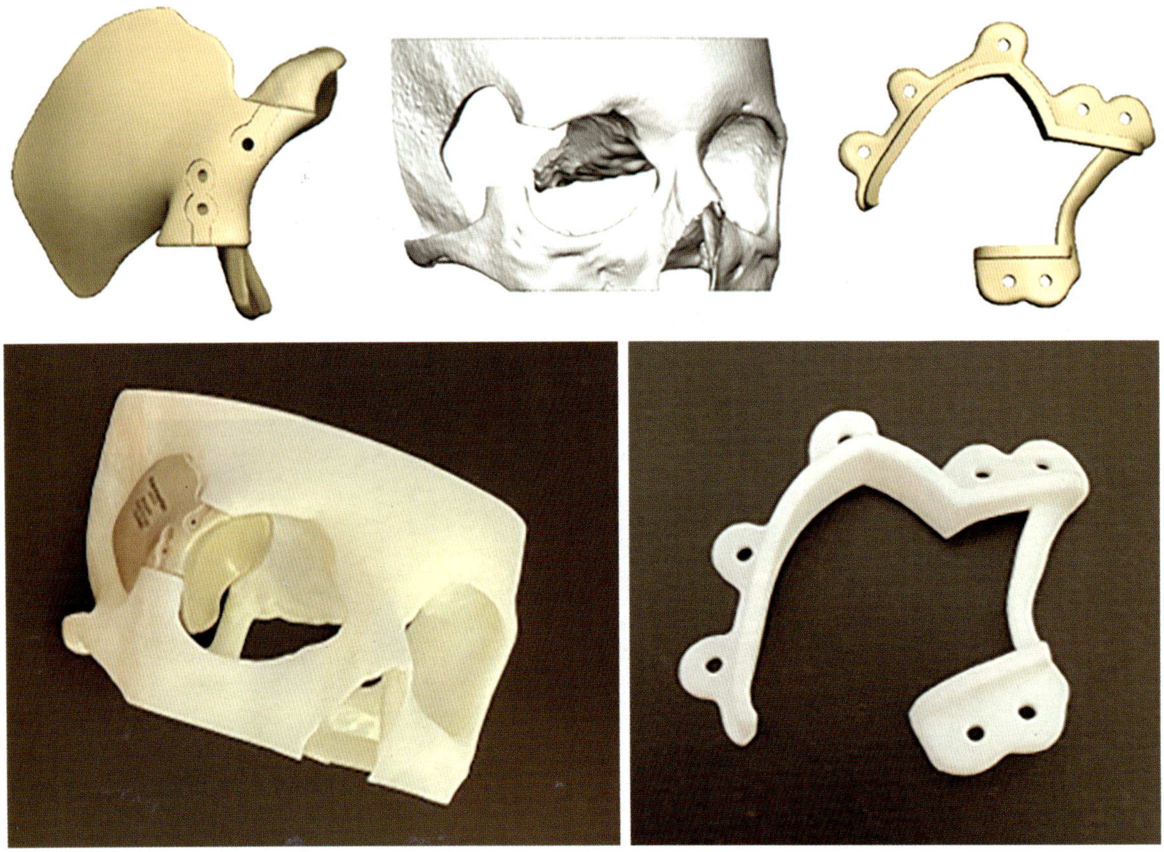

**Fig. 21.3** Computer-assisted planning and three-dimensional printed model.

skull base, navigation-assisted surgery contributes to the transfer and further execution of the previous planning (Fig. 21.2B).

## Operative technique

The operative steps of the procedure vary depending on the location and type of the tumor and the surgeon's preferred technique.

Steps:

- Registration of the patient with the navigation system.
- Approach: Endoscopic approaches, including recently the transorbital endoscopic approaches, are commonly used particularly for the resection of lesions affecting the central skull base and have also been described to excise tumors located in the infratemporal fossa and other locations.[16-18] In cases of complex resections, such as those involving the skin, extensive orbital resections, or where there is need for a complex reconstruction, open approaches are indicated. A coronal or an antero-lateral craniofacial approach is usually used for access to complex cranio-orbital resections. A temporary osteotomy of the lateral orbital wall, including the lateral orbital rim (orbitozygomatic approach), provides access to the orbital contents while preserving the bone anatomy of the orbit once the osteotomized fragment is replaced. A pterional craniotomy is frequently used by the neurosurgeon to access the intracranial component of the lesion. Combined approaches, such as the intraoral or transmandibular approaches, could be necessary in cases of extended resections, including maxillectomy or orbital exenteration.
- Coronal approach
  - Anesthetic solution with lidocaine, adrenaline, and saline solution can be infiltrated to reduce bleeding and facilitate separation of the subgaleal plane.

- A coronal incision is performed 2 to 3 cm behind the hairline, extending into the preauricular area if needed. If a hemicoronal incision is chosen (in cases of orbitozygomatic approaches, for example) the incision can be slightly curved anteriorly in the midline.
- The subgaleal plane is reached and the loose areolar tissue bluntly dissected. Raney clips are placed along the incision edges for hemostasis. The dissection is carried supraperiostally to preserve an anteriorly based pericranial flap that can be later used to seal the frontal sinus or intracranial structures or to cover the repaired defect.
- A change to a deeper plane at the level of the zygomatic arch and an angulation of 45 degrees anteriorly is needed in order to avoid damage to the frontalis branch of the facial nerve. Dissection is then carried as far as needed, reaching even the frontonasal suture, the supraorbital rim, the zygomatic bone, and the lateral aspect of the floor of the orbit, completely exposing the zygomatic arch.

- Combined coronal and transconjunctival approach
  - This is the authors' preferred approach for maxillary tumors or skull base tumors extended to an orbit needing exenteration while the eyelids and conjunctiva can be preserved. This technique, recently published, avoids midfacial cutaneous incisions combining a coronal or intraoral approach with a perilimbic-transconjunctival incision, sparing the eyelids and the conjunctiva to eventually fit an ocular prosthesis.[19]
- Intraoral approach
  - In cases of mid-facial tumor resections combined with orbitocranial tumors, intraoral is usually the approach of choice. It can be combined, if needed, with a coronal or an antero-lateral craniofacial approach.
  - An incision in the oral vestibule is performed followed by the subperiosteal exposure of the maxillary bone. A conventional or piezoelectric saw can be used to cut through the maxillary bone to carry out an osteotomy to access the deep retromaxillary regions, or in case of tumors affecting the upper jaw, to perform the resection with adequate margins.
  - If the eye globe is to be spared, care must be taken to protect the orbital contents with a soft tissue retractor.

- Tumor resection. Following the approach, the excision of the tumor is executed. Resection guides and/or navigation-assisted surgery ensure that the resection is performed according to the preoperative planning.
- Immediate reconstruction is performed after tumor resection based on the preoperative planning. Depending on the size of the defect, isolation of the intracranial contents can be achieved with the use of regional or microvascular flaps. In case of bone reconstruction, fixation of the PSI or the bone flap is performed with low-profile miniplates. A lateral canthopexy can be necessary in cases of lateral orbit reconstruction with eyelid preservation. Finally, the reconstructed area is covered with a galeal-pericranial flap, if possible, to provide a uniform surface over the reconstruction. Drains are placed and, finally, the skin incision is sutured.

## Clinical case

Our protocol for computer-assisted surgery including CAD/CAM procedures and navigation has been described in this chapter based on the description of a case of a 38-year-old female affected by relapsing spheno-temporo-orbital fibrous dysplasia with extensive orbital involvement with severe exophthalmos and diplopia after four previous limited surgeries. Since complete excision of the lesion at the skull base was considered impossible, a subtotal resection was planned, aiming to remove the orbital component and to perform orbital decompression (Fig. 21.2A, 2B). Fig. 21.2C shows the intraoperative aspects of the navigation-guided resection followed by immediate repair of the defect with a PEEK PSI fixed with miniplates. Intraoperative checking of the implant positioning was carried out, as will be described in the next section (Fig. 21.2D) and coverage of the reconstructed area was performed with the temporalis muscle and a galeal-pericranial flap without any complication and with a good postoperative result.

Fig. 21.4 shows a case of orbitocranial meningioma from computer-assisted planning to reconstruction with a PSI. A case of orbital adenoid cystic carcinoma with craniofacial surgical resection and reconstruction with a microvascular fibula flap is shown in Fig. 21.5.

## Fidelity/verification

Checking of the accuracy of the resection and the reconstruction implant positioning should ideally be carried out intraoperatively in craniofacial tumor surgery. This is accomplished in our protocol by checking in the navigation system the resection margins compared with the previously planned resection. Intraoperative CT imaging can also contribute to checking the accuracy of the bone resection and the reconstruction results (Fig. 21.2D,

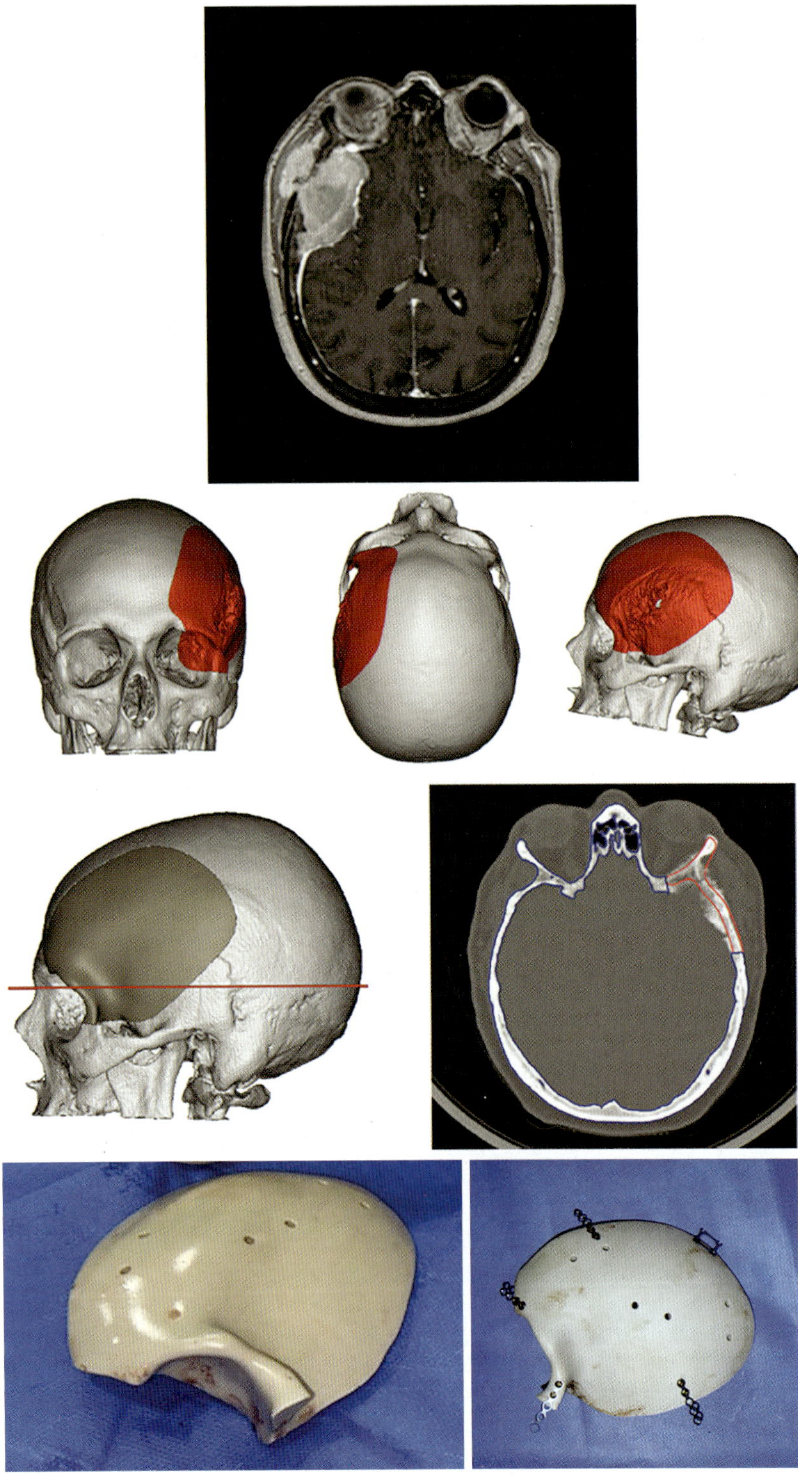

Fig. 21.4 Orbitocranial meningioma case.

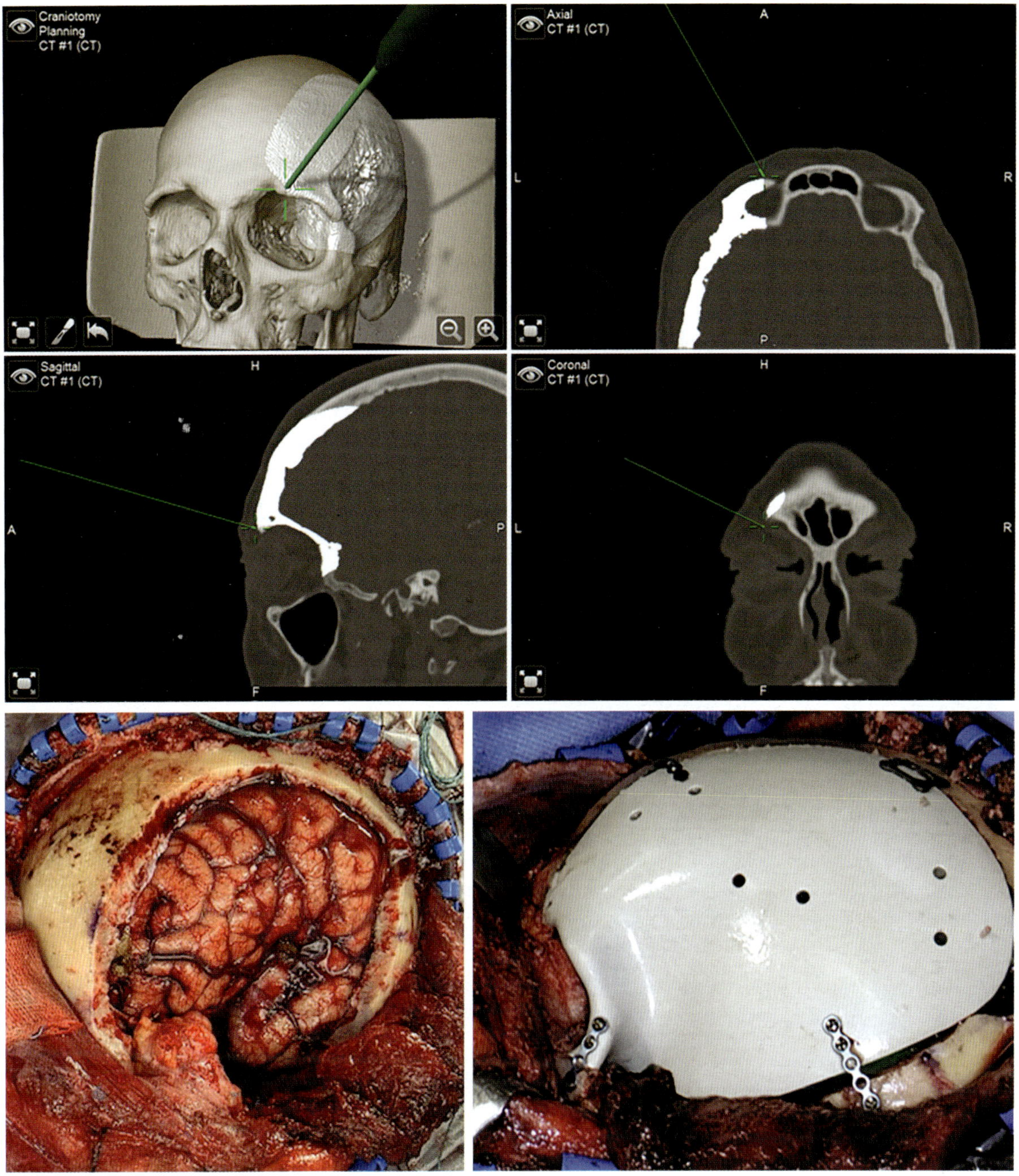


Fig. 21.4, cont'd

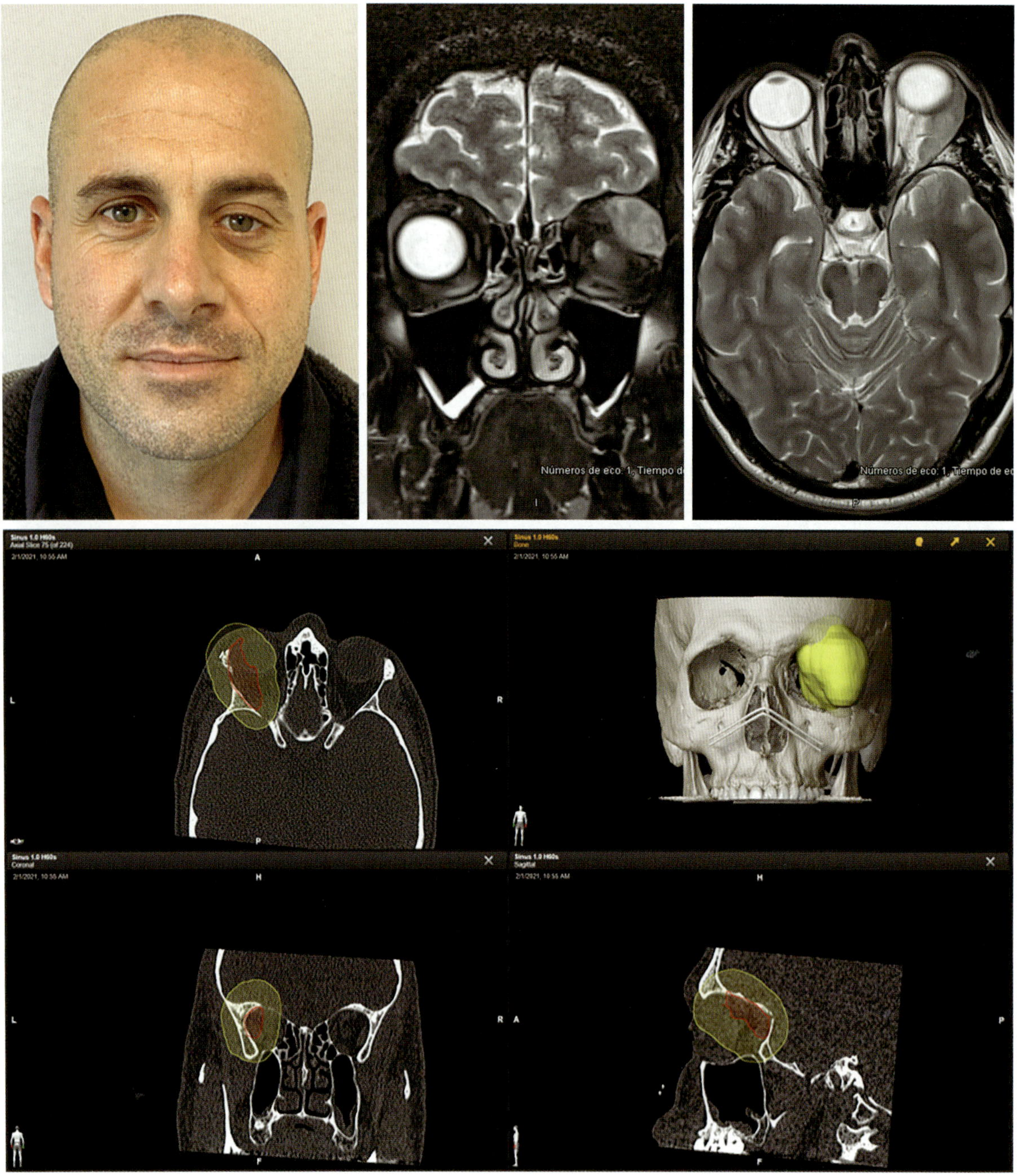


**Fig. 21.5** Orbital adenoid cystic carcinoma. Craniofacial resection and fibula flap microvascular reconstruction.

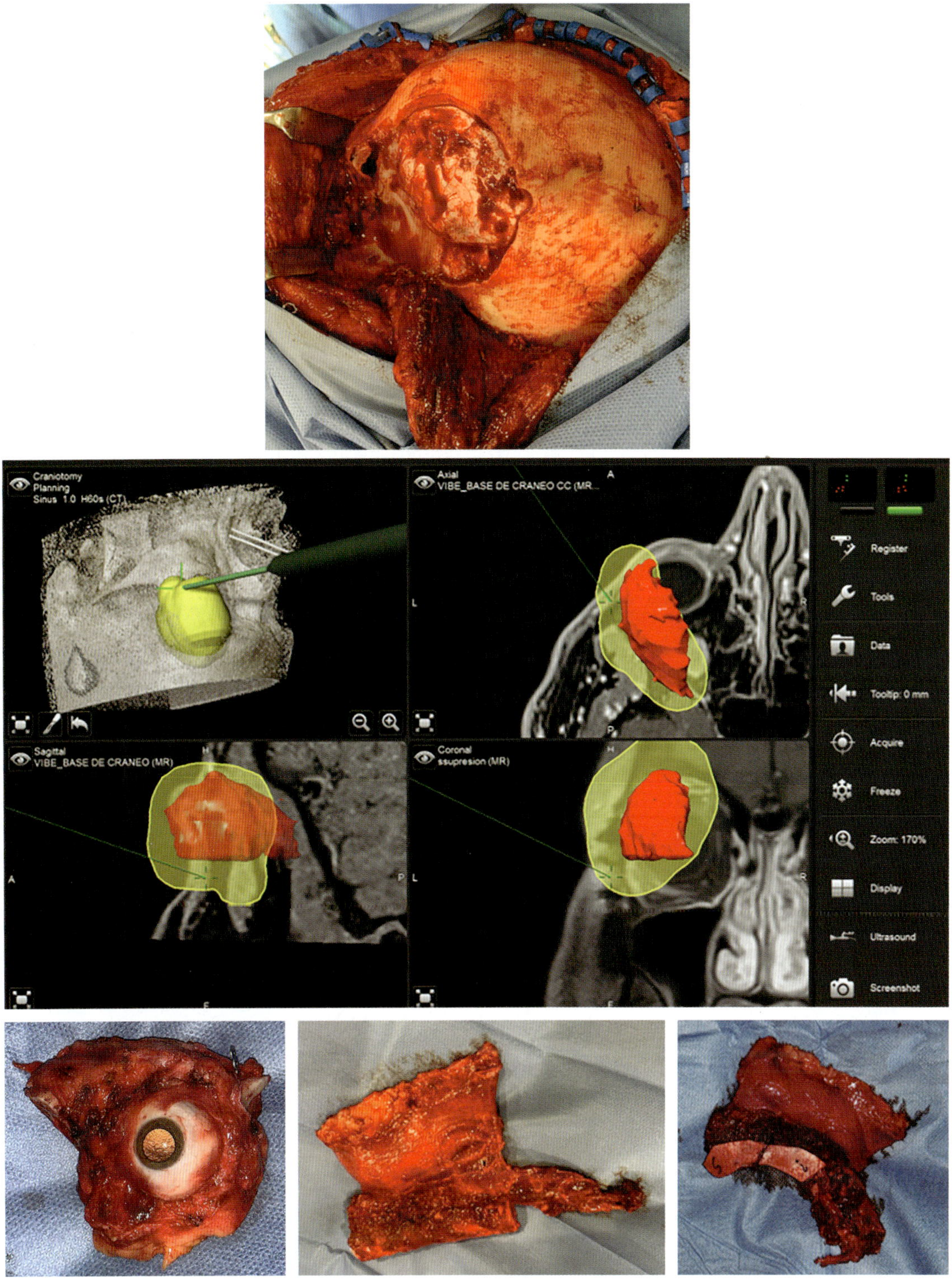


Fig. 21.5, cont'd

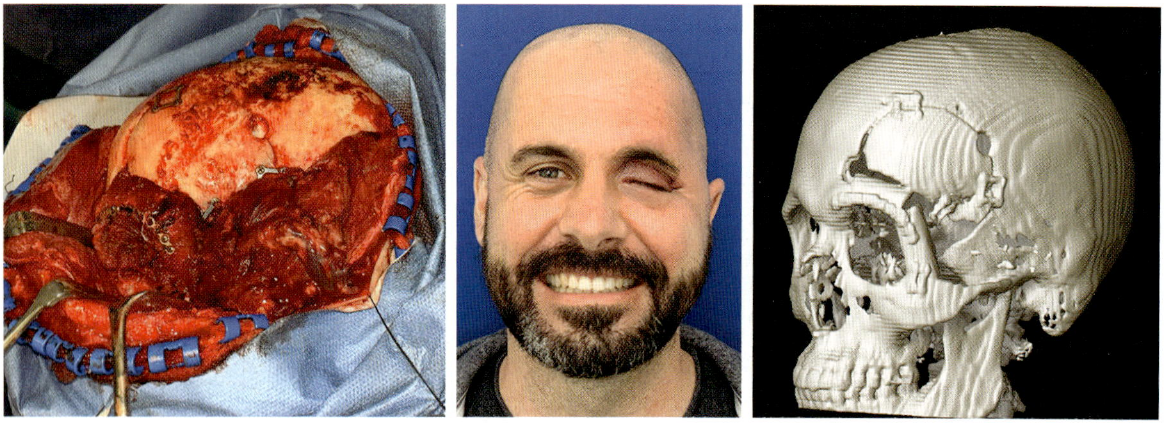

Fig. 21.5, cont'd

Video 21.3). Superimposition of the intraoperative CT image with the computer-assisted planning of the resection and reconstruction shows the consistency of the final result with the planned operation. Fig. 21.6 shows the malposition of an implant at the intraoperative control after reconstruction of another case of spheno-orbital meningioma, allowing for the intraoperative correction of the implant situation. If intraoperative imaging is not available, a postoperative CT should be performed, which could also be necessary in case of

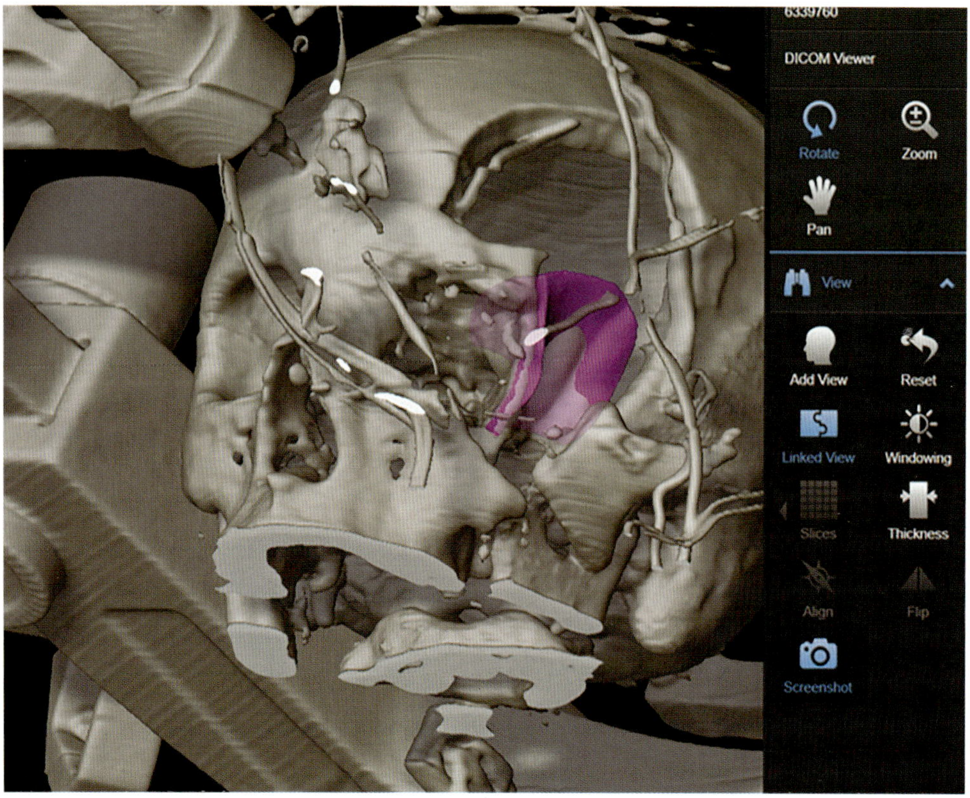


**Fig. 21.6** Verification 2.

intracranial combined procedures in order to control the postoperative evolution.

## Pearls/pitfalls

- CaSP allows a better understanding of the tumor outline, its relationship with vital structures, and the best surgical approach. The desired tumor margins can also be designed and later navigated.
- CAD implants or flaps enhance the reconstruction results.
- Computer-assisted surgery and navigation provide a better orientation of the surgeon in the surgical field allowing the accurate visualization of the actual position of a surgical instrument in the surgical field while resecting a tumor in the craniofacial region.
- Patients' safety increases since vital structures can be securely avoided.
- Achievement of the planned resection margins can be checked intraoperatively.
- Accuracy of reconstruction according to the preoperative plan can be checked intraoperatively and adjustments made if needed.
- Computer-assisted surgery and navigation devices are expensive tools, which means this technology is not available everywhere.
- CaSP can be lengthy, requiring investment in additional preoperative time.
- The manufacturing process can result in delays in the delivery of implants/guides.

## Outcomes/complications

Traditional procedures to excise tumors in the complex orbitocranial region are mainly based on the surgeon's experience, and the resection and repair of the defect can be unpredictable. Preoperative computer design, 3D modeling, and intraoperative navigation provide a useful guide for more accurate and safe tumor excision and true-to-plan reconstruction. Computer-assisted designed and manufactured implants can avoid the use of autogenous bone grafting, thus reducing morbidity and operating time. Surgical navigation is a time-consuming tool, and where the surgeon is on the learning curve in the use of this technique can affect the implementation of this technology, even though at some point in the learning curve the overall operation time will speed up.[20,21]

Surgical navigation accuracy depends on preoperative calibration. The optimal method for the most accurate triangulation has been suggested to be fixed registration points. It should be mentioned that an acceptable margin of error is less than 1 mm and for this, a fixed skeletal reference tool is recommended. During surgery the reference array could accidentally lose its fixation and the registered configuration of the system can be altered causing a loss of accuracy that can lead to errors, therefore the surgeon must continuously check the accuracy of the system configuration.[22]

Tumors with soft tissue involvement are a challenging indication for surgical navigation as they are bound to deformation.

## Conclusion

Computer-assisted surgery, including preoperative planning of tumor excision and reconstruction, design and manufacturing of 3D models or patient-specific implants, navigation, and digital intraoperative imaging allow the surgeon to achieve more accurate and safer results in cranio-orbital tumor surgery, as well as to obtain an optimal aesthetic and functional result. In addition, surgical time can be reduced with these tools, minimizing patient exposure and general anesthesia and associated complications.

Intraoperative CT imaging and navigation can help to check the correct resection margins as well as the accuracy of the reconstruction.

## Take-home points

- CAD/CAM technology provides excellent tools to visualize and predict an effective surgical approach and reconstructive plan in resection of cranio-orbital tumors.
- Computer-assisted surgery contributes to improve surgical efficiency and safety, helping to identify and protect vital structures, minimizing complications, and reducing operating time.
- Although each step of the workflow process is critical, meticulous planning procedures will increase success and accuracy in the operating room.

## References


1. Brown JS, Shaw RJ. Reconstruction of the maxilla and midface: Introducing a new classification. *Lancet Oncol*. 2010;11(10): 1001-1008.
2. Acero J, Maza C, Salmerón J, Ochandiano S. In: Vila CN, ed. *Reconstructive Oral and Maxillofacial Surgery*. Switzerland: Springer International Publishing; 2015:228.
3. Alokby G, Casiano RR. Endoscopic resection of sinonasal and ventral skull base malignancies. *Otolaryngol Clin North Am*. 2017;50(2):273-285.
4. Hanna E, DeMonte F, Ibrahim S, Roberts D, Levine N, Kupferman M. Endoscopic resection of sinonasal cancers with and without craniotomy: oncologic results. *Arch Otolaryngol Head Neck Surg*. 2009;135(12):1219-1224.
5. Acero J, de Leyva P. Computer assisted surgery and navigation in cranio-orbital resection and reconstruction. In: Acero J, ed. *Innovations and New Developments in Craniomaxillofacial Reconstruction* [Internet]. Switzerland: Springer Nature; 2021:240. doi:10.1007/978-3-030-74322-2_9.
6. Bell RB. Computer planning and intraoperative navigation in cranio-maxillofacial surgery. *Oral Maxillofac Surg Clin N Am*. 2010;22(1):135-156.
7. Schmitt PJ, Barrett DM, Christophel JJ, Leiva-Salinas C, Mukherjee S, Shaffrey ME. Surgical perspectives in craniofacial trauma. *Neuroimaging Clin N Am*. 2014;24(3):531-552.
8. Yu H, Shen SG, Wang X, Zhang L, Zhang S. The indication and application of computer-assisted navigation in oral and maxillofacial surgery – Shanghai's experience based on 104 cases. *J Cranio-Maxillofac Surg*. 2013;41(8):770-774.
9. Wilkat M, Kübler N, Rana M. Advances in the resection and reconstruction of midfacial tumors through computer assisted surgery. *Front Oncol*. 2021;11:719528.
10. Wang YY, Fan S, Zhang HQ, Lin ZY, Ye JT, Li JS. Virtual surgical planning in precise maxillary reconstruction with vascularized fibular graft after tumor ablation. *J Oral Maxillofac Surg*. 2016;74(6):1255-1264.
11. Macía G, Picón M, Nuñez J, Almeida F, Alvarez I, Acero J. The use of free flaps in skull base reconstruction. *Int J Oral Maxillofac Surg*. 2016;45(2): 158-162.
12. Lv M, Yang X, Gvetadze SR, Gupta A, Li J, Sun J. Accurate reconstruction of bone defects in orbital–maxillary–zygomatic (OMZ) complex with polyetheretherketone (PEEK). *J Plast Reconstr Aesthet Surg*. 2022; 75(5):1750-1757.
13. Jalbert F, Boetto S, Nadon F, Lauwers F, Schmidt E, Lopez R. One-step primary reconstruction for complex craniofacial resection with PEEK custom-made implants. *J Craniomaxillofac Surg*. 2014;42(2):141-148.
14. Powcharoen W, Yang WF, Yan Li K, Zhu W, Su YX. Computer-assisted versus conventional freehand mandibular reconstruction with fibula free flap: A systematic review and meta-analysis. *Plast Reconstr Surg*. 2019;144(6):1417-1428.
15. Saad A, Winters R, Wise MW, Dupin CL, St Hilaire H. Virtual surgical planning in complex composite maxillofacial reconstruction. *Plast Reconstr Surg*. 2013;132(3):626-633.
16. Abdelmeguid AS, Raza SM, Su SY, et al. Endoscopic resection of sinonasal malignancies. *Head Neck*. 2020;42(4):645-652.
17. Reshef ER, Bleier BS, Freitag SK. The endoscopic transnasal approach to orbital tumors: A review. *Semin Ophthalmol*. 2021; 36(4):232-240.
18. Krischek B, Carvalho FG, Godoy BL, Kiehl R, Zadeh G, Gentili F. From craniofacial resection to endonasal endoscopic removal of malignant tumors of the anterior skull base. *World Neurosurg*. 2014;82(suppl 6):S59-S65.
19. Acero J, de Leyva P, Almeida F, Núñez J, Picón M. The combined coronal–transconjunctival approach: An innovative surgical access for orbital exenteration in craniofacial resection. *Int J Oral Maxillofac Surg*. 2022;51(3): 300-306.
20. Goertz L, Stavrinou P, Stranjalis G, Timmer M, Goldbrunner R, Krischek B. Single-Step Resection of Sphenoorbital Meningiomas and Orbital Reconstruction Using Customized CAD/CAM Implants. *J Neurol Surg Part B Skull Base*. 2020;81(2):142-148.
21. Jalbert F, Boetto S, Nadon F, Lauwers F, Schmidt E, Lopez R. One-step primary reconstruction for complex craniofacial resection with PEEK custom-made implants. *J Cranio-Maxillo-fac Surg Off Publ Eur Assoc Cranio-Maxillo-fac Surg*. 2014;42(2):141-148.
22. Yang M, Wu Z, Yu H, Cheng J. Reconstruction for diverse fronto-orbital defects with computer-assisted designed and computer-assisted manufactured PEEK implants in one-stage operation: Case reports. *Medicine (Baltimore)*. 2021 8;100(40).

Chapter 22

# Computer-assisted surgical planning and navigation in maxillo-mandibular tumor resection

Max Wilkat, Majeed Rana

CHAPTER OUTLINE



## Introduction

Surgical treatment of maxillo-mandibular tumors aims for in-sano resection. Besides information about dignity (benign/malignant) and entity of the tumor provided via specimen taking and histopathological examination, the extent of the tumor is crucial for surgical treatment planning. Tumor extent is typically based on the clinical picture and radiological imaging. While localized and sharply circumscribed tumors can be resected relying on the clinical picture alone, more advanced tumor disease challenges the surgeon: the urge for a more extensive resection can be in conflict with the maintenance of important anatomical structures.

Computer-assisted surgical planning (CaSP) can help extract all the relevant information from radiological data sets by displaying the complex three-dimensional (3D) anatomy of the head and neck region and visualizing the tumor extent. In localizations where the radiological imaging is not certain, further pathohistological examination might be needed to elucidate the true tumor extent via tumor mapping. A trajectory-based surgical specimen taking using intraoperative navigation tools allows a minimally invasive approach combined with a precise localization of the uncertain anatomical areas marked in the CaSP. The pathological examination results, which are linked to the coordinates of the navigated specimen taking, can be transferred to the CaSP, thus enhancing the information content even further.

Segmentation of the tumor extent can be performed on the basis of these enhanced data sets. Adding a sufficient 3D resection margin depending on the tumor entity, while respecting critical anatomical structures, results in the display of the needed resection "wall" for both the soft and hard tissue. Regarding the bony part of the resection, cutting guides can be virtually designed and fabricated via rapid prototyping to transport the information of the virtually defined resection border into the theater. In cases of primary reconstruction, vector-based drilling guides for indexing the fixation holes for the patient-specific reconstruction plates can be added to these guides. Also, bony flap raising can be facilitated by designing and manufacturing harvesting guides, which help with the contouring and fixation of the transplant.

Compared to conventional "free-hand" resection, CaSP provides some advantages in facilitating the surgery (see Table 22.1). As long as high-quality 3D radiological data sets can be obtained, there is no medical contraindication for the use of CaSP in tumor resection. However, these techniques do not reflect the gold standard of pathohistology, which limits their use regarding the aim of curative oncological surgery: pathohistological R0-resection.

**Table 22.1 Advantages and disadvantages of using computer-assisted surgical planning and navigation in maxillo-mandibular tumor resection**

| Advantages | Disadvantages |
|---|---|
| Higher extraction rate of relevant information out of radiological imaging data sets | Limited by quality of radiological data sets/artifact disturbances |
| High accuracy for navigation and resection of bony tissue | Limited accuracy for navigation and resection of soft tissue |
| Better predictability of reconstruction result | Limited flexibility in cases of unforeseen tumor extent |
| Shorter operation time, shorter hospitalization | Higher preoperative planning time, higher preoperative personnel expenses during planning sessions |
| Overall cost might be balanced or even reduced | Higher costs for software licenses, computing devices, and manufacturing of guides and plates |
| Virtual operation procedure offers best preparation for actual surgery including recognition of complicated steps | Need for training in this new procedure |
| Demonstration of treatment plan offers higher transparency toward patients | Some patients might be intimidated by too much information/transparent treatment plan |
| Passing on of computer-assisted surgical planning (CaSP) treatment plan to radiotherapist or other treating disciplines offers better interdisciplinary exchange | Technical platform for interdisciplinary exchange needed |
| Valuable for younger surgeons with less experience, usable for medical teaching of students | Need for sufficient equipment, software licenses, etc. |
| Better quality control as surgical aim has been defined preoperatively | Surgery can only be as good as the CaSP has been |

## Clinical considerations

In the treatment of head and neck cancer a comprehensive staging is mandatory. This involves a complete history of other diseases, especially other entities of cancer, previous cancer treatments, or side diseases that limit the cancer treatment options, such as advanced cardiovascular or neurological disease. Clinical examination involves the inspection and palpation of the primary tumor formation, exclusion of second tumor formation, and palpation and ultrasound of the neck looking for lymph node metastasis. For completion of the staging with regard to primary tumor extent and cervical lymph node metastasis, further 3D radiological imaging of the head and neck region, from the skull base to the upper thoracic aperture, is needed. In cases of advanced disease a scan of the thorax and abdomen is recommended to rule out distant metastasis.

When it comes to CaSP, radiological scanning is key, as the whole procedure is based on these examinations. Therefore, a high-quality computed tomography (CT) scan following a standardized protocol is recommended, fulfilling certain criteria for tumor resection planning:

- Complete coverage of the relevant regions.
- Removal of all foreign bodies (dental prostheses, jewelry, face masks) to reduce artifacts.
- In case navigation is required, ensure correct prescan insertion of navigation markers.
- Reduction of movement artifacts in patients with neurological disorders, anxiety diseases, mental disabilities, dementia and children by use of sedation/narcosis.
- Biphasic contrast medium administration protocol (split bolus).
- Reconstruction of thin slices with a thickness of 1 mm or less.
- Means of reduction of metal artifacts (e.g., using single-energy-based metal artifact reduction).

A high-quality CT scan is the prerequisite for a high-resolution 3D surface model of the facial skull, which serves as the basis for the design of resection guides. Enhanced by contrast medium, this offers a good enough soft tissue contrast for differentiating tumor tissue. In cases of severe artifacts due to metallic dental restorations overshadowing the region of the tumor formation, information content is limited and has to be completed by the clinical picture. In case of reduced soft tissue contrast, a magnetic resonance imaging (MRI) scan should be obtained, which can be merged with the CT scan to combine the information content of both modalities.

In cases of planned navigated procedures, reference markers are needed either as transcutaneous bone-fixed screws (e.g., mandibulo-maxillary fixation [MMF] screws made of steel or titanium) or removable dental splints with osteosynthesis screws attached to the splint. If these reference markers have not been in place during the initial scan, another cone-beam CT scan with inserted reference markers is sufficient and can be merged with the initial scan. If navigation is needed for the region of the mandible, a fixed reproducible position of the lower jaw in relation to the upper jaw and skull base is obligatory. This can be achieved by fixation in occlusion (habitual if well defined or with a bite splint) or, if an open mouth is needed during navigation, inserting a patient-specific bite wedge during the CT scan and during surgery.

In cases of primary bony reconstruction, a CT scan of the donor site is needed, which has to match similar criteria mentioned above. In particular, a reconstruction of thin slices with a thickness of 1 mm or less is needed for well-fitting harvesting guides. Moreover, contrasting in the arterial phase gives insight into potential peripheral artery disease which might expel transplant harvesting due to insufficient vascular supply of the donor region.

In summary, close cooperation with the radiologist is recommended to prevent unnecessary repetition of examinations and thus minimize radiation exposure, avoid unnecessary delay of treatments, save costs and time, and avoid staff overload and patient frustration.

## Workflow of computer-assisted design/computer-assisted manufacturing

Please see Fig. 22.1 and ppt 22.1.

## Computer-assisted design

Please see Figs. 22.2–22.4,Video 22.1, and ppt 22.2.

## Computer-assisted manufacturing

Please see Figs. 22.5–22.8 and Video 22.1.

## Operative technique

Please see Figs. 22.9–22.14, ppt 22.1 and 22.2, and Video 22.2.

## Fidelity/verification

Please see Fig. 22.15.

## Pearls/pitfalls

- Low-quality data sets insufficient for the anatomical region with artifacts or inappropriate examination protocol (slices too thick, wrong modality) are no basis for CaSP and CAD/CAM leading to bad fitting of guides and plates for tumor resection and reconstruction and should therefore be avoided.
- Other reasons for poor fit of the guides can be:
  - Imprecise segmentation of bone.
  - Design error, such as too few undercuts defining correct positioning.
  - Insufficient surgical exposure of positioning area.
  - Soft tissue interference.
- Surgical procedure and approach has to be kept in mind during computer-assisted designing: if too bulky, guides and plates might not be able to be put in place via the desired surgical approach. If too steep, posteriorly angulated drilling vectors might not be feasible if they interfere with overlying soft tissue.
- Limitation of the procedure must be kept in mind as it is still based on radiological data sets resulting in radiological resection margins, which do not equal pathohistological margins. The following tactics might help to balance this problem:
  - Further specimen taking at the periphery of the tumor mass as a diagnostic step before definitive tumor surgery, can be combined with means of navigation. Thus, the results of tumor mapping are transferred to CaSP leading to an enhanced data set comprising pathohistological information.
  - Taking frozen sections of the margins of the resection cavity.
  - The reconstruction plan should include some space for extending the resection if the margins are affected.

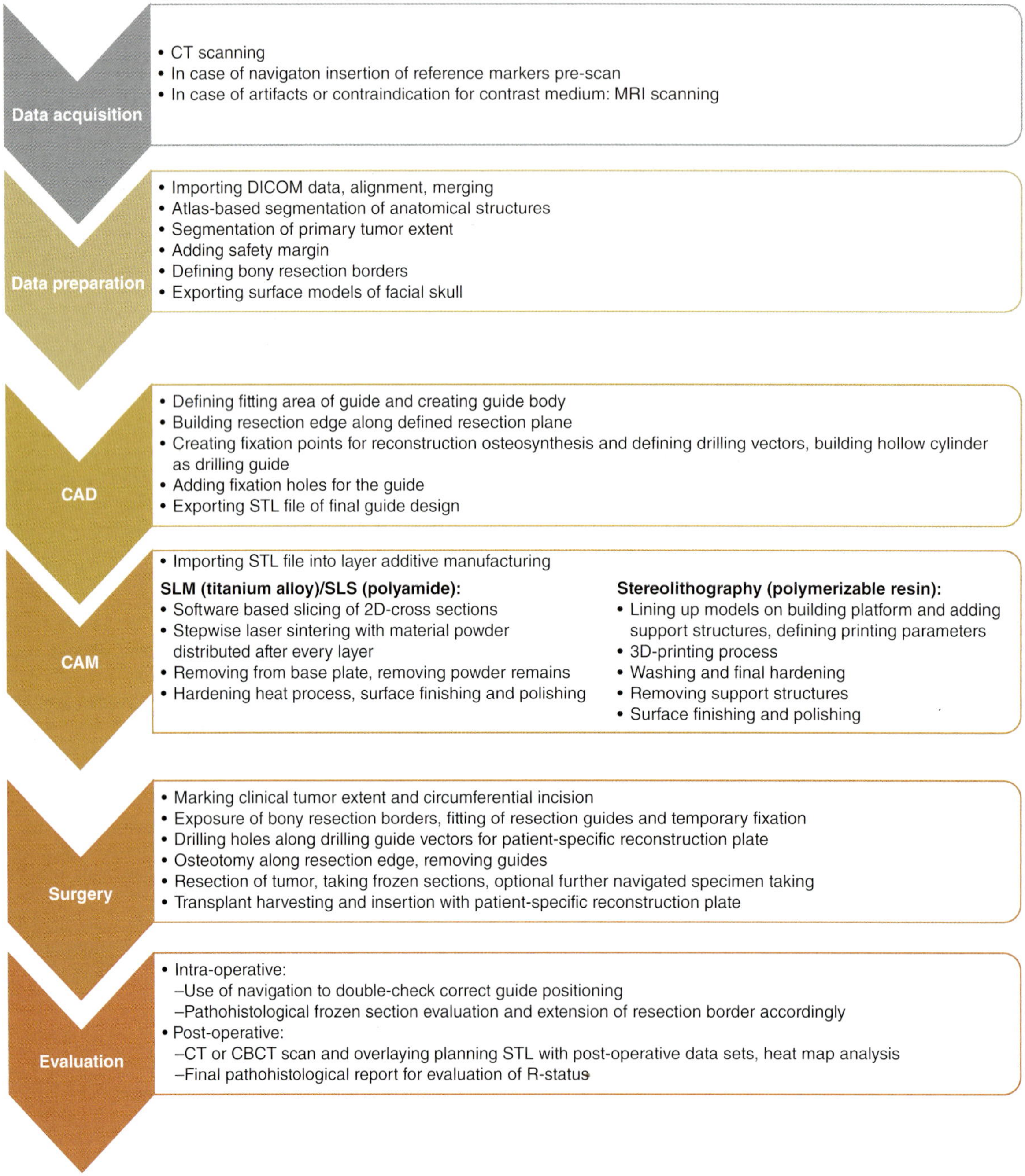


**Fig. 22.1** Flowchart for computer-assisted design/computer-assisted manufacturing (CAD/CAM) procedure of computer-assisted tumor resection. Some of these steps (data preparation, CAD/CAM) can conveniently be provided by an external company, and explicit planning steps can be discussed via a web-based communication platform or virtual meeting.

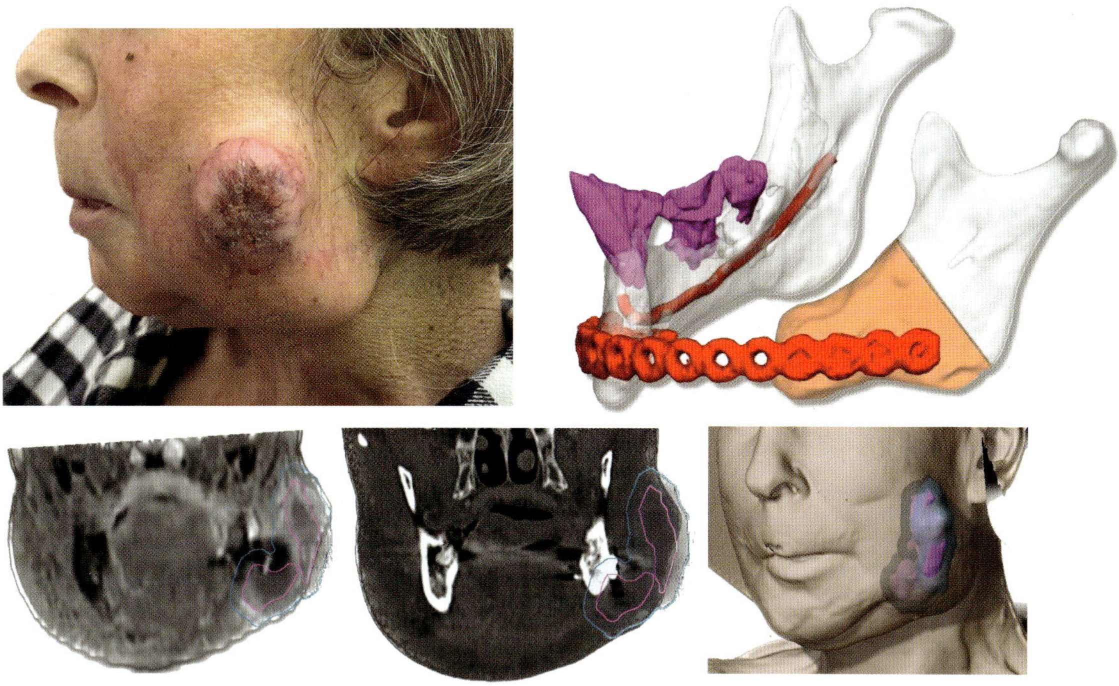

**Fig. 22.2** From clinic to computer-assisted surgical planning (CaSP). A 68-year-old patient with a fast growing, early recurrence of an oral squamous cell carcinoma located para- and submandibular on the left side with extension into the cheek. After a history of partial mandible resection on the left side with insertion of a pre-bent reconstruction plate and neck dissection level I–V left and level I–III right with adjuvant radiochemotherapy it was decided to perform salvage surgery using CaSP and computer-assisted design/computer-assisted manufacturing resection guides without primary bony reconstruction efforts. Acquired and merged magnetic resonance imaging and computed tomography scans enabled segmentation of the extension of the tumor mass (*purple*). After adding a three-dimensional (3D) safety margin (*blue*) the required resection borders were marked on a 3D surface model of the mandible. The orange part of the mandible was in need of resection along with removal of the former reconstruction plate (*red*).

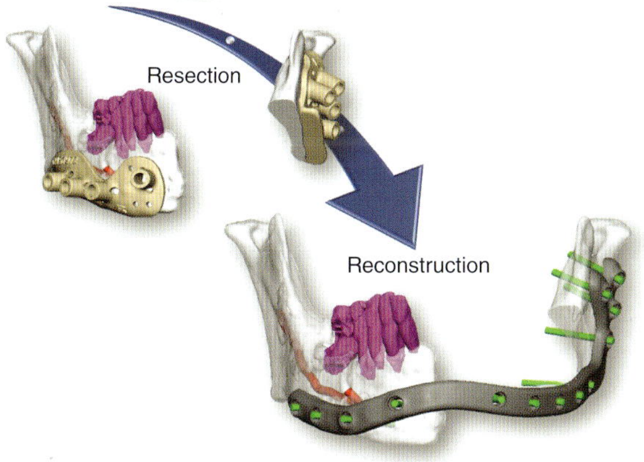


**Fig. 22.3** Planning steps for designing resection guides and reconstruction plate. Segmentation of certain structures is the first step in guide design, such as the bone to be resected (*orange*), osteosynthesis to be removed (*light red*) and anatomical structures to be preserved (teeth in *pink* and canal of the right inferior alveolar nerve in *dark red*). The guides are designed to cover the bone adjacent to the resection area to indicate the line of osteotomy. Guides should be extended to cover enough area for fixation of the reconstruction plate. The drilling holes need to follow certain vectors (*green*) which are designed to spare important anatomical structures, like teeth roots and nerves, yet traverse enough solid bone to ensure a fixation of the load-bearing fixation plate. The screw holes in the reconstruction plate need to follow the same vectors and offer enough thread height while maintaining a flat profile.

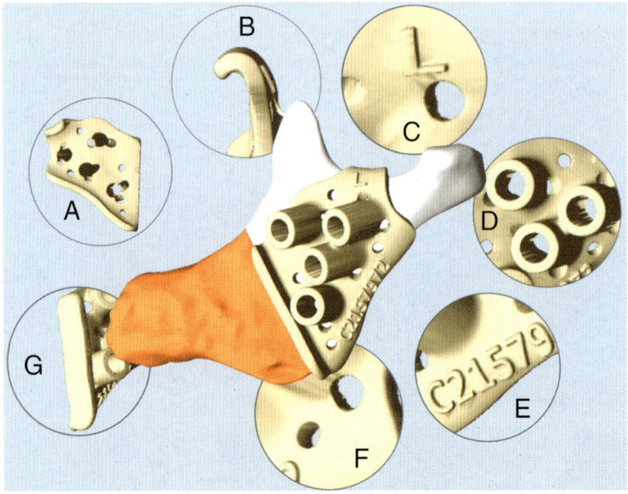


**Fig. 22.4** Features of computer-assisted design/computer-assisted manufacturing resection guides. (A) Back of the guide featuring the anatomical shape of the part of the bone that will not be resected. (Orange color indicates the bony part that needs to be resected). (B) Back spin as orientation for positioning the guide. (C) Labeling of the guide for differentiation of the particular guides. (D) Vector-guided drill holes for predrilling the fixation holes for the patient-specific reconstruction plate. (E) Labeling for identification of the correct case number. (F) Fixation holes for temporary fixation of the resection guide. (G) Cutting edge indicating the guided osteotomy line.

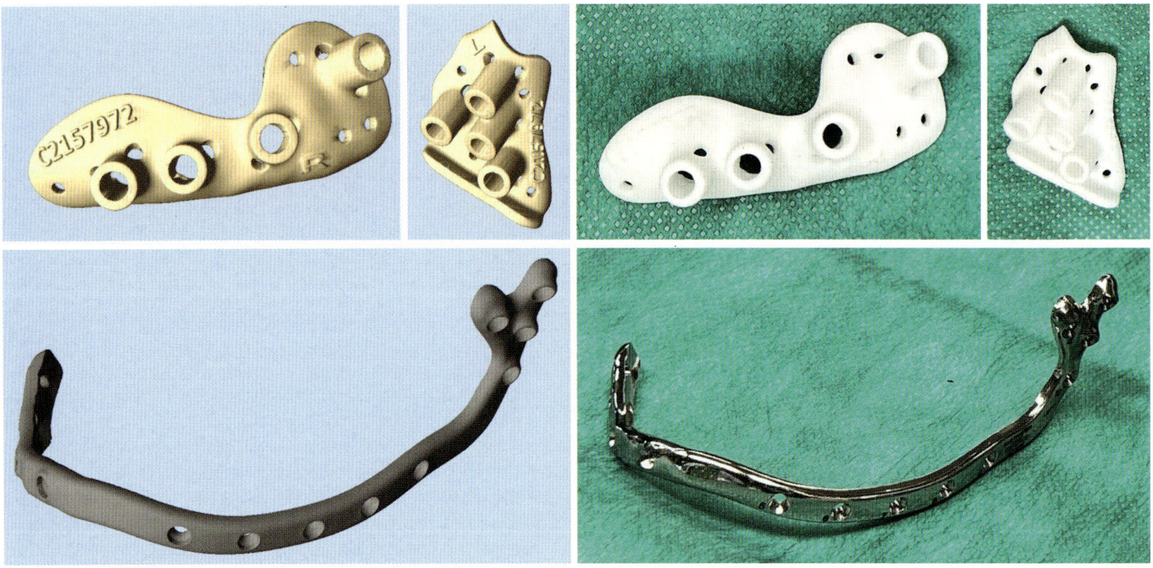

**Fig. 22.5** From computer-assisted design to manufactured workpieces. The final design can be exported as an STL file and serves as the three-dimensional building plan during the process of layer additive manufacturing. The resection guides were produced out of polyamide (PA12) via selective laser-sintering. The reconstruction plate was made of high-strength titanium alloy (Ti6Al4V) by selective laser-melting.

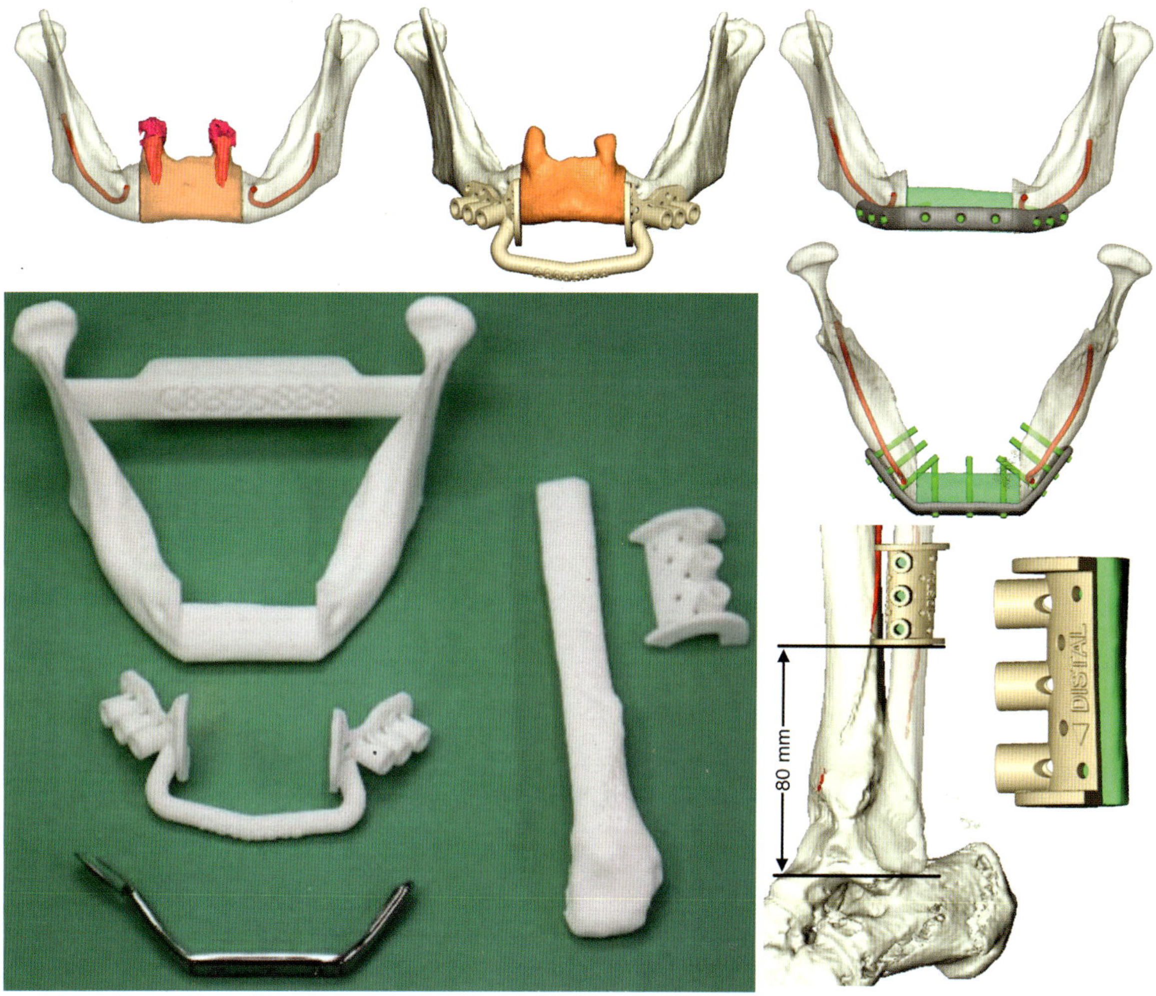


**Fig. 22.6** Case planning #1. A case of a squamous cell carcinoma of the alveolar ridge in-between the lower canines. After segmentation of the tumor and anatomical structures including the mandible and the inferior alveolar nerve (*red*), the segment in need of resection could be defined (*orange*). Design of the resection guides included grooves to spare the mental nerve at its bony exit point and a connection brace to ensure correct positioning, as single guides for each side might not find a reproducible fit. Drilling vectors are angulated to spare the nerves. Reconstruction with a fibula transplant was facilitated by introducing a harvest guide, which needed positioning with a distance of 80 mm from the lateral malleolus and allowed predrilling to fit the patient-specific reconstruction plate. Manufactured guides and reconstruction plate were accompanied by anatomical models of the mandible and distal fibula, which were produced via stereolithography out of polymerizing resin.

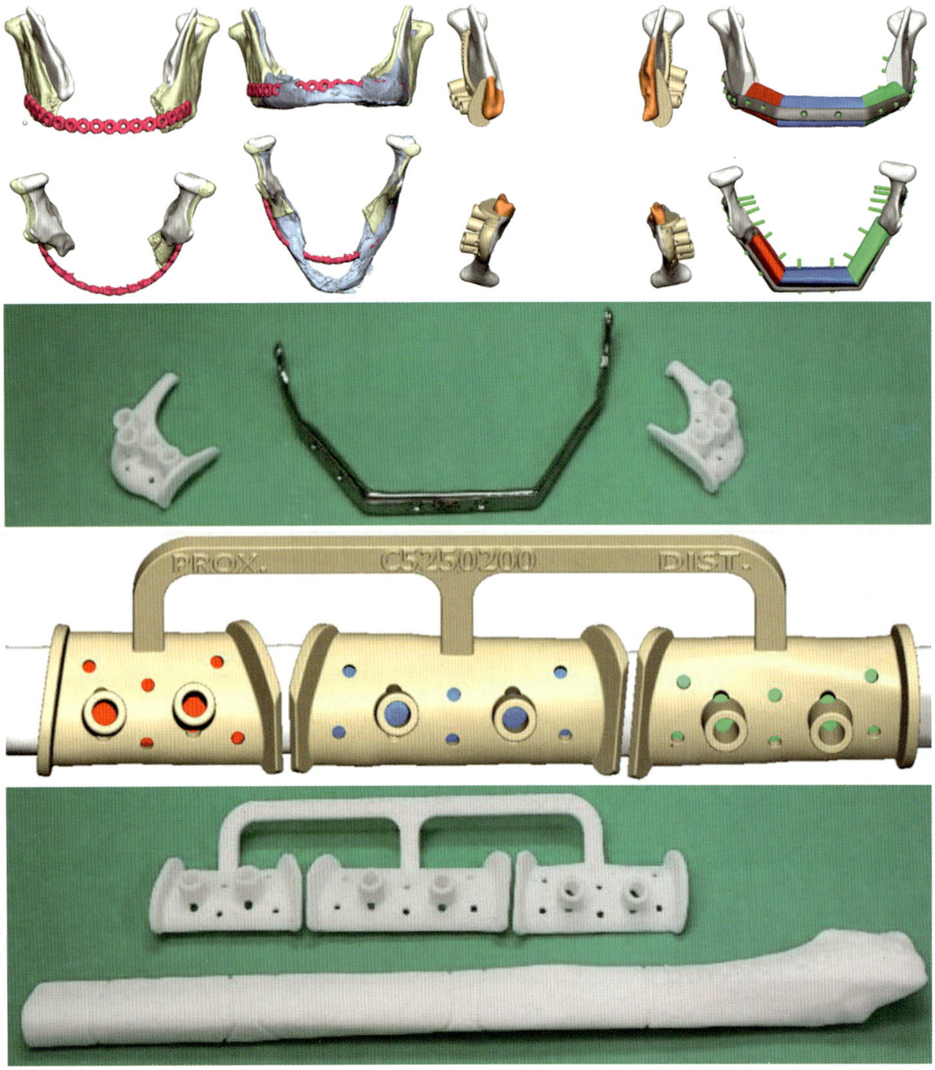


**Fig. 22.7** Case planning #2. With a history of partial resection of the mandible due to squamous cell carcinoma and primary reconstruction via a prebent reconstruction plate, this patient required a secondary reconstruction with a fibula graft to pave the way to dental rehabilitation. As the current situation (bone shown in *yellow*, prebent plate in *pink*) does not fit the starting position, visible by superimposing the initial mandible (*blue*), virtual repositioning of the mandibular condyles (*white*) was conducted to enable true-to-origin reconstruction. Guide and plate design were fitted accordingly with a three-segmented fibula graft to enable a profile resembling the anatomical alveolar arch.

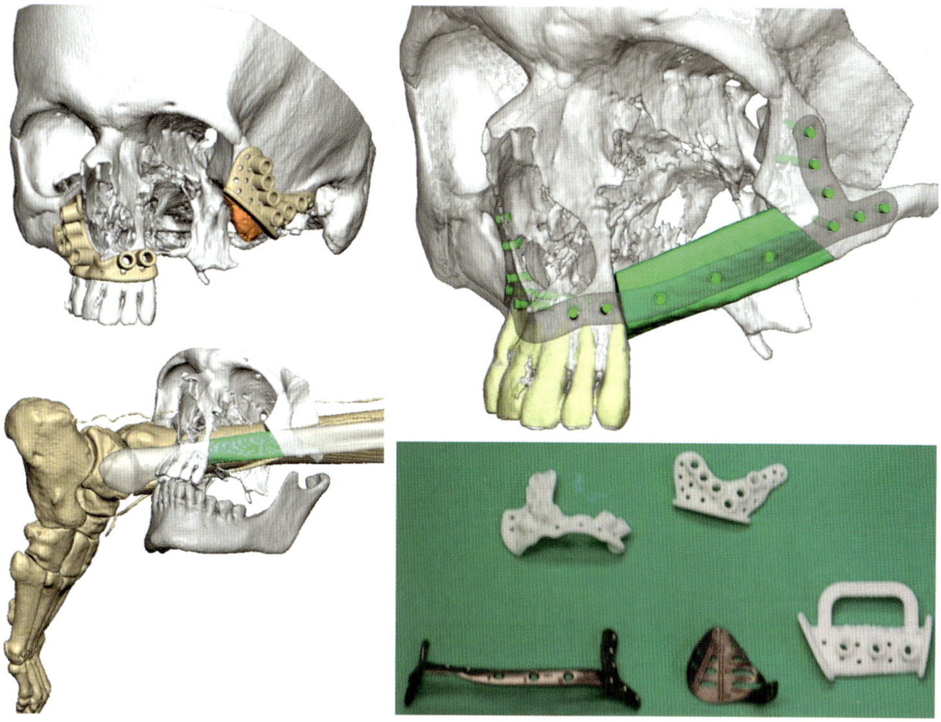

**Fig. 22.8** Case planning #3. This case of secondary reconstruction of the left maxilla demonstrates the design requirements for guides in the midface. Former Weber-Ferguson approach facilitated the exposure of the left zygoma to position the guide in this area. Drilling vectors were designed to fit the local bone quality and to spare dental roots. Virtual transplantation of the fibula graft provided the necessary information for the angulation of the cutting edge of the harvesting guide. The manufactured guides and reconstruction plate were accompanied by a patient-specific implant for reconstruction of the orbital floor which had been designed with recesses for drainage and grooves for intraoperative positioning control by trajectory navigation.

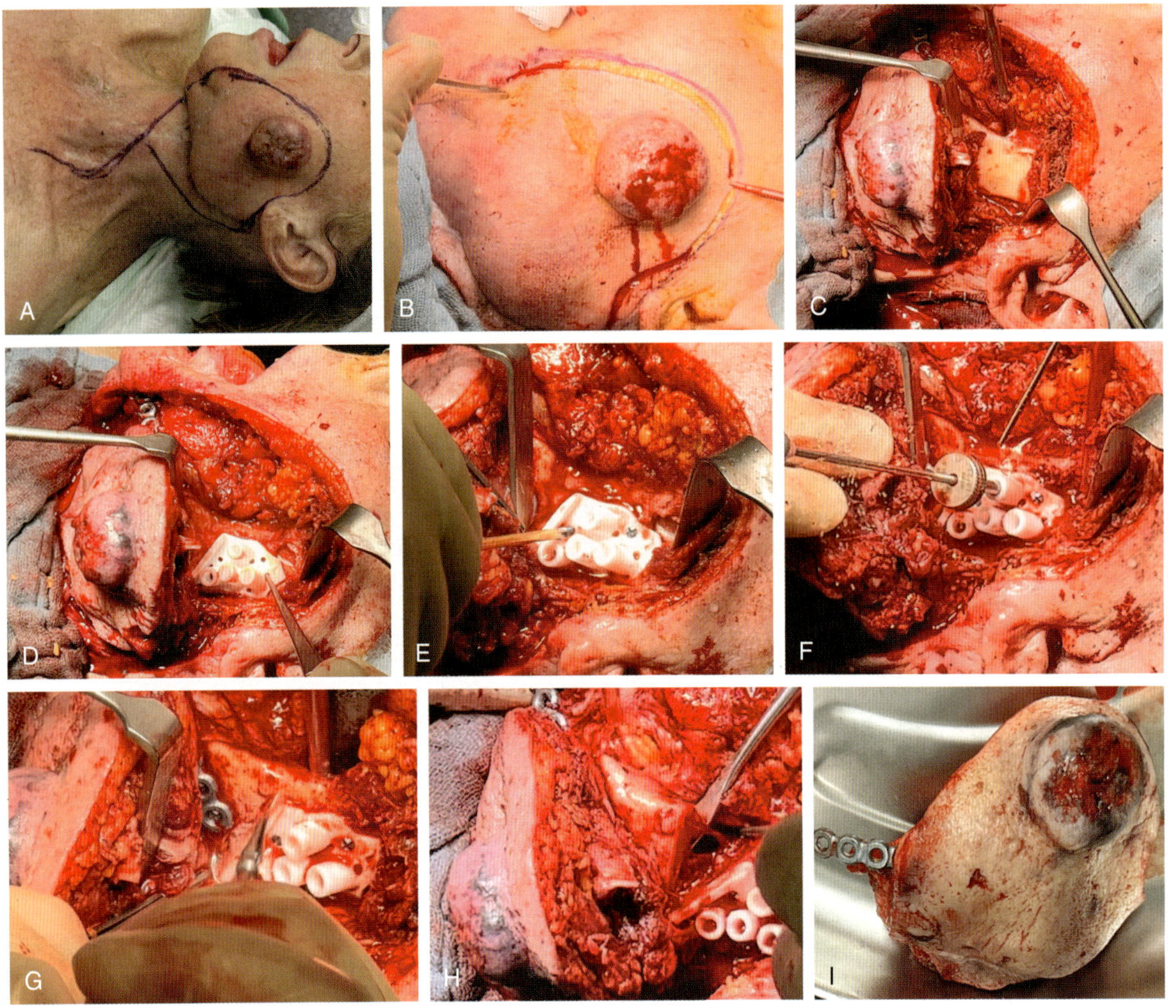


**Fig. 22.9** Steps of tumor resection using computer-assisted design/computer-assisted manufacturing resection guides during the surgical procedure of the previously mentioned case of recurrent oral squamous cell carcinoma – Part 1. computer-assisted design/ computer-assisted manufacturing (A) Marking of the incision line with a safety margin of 10 mm around the clinically visible and palpable tumor formation with the three-dimensionally tumor extent visualized in computer-assisted surgical planning in mind. (B) Skin incision. (C) Tissue preparation with exposure of the left ascending ramus. (D) Fitting of resection guide with special attention to prevent soft tissue interference. (E) The guide is fixed in its reproducible position. (F) Predrilling the holes for reconstruction plate according to the defined vectors using drilling guide. (G) Osteotomy along the cutting edge of the resection guide. (H) After bony resection further soft tissue resection is performed. (I) En-bloc tissue resection consisting of bony resection stump, old prebent reconstruction plate, and soft tissue coat.

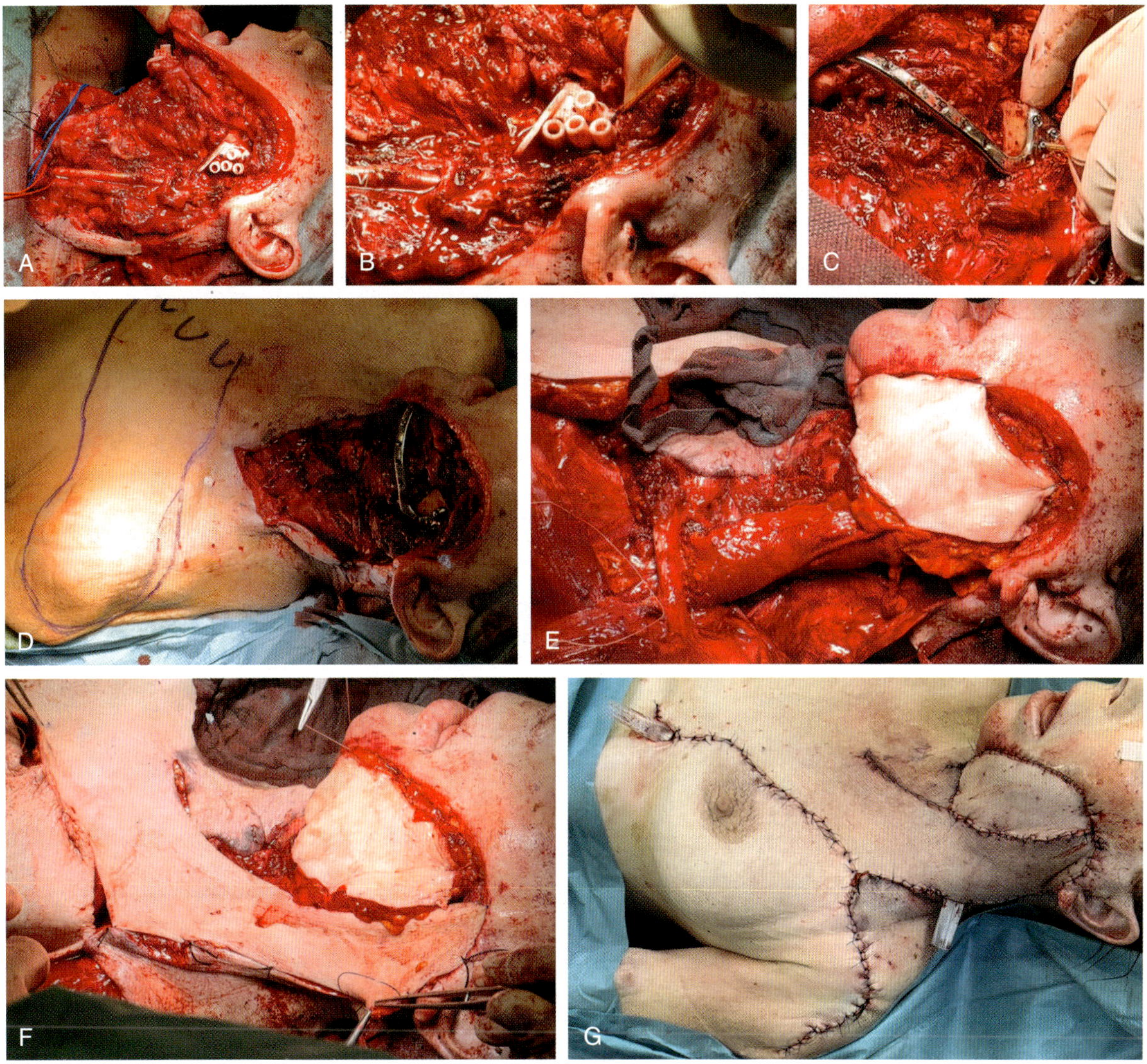


**Fig. 22.10** Steps of tumor resection using computer-assisted design/computer-assisted manufacturing resection guides during the surgical procedure of the previously mentioned case of recurrent oral squamous cell carcinoma – Part 2. (A) Resection cavity with guide still in situ. (B) Removing fixation screws of resection guide. (C) Fixation of patient-specific reconstruction plate for restoration of mandibular continuity using the vector-guided, predrilled screw holes. (D) Marking of deltopectoral and pectoralis major flap for soft tissue covering of the resection defect. Local flap raising was preferred and initially planned bony reconstruction via fibula transplant was deferred due to acute worsening of the patient's condition preoperatively. (E) Skin island of pectoralis major flap sewn into recipient site covering the reconstruction plate after tunneling beneath the clavicle for extension of the flap pedicle. (F) Deltopectoral flap rotated to cover rest of defect of cervical skin. (G) Wound closure with inserted drainage.

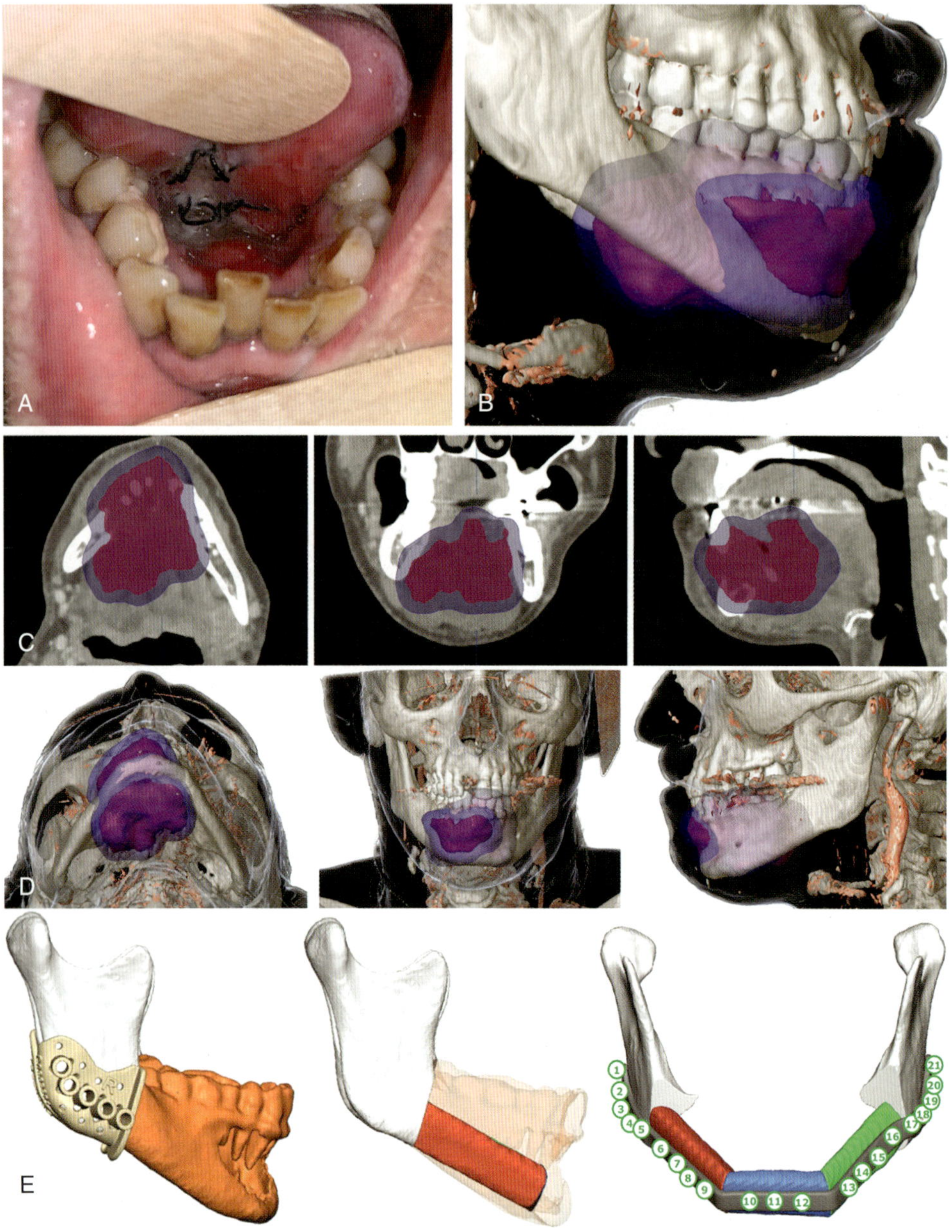


**Fig. 22.11** Primary advanced oral squamous cell carcinoma of the floor of the mouth – Part 1. (A) Clinical photograph of the sublingual tumor formation after specimen taking. (B) Segmented three-dimensional (3D) model of the tumor formation (*purple*) with calculated safety margin (*transparent blue*) from the right-side view. Interference with the anterior bone model indicates bony invasion while the mental skin has not yet been infiltrated. (C) Segmenting the tumor mass of the mouth's floor with the 3D-SmartBrush tool in the multiplanar view and adding a safety margin of 10 mm. (D) A 3D image of tumor formation, safety margin, facial bone, contrasted vessels and overlying skin from caudal, frontal, and left-side view giving an idea of the spatial tumor and resection extension. (E) Computer-assisted surgical planning with part of the mandible for resection (*orange*) and designed resection guides. Superimposing the neo-mandible composed of planned fibula segments with the former mandible shows the preserved profile of the alveolar arch without contouring the chin to prevent plate exposure. All 21 screw holes of the reconstruction plate are related to a determined screw length to use the bony anchorage without penetrating into the soft tissue.

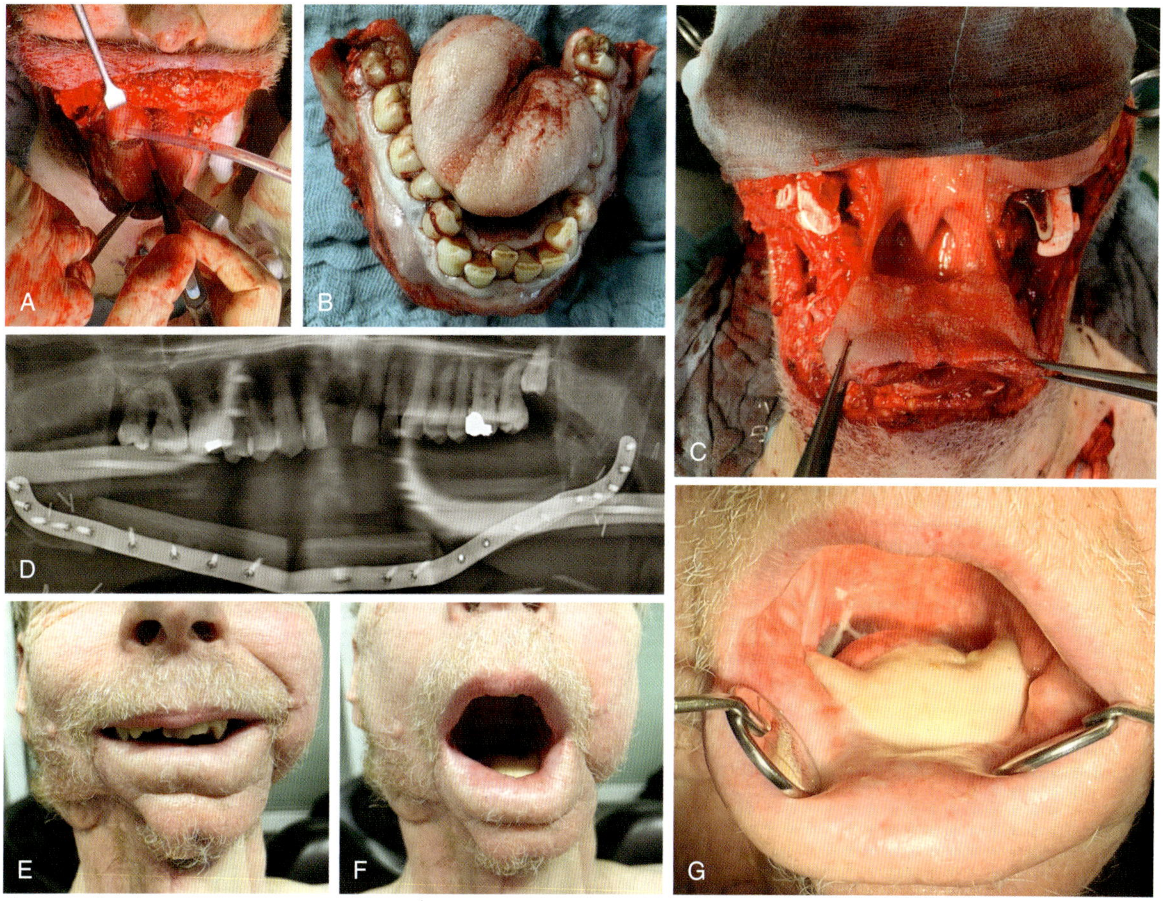


**Fig. 22.12** Primary advanced oral squamous cell carcinoma of the floor of the mouth – Part 2. (A) First incision in the area of the dorsal tongue for tumor resection after exposure by visor approach. (B) En-bloc tissue resection. (C) Resection cavity: resection guides are still in situ at the bony margins of the mandibular angles. (D) Postoperative panoramic radiograph showing the three-segmented fibula transplant fixed by computer-assisted design/computer-assisted manufacturing reconstruction plate. (E–G) Clinical photographs 15 recurrence-free months after tumor resection showing the fibula transplant with its skin island covering the floor of the mouth, while functions like mouth-opening and facial expression have been preserved.

## Outcomes/complications

With the introduction of CaSP, the aim of ablative oncological surgery and its reconstructive efforts can be formulated and displayed in all transparency for the first time because of the capabilities of the planning software. Thanks to modern 3D additive manufacturing processes, anatomical models, guides and patient-specific implants can be produced that enable the surgeon to precisely put the plan into practice. In addition, the process of evaluation has also significantly been improved by means of CaSP because previously there was no way to superimpose the preoperative planning on the postoperative result. Thus, CaSP techniques have improved the possibilities of quality control leading to a greater urge for precision in reconstructions.

Besides improved accuracy, computer-assisted surgery results in greater efficiency and reduced operative time compared with traditional techniques. The decreased operation room time comes along with a decrease in exposure time to general anesthesia, wound exposure, and decreased blood loss, with a more precise surgical procedure reported for both the maxilla and mandible.

Many authors argue against CaSP and computer-assisted surgery because of the higher costs. Ballard et al. calculated that at a yearly usage of a minimum of 63 models or

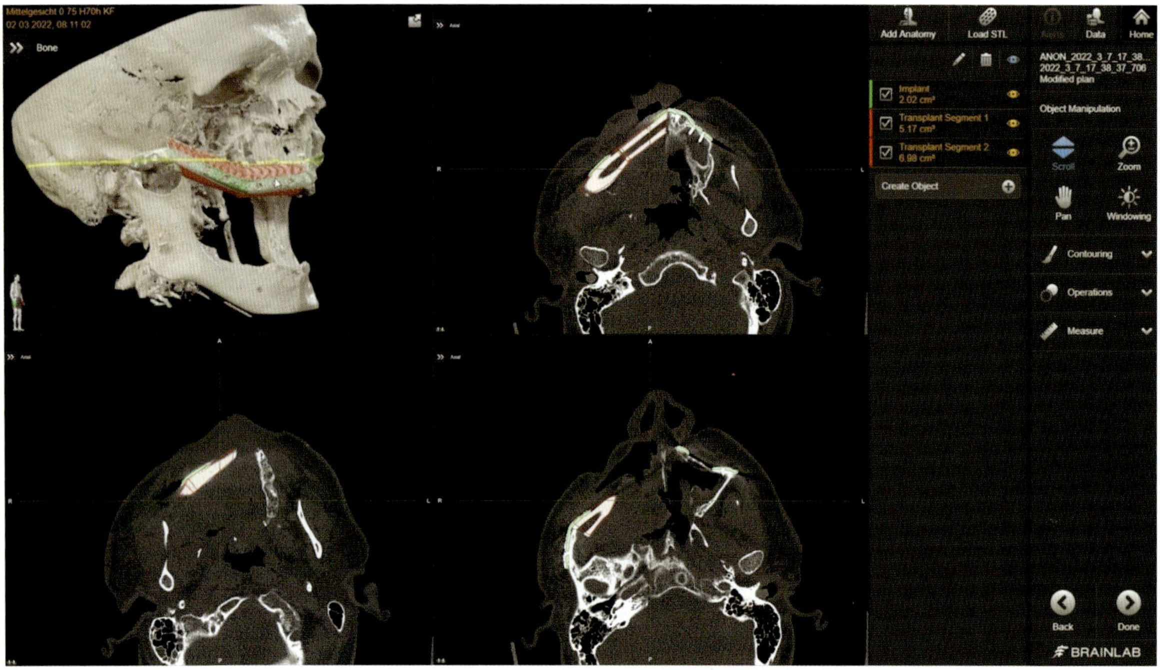


**Fig. 22.15** Postoperative evaluation. Postoperative data set of native computed tomography scan (0.75-mm slice thickness) imported into planning software with the STL-file of the preoperative planning superimposed showing the exact match of virtual surgical planning with the postoperative reconstruction result. If the STL-files are loaded into the navigation data set, intraoperative positioning control of the guides and the reconstruction plates can also be achieved by real-time navigation.

modern 3D additive manufacturing, a 3D virtual plan can be very precisely executed by the use of 3D-printed guides. Patient-specific implants can be designed in any desired shape but should be applied with the proper knowledge of load distribution models and biomechanical considerations obtained during the development of modern osteosynthesis systems.

The higher costs of 3D-guided surgery may prohibit its use in some countries, but this should not be used as an argument against it, as shorter surgery duration and a higher degree of reconstructive precision provide clear advantages for the patient.

The perceived problem of tumor margin control, when surgery is preoperatively planned by 3D technology, must be taken into control. Several solutions, such as frozen sections or navigated specimen-taking, have been developed to ensure margin control and should be used during computer-assisted surgery.

## Take-home points

- Computer-assisted surgery with CaSP and CAD/CAM technology relies on radiological data sets, and therefore should be based on standardized high-quality scans matching the required prerequisites.
- Tumor segmentation determines the extent of resection and should therefore be carried out carefully. If there are uncertainties in the radiological imaging, other examination modalities, such as MRI or further navigated specimen-taking with coordinate-linked pathohistological examination, can enhance the data sets.
- CADs of guides and implants can easily be modified, but have to match certain design features to meet the requirements.
- 3D additive manufacturing can be carried out in-house for anatomical models with the purpose of prebent plates as these are not considered to be medical devices. However, typical resection guides and implants for maxillo-mandibular reconstruction are mainly manufactured by industrial companies, which entails a certain cost effort and presurgical lead time, which have to be taken into account.
- High planning transparency with the ability for postoperative quality control, shorter operation times and higher precision with regard to reconstruction

results are clear advantages of computer-assisted oncological surgery.

- Surgical outcome with regard to margin control, recurrence, and survival match the conventional free-hand method. Tools such as frozen section and evaluation of the definitive pathohistological report remain fixed components of surgical oncological treatment.

## References


1. Aponte-Tinao L, Ritacco LE, Ayerza MA, Luis Muscolo D, Albergo JI, Farfall GL. Does intraoperative navigation assistance improve bone tumor resection and allograft reconstruction results? *Clin Orthop Relat Res*. 2015;473:796-804.
2. Ballard DH, Mills P, Duszak R, Weisman JA, Rybicki FJ, Woodard PK. Medical 3D printing cost-savings in orthopedic and maxillofacial surgery: cost analysis of operating room time saved with 3D printed anatomic models and surgical guides. *Acad Radiol*. 2020;27:1103-1113.
3. Bittermann G, Wiedenmann N, Voss P, Zimmerer R, Duttenhoefer F, Metzger MC. Marking of tumor resection borders for improved radiation planning facilitates reduction of radiation dose to free flap reconstruction in head and neck cancer surgery. *J Craniomaxillofac Surg*. 2015;43:567-573.
4. Essig H, Rana M, Meyer A, et al. Virtual 3D tumor marking-exact intraoperative coordinate mapping improve post-operative radiotherapy. *Radiat Oncol*. 2011;6:159.
5. Farfalli GL, Albergo JI, Ritacco LE, Ayerza MA, Milano FE, Aponte-Tinao LA. What is the expected learning curve in computer-assisted navigation for bone tumor resection? *Clin Orthop Relat Res*. 2017;475:668-675.
6. Flukes S, Lohia S, Barker CA, et al. Primary tumor volume as a predictor of distant metastases and survival in patients with sinonasal mucosal melanoma. *Head Neck*. 2020;42:3316-3325.
7. Guijarro-Martínez R, Gellrich NC, Witte J, et al. Optimization of the interface between radiology, surgery, radiotherapy, and pathology in head and neck tumor surgery: a navigation-assisted multidisciplinary network. *Int J Oral Maxillofac Surg*. 2014;43:156-162.
8. Heffler MA, Le LQ, Xi Y, Chhabra A. Tumor segmentation of whole-body magnetic resonance imaging in neurofibromatosis type 1 patients: tumor burden correlates. *Skeletal Radiol*. 2017;46:93-99.
9. Heidkamp J, Weijs WLJ, van Engen-van Grunsven ACH, et al. Assessment of surgical tumor-free resection margins in fresh squamous-cell carcinoma resection specimens of the tongue using a clinical MRI system. *Head Neck*. 2020;42:2039-2049.
10. Rana M, Modrow D, Keuchel J, et al. Development and evaluation of an automatic tumor segmentation tool: a comparison between automatic, semi-automatic and manual segmentation of mandibular odontogenic cysts and tumors. *J Craniomaxillofac Surg*. 2015;43:355-359.
11. Ricotta F, Cercenelli L, Battaglia S, et al. Navigation-guided resection of maxillary tumors: Can a new volumetric virtual planning method improve outcomes in terms of control of resection margins? *J Craniomaxillofac Surg*. 2018;46:2240-2247.
12. Ritacco LE, Milano FE, Farfalli GL, Ayerza MA, Muscolo DL, Aponte-Tinao LA. Accuracy of 3-D planning and navigation in bone tumor resection. *Orthopedics*. 2013;36(7):e942-e950.
13. Schramm A, Suarez-Cunqueiro MM, Barth EL, et al. Computer-assisted navigation in craniomaxillofacial tumors. *J Craniofac Surg*. 2008;19:1067-1074.
14. Sternheim A, Rotman D, Nayak P, et al. Computer-assisted surgical planning of complex bone tumor resections improves negative margin outcomes in a sawbones model. *Int J Comput Assist Radiol Surg*. 2021;16:695-701.
15. Tang ZN, Hu LH, Soh HY, Yu Y, Zhang WB, Peng X. Accuracy of mixed reality combined with surgical navigation assisted oral and maxillofacial tumor resection. *Front Oncol*. 2022;11:715484.
16. Wang Y, Fan S, Zhang H, Lin Z, Ye J, Li J. Virtual surgical planning in precise maxillary reconstruction with vascularized fibular graft after tumor ablation. *J Oral Maxillofac Surg*. 2016;74:1255-1264.
17. Wilkat M, Kübler N, Rana M. Advances in the resection and reconstruction of midfacial tumors through computer assisted surgery. *Front Oncol*. 2021;11:719528.

Chapter 23

# Virtual surgical planning and computer-assisted design/computer-assisted manufacturing in facial feminization surgery

Brendan J. Cronin, Harsh Patel, Justine C. Lee

CHAPTER OUTLINE



## Introduction

### Background

Facial feminization surgery (FFS) is an essential component of the multidisciplinary treatment of gender dysphoria. First described by Ousterhout in the 1980s,[1-3] FFS has become increasingly common following recent approval of Medicare reimbursement for gender confirming surgery.[4,5] Precision and careful preoperative planning are paramount in FFS due to transformation of normal preoperative masculine anatomy into a feminine appearance rather than restoration of normal from abnormal form in congenital or traumatic craniofacial conditions.

A range of preoperative planning techniques and intraoperative "guides" have been used to determine the location of osteotomies for FFS osseus manuevers. These include transillumination of the frontal sinus on perioperative clinical exam,[6] preoperative assessment of sinus dimensions on radiograph[7] or computed tomography (CT) scan,[8,9] as well as measurements of various anthropometric landmarks.[1] Intraoperative assessment alone based on surgeon experience without preoperative imaging,[10,11] three-dimensional (3D) printing of patient skulls to simulate maneuvers prior to surgery,[12,13] and 3D photogrammetry[12] have also been described. However, once planned by the aforementioned methods, osseus maneuvers-such as frontal setback, reduction genioplasty, and gonial angle reduction-were traditionally performed entirely freehand. The advent of computer-assisted design/computer-assisted manufacturing (CAD/CAM) and its widespread application in pediatric craniofacial and orthognathic surgery marked the transition to guide-directed osteotomies,[14,15] which were then adopted in the growing field of gender confirming facial surgery.

## Indications

Facial gender affirmation surgery is an essential component in the treatment of gender dysphoria. Similar to all other aspects of gender transition, the need and the anatomical areas treated in facial surgery are highly individualized and dependent upon the triggers for dysphoria in each patient. Although WPATH Standards of Care V7 does not outline specific criteria for FFS,[16] our typical preoperative protocol for proceeding with facial feminization surgery include the following for all patients:

- Evaluation by a multidisciplinary group of gender health specialists
- Two letters of support from gender health specialists with at least one from a licensed mental health provider
- Robust patient support network
- 12-month trial in the gender-identity congruent role ± medical transition
- Agreement from the senior surgeon that the patient is medically, socially, and psychologically ready for surgery
- Patient must be at skeletal maturity

Indications for CAD/CAM in FFS have been subject to debate.[2,10-13,17] Certain authors advocate against the use of CAD/CAM under the pretense that a "color by number" approach risks a standardized process lacking consideration of individualized anatomy and aesthetic.[10,11] Critics also comment that CAD/CAM relegates the surgeon to a technician that "cuts along the dotted lines" and inhibits learning.[10,11] However, multiple authors report using computer-assisted planning of some kind for FFS.[2,12,17] Deschamps-Braly et al. routinely obtain 3D CT face and panorex imaging prior to reduction genioplasty, but utilize CAD/CAM for challenging cases to achieve the most feminine results.[3] Interestingly, Capitán et al. even reported designing specific FFS-related CAD/CAM software.[12]

In our practice, we perform CAD/CAM for all patients prior to FFS for intraoperative precision, safety, and speed of all skeletal moves. Decision-making during the CAD session is based on clinical exam, cephalometric measurements, and are secondarily double-checked using a reference female skull.[18] Because FFS is a combination of hard tissue and soft tissue maneuvers, one note of caution is that precision planning and execution of the bony maneuvers is not the only factor necessary to achieve optimal results.

## Contraindications

Patient factors:

- Unrealistic expectations[2]
- Inappropriate motivation for gender affirming surgery
  - Ulterior motives or possible comorbid psychiatric conditions, such as body dysmorphia[2]

Surgical contraindications:

- Medical comorbidities that preclude prolonged surgery/general anesthesia
- Skeletal immaturity
  - Skeletally immature bone lacks the rigidity required for the precise osseus maneuvers[2]
  - Delaying surgery until skeletal maturity reduces disruption of normal facial skeletal growth and maximizes postoperative symmetry
- Older age, independent of surgical candidacy, is *not* a contraindication

Contraindications to CAD/CAM:

- No specific contraindications
- Cost of CAD/CAM and custom guide manufacturing can be significant, and may not be available depending on the practice setting and institution

## Clinical considerations

Naturally, the key anatomical considerations in FFS center around the differences between the male and female facial skeleton and soft tissues.[1,19] In regard to underlying skeletal framework, masculine faces tend to have more prominent and angular features, while females tend to have obtuse, softer features. Table 23.1 provides a review of the key anatomical differences of the underlying facial skeleton and overlying soft tissues in male and female patients, as well as the relevant maneuvers to address these differences in FFS.

As described by Ousterhout, forehead morphology can be further divided into four types based on radiographic findings and corresponding surgical treatment (Table 23.2).[1] Lateral orbital hooding, gonial angle/lower facial width, and chin width/height can also be stratified by severity; Hoang et al., for example, utilized a classification scheme of mild (1), moderate (2), and severe (3).[18] However, management of these regions is less influenced by severity and requires consideration of other variables, such as the need for chin advancement rather than reduction alone, for appropriate operative planning.

Key features of the clinical and radiographic examination of the patient considering facial feminization surgery are outlined in Fig. 23.1 and Table 23.1.

## Clinical examination

- Systematic facial analysis
  - Evaluation of the hairline
    - Hairline position
    - Hairline shape and temporal recession
  - Evaluation of the forehead
    - Length at the midline and above the lateral brow
    - Eyebrow position/symmetry

**Table 23.1** Differences in male/female facial characteristics and their management in facial feminization surgery

| Characteristic | Male | Female | Procedure |
|---|---|---|---|
| Frontal bone | • Larger, broader frontal bone<br>• Larger frontal sinus<br>• Flat and retroclined frontal bone on lateral view | • Smaller frontal bone<br>• Smaller frontal sinus<br>• Gentle curve from frontonasal junction to hairline on lateral view | • Anterior table setback<br>• Brow recontouring |
| Orbits | • Prominent supraorbital bossing/lateral orbital hooding | • No supraorbital bossing/lateral orbital hooding | • Supraorbital recontouring<br>• Lateral orbital recontouring/ ostectomy |
| Zygoma | • Flatter, lower and less prominent zygomatic arch | • Higher and more projecting zygomas | • Zygomatic implants<br>• Fat grafting |
| Mandible | • Wider lower facial width<br>• Acute gonial angle | • Narrower lower facial width<br>• Gentler, less defined gonial angle | • Gonial angle reduction |
| Chin | • Wider and "boxier" chin with increased height and projection | • Narrow, pointed chin, generally shorter and less projected | • Chin recontouring<br>• Reduction genioplasty |
| Forehead hairline brow | • Higher "M" shaped hairline with bitemporal recession<br>• Flatter brows that sit lower across the orbital ridge | • Lower "O" shaped hairline without recession<br>• Curved brows that arch above the supraorbital rims | • Hairline lowering<br>• Hair transplant<br>• Brow lift |
| Nose | • Larger nose with acute glabellar and nasolabial angles<br>• Prominent dorsal hump or straight dorsum | • Smaller nose with more obtuse nasolabial and glabellar angles<br>• Narrower with possible concavity or supratip break | • Reduction rhinoplasty |
| Lips | • Longer and thinner lips<br>• Minimal incisal show in repose | • Fuller and shorter lips with increased visibility of the vermilion<br>• Greater incisal show in repose | • Dermal lip augmentation<br>• Lip lift |

**Table 23.2** Ousterhout classification of forehead types

| Forehead type | Defining features | Techniques for transformation |
|---|---|---|
| Type I | • Mild bossing, no or minimum frontal sinus<br>• Thick anterior wall | • Burring |
| Type II | • Moderate bossing, midforehead flattening<br>• Normal forehead protrusion | • Burring plus cement filling |
| Type III | • Significant bossing, large projection<br>• Large frontal sinus with thin anterior table | • Anterior frontal sinus wall setback |
| Type IV | • Severe forehead slope not amenable to setback | • Cement filling to create aesthetic forehead profile without setback |

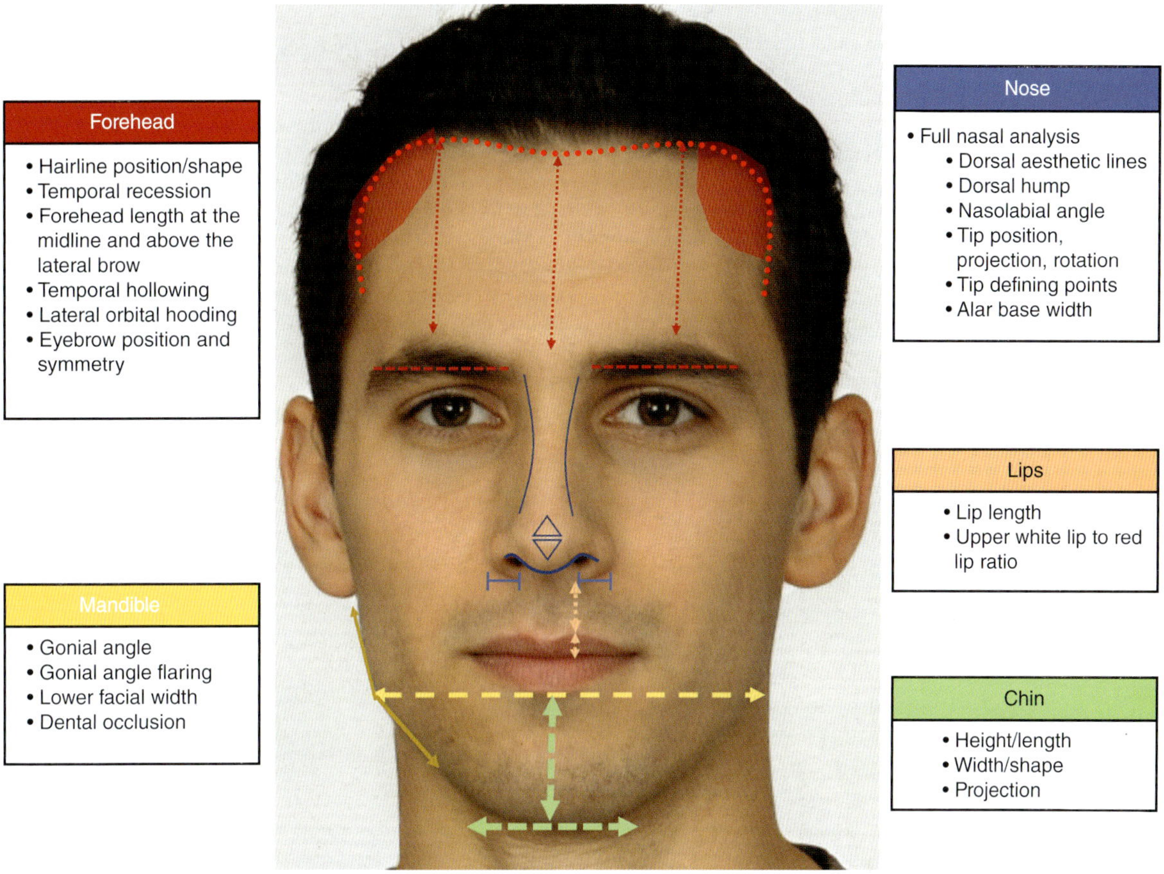


**Fig. 23.1** Key clinical examination features in patients considering facial feminization surgery. Vital elements of the facial analysis are displayed and annotated above. A systematic method of clinical examination should be developed to ensure all elements of the facial aesthetic are taken into consideration during consultation. Critical elements to note for computer-assisted design/computer-assisted manufacturing are forehead contour and supraorbital bossing, lower facial width with gonial angle severity and chin position, width, and projection. (Photograph provided by www.generated.photos, an open-access platform using artificial intelligence software to generate realistic human portraits.)

- Frontal bone
    - Frontal view
        - Lateral orbital hooding
    - Lateral view
        - Supraorbital bossing
        - Contour
    - Mandible
    - Gonial angle
    - Gonial angle flaring
    - Lower facial width
    - Dental occlusion
- Chin
    - Length/height
    - Position/projection
- Lip length
    - Upper white lip to red lip ratio
    - Full nasal analysis

## Radiographic workup

Fine-cut CT face (section thickness of 0.6 mm) + 3D reconstruction

- Obtain in all patients undergoing FFS for virtual planning
- Assess for:
    - Forehead type (see Table 23.2)
    - Frontal sinus size and dimensions
    - Sagittal distance between the anterior globe and the anterior most portion of the forehead
    - Course of the inferior alveolar nerve

Standard cephalometric measurements:

- Upper facial height to lower facial height ratio + Holdaway ratio (Fig. 23.2)
  - Used to determine the need for and magnitude of chin repositioning
- Relationships of the maxilla and mandible to each other and the skull base
  - Reveal any underlying skeletal discrepancies or malocclusion that would indicate the need for orthognathic surgery (if necessary, this is performed prior to all other feminization procedures as a separate surgery)

## Computer-assisted design

Preoperative planning of the osseous maneuvers of FFS are performed using a standard female skull as a reference. Some 3D CT scans of a representative patient's skull and the skull of a reference female are shown (Fig. 23.3A, left).

These reconstructions are subsequently superimposed to identify the precise areas of reduction at the forehead *(red dotted line)*, gonial angles *(blue dotted line)*, and chin *(yellow dotted line)*. The reference skull (Fig. 23.3B, *orange*

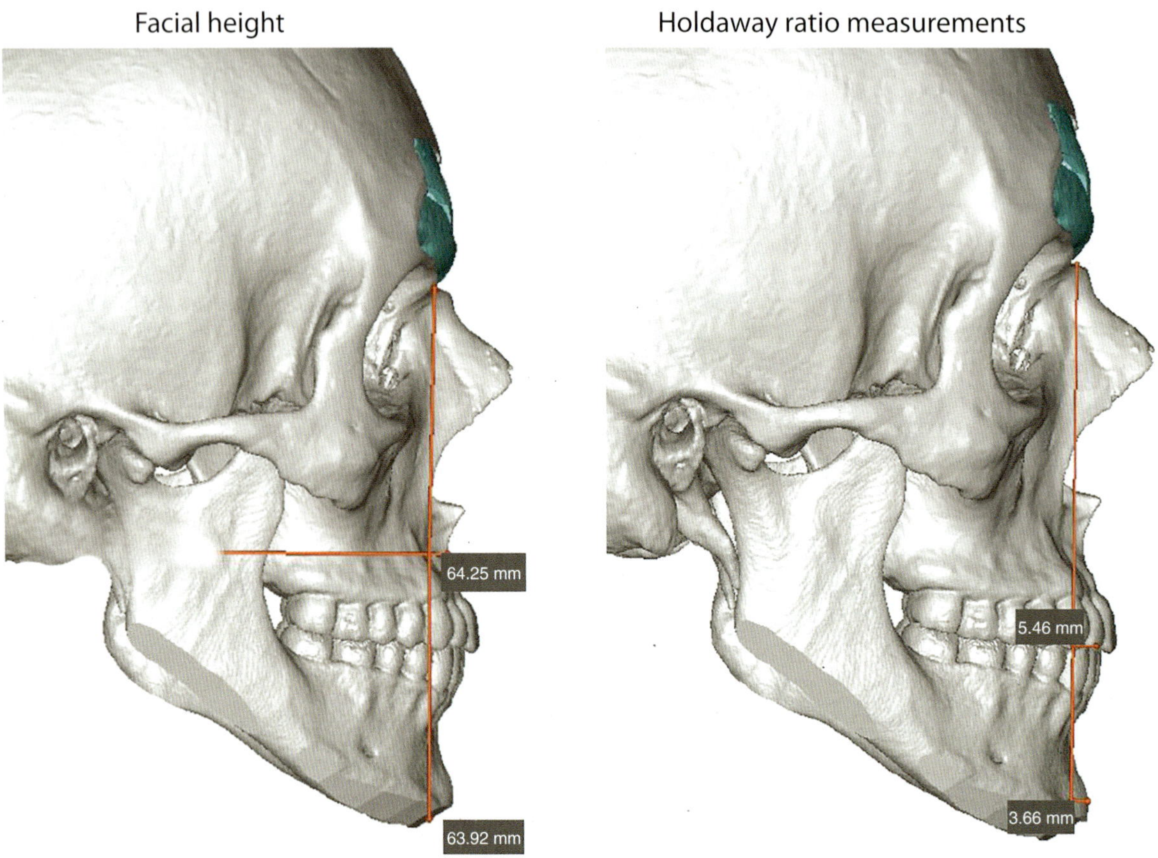


**Fig. 23.2** Key measurements in computer-assisted design/computer-assisted manufacturing. Orthognathic and dentofacial analysis ratios, including the facial height and Holdaway ratio, are mapped preoperatively to guide operative maneuvers. Facial height (distance from glabella to menton) is used to calculate the ratio of upper (glabella to subnasale) and lower (subnasale to menton) facial height and informs need for vertical chin repositioning. Holdaway ratio is defined by the ratio of (1) the horizontal distance from vertical plane NB to the anteriormost aspect of the lower incisor (NB–LI) and (2) the horizontal distance from vertical plane NB to the anteriormost aspect of the bony chin or pogonion (NB–Po). This ratio informs the need for chin repositioning in the horizontal plane (sliding genioplasty). Above, an NB–LI of 5.46 mm and NB–Po of 3.66 yields a Holdaway ratio of 1.5, indicating the need for chin advancement.

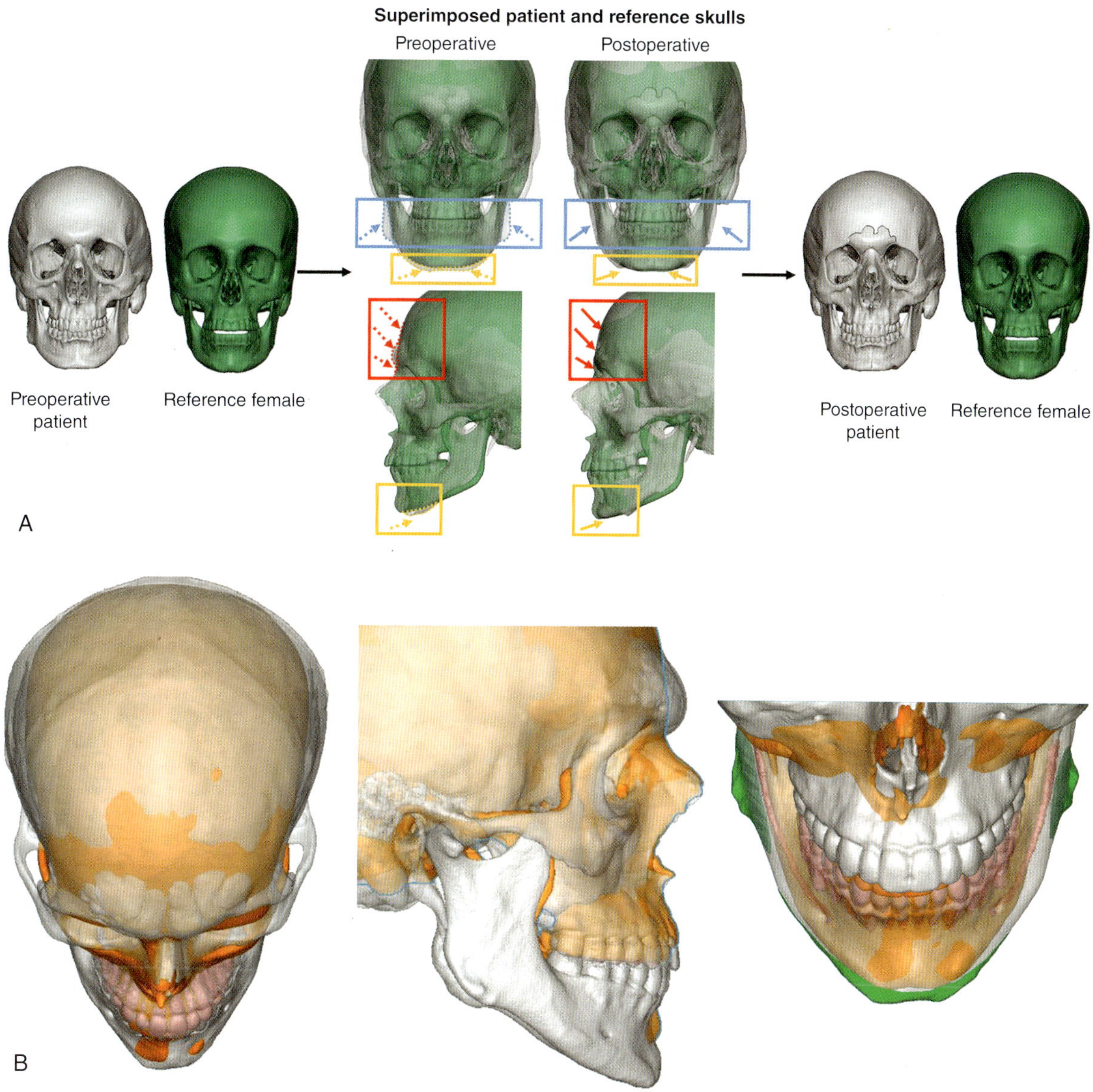


**Fig. 23.3** Modeling osseous maneuvers on a female skull. Superimposed reference and patient skulls identify the precise areas of reduction at the forehead *(red dotted line)*, gonial angles *(blue dotted line)*, and chin *(yellow dotted line)*. The reference skull (Fig. 23.3B, *orange "mask"*) is scaled relative to the patient skull (*white "mask"*) based on the position of the nasion and overlap of the anterior aspect of the maxilla and zygomatic arches. Vertical position is set via alignment of the infraorbital rims and apex of the skull. Horizontal position is set based on symmetry of the zygomatic arches. The images are "zeroed" and the volumetric difference between patient and reference skull is mapped *(green)*.

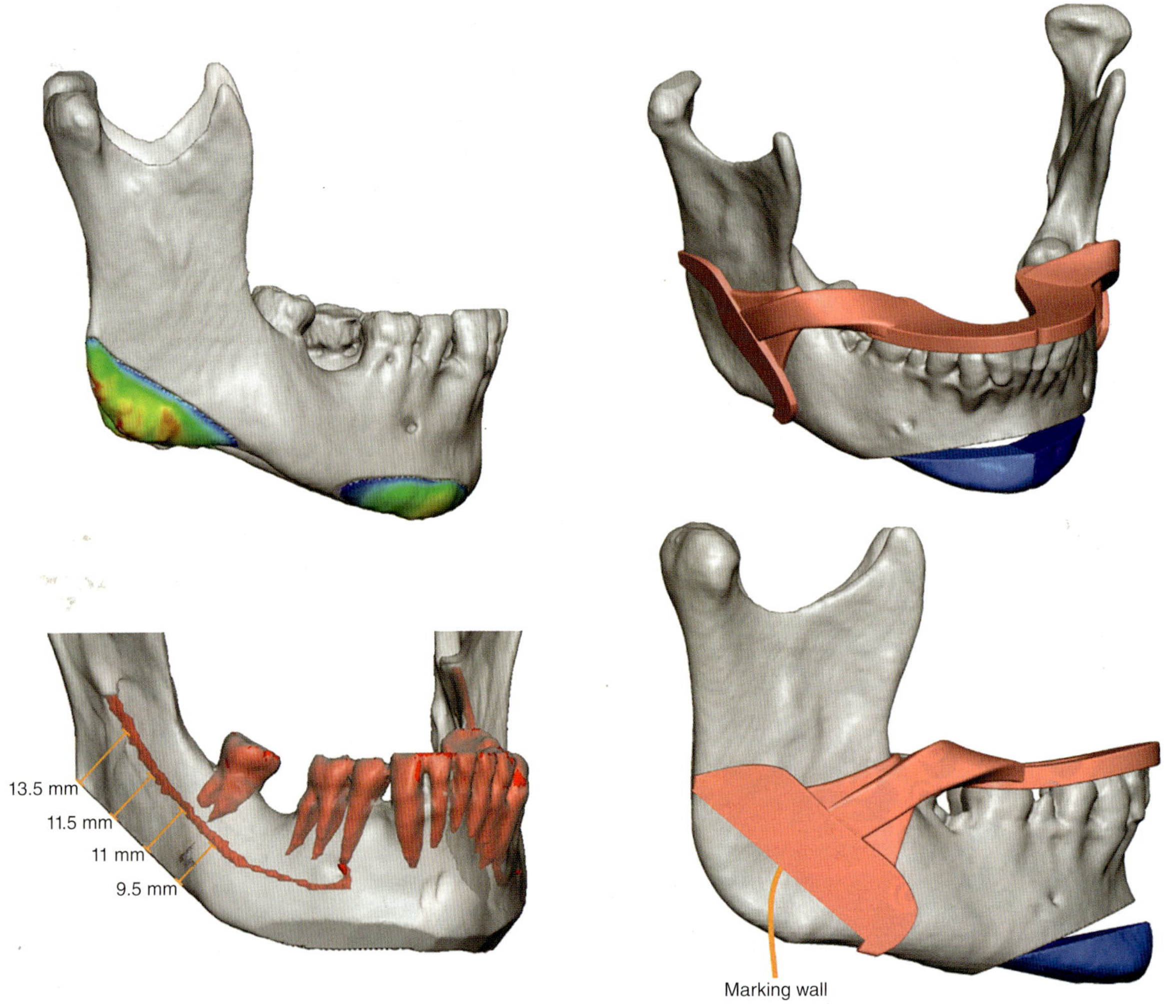


**Fig. 23.6** Computer-assisted design/computer-assisted manufacturing and cutting guide for gonial angle reduction. The excess height and projection of the mandibular angles (top left) as well as the course of the inferior alveolar nerve in relation to planned ostectomy (bottom left) are virtually planned. The gonial angle cutting guide is seated via the mandibular dentition and the contour of the inferior mandibular border. The marking wall delineates the ostectomy line to achieve the planned resection.

- Any need for chin repositioning (excess lower facial height, chin retrusion or prominence, abnormal Holdaway ratio) → single or two-piece genioplasty
  - One-piece genioplasty + plate fixation: indicated for increasing projection, reducing chin height
  - Two-piece genioplasty + plate fixation: when chin narrowing required.

## Operative technique

All cases were performed by the same senior surgeon (JCL). Videos 23.2 and 23.3 demonstrate our operative planning and surgical technique for feminization of the forehead and lower face, respectively.

In patients requiring forehead reduction, a hairline-lowering pretrichial incision is marked in the midline and

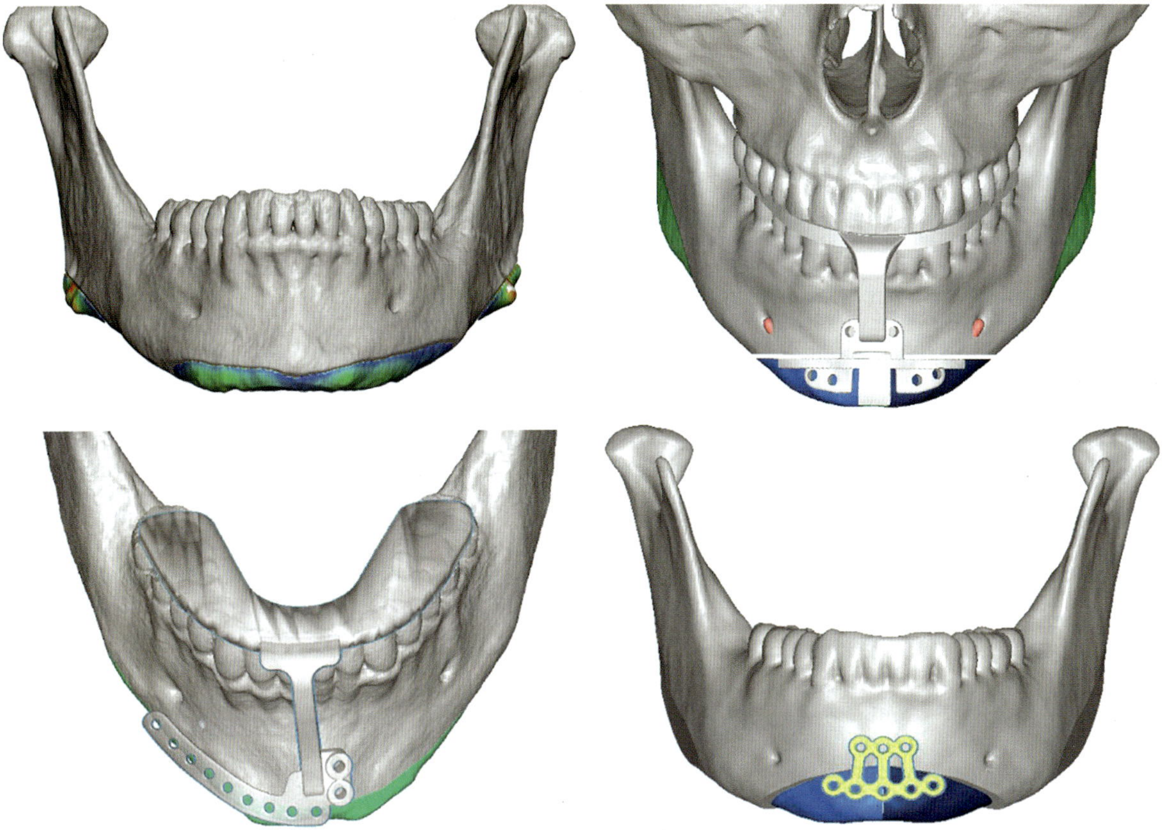

Fig. 23.7 Chin reduction/repositioning via burring or three-piece osseus genioplasty. The desired chin contour is planned. In the case of moderate to mild masculine features or those without need for significant chin repositioning via genioplasty, we use burring alone. Burring is directed via guides with preplanned holes outlining the areas of bone to be removed. Guides are designed for either side and the bone taken down with a burr until the drill holes are no longer visible. In patients who require more aggressive chin manipulation (severe masculine features, inadequate or excessive chin projection, abnormal Holdaway ratios), we perform a three-piece genioplasty via a T-shaped cutting guide. Our guide incorporates prepositioned drilling holes for postgenioplasty osteosynthesis as well as guides for the horizontal and vertical osteotomies with removal of the central bone wedge. Cuts are made along the top of the horizontal guide, appropriately below the mental nerve foramen, and vertically, adjacent to the central bone wedge to be removed.

extended to a coronal incision posterolaterally. In patients with appropriate forehead length, a bicoronal incision is planned. The abdomen and submental region are infiltrated with tumescent solution in anticipation of autologous fat harvest. The patient is positioned supine in a horseshoe headrest and prepped and draped in the usual fashion.

Autologous fat is harvested from the abdomen using a nontraumatic aspiration technique with a Coleman canula. Fat is then injected in 1-mL aliquots at various depths into the bitemporal, malar, geniomandibular, and chin regions.

Attention is then turned to the frontal exposure. The pretrichial or coronal mark is incised through skin and galea and subperiosteal dissection is performed to expose the frontal bone, superior orbit, and zygomaticotemporal suture. Laterally, dissection is performed on the surface of the deep temporal fascia to protect the frontal branch of the facial nerve. Osteotomies may be required to release the supraorbital neurovascular bundle to achieve complete orbital dissection.

## Frontal setback

If the patient has a type III forehead, the virtually planned osteotomy cutting guide is placed on the frontal bone and secured with 5-mm screws. Footplates extend into and hook under the orbital rims allowing facile and accurate positioning of the custom 3D-printed guide. Oblique osteotomies based on the cutting guide are then performed to remove the anterior table, which is recontoured. Vertical and, occasionally, both vertical and horizontal osteotomies, are performed to achieve adequate flattening of the osteotomized frontal table for smooth forehead contour upon replating. The porcupine guide is then seated and secured in a similar manner. A 2.7-mm drill guide and 2.7-mm drill are used to drill into the frontal bone at varying depths based on the guide. The holes are infiltrated with Bonny blue dye to clearly demonstrate depth of desired reduction. A pineapple burr is then used to burr down the forehead, superior orbital rims, and lateral orbital rims. Care is taken to prevent dural violation or contour deformity. The radix is also burred to ensure a smooth transition to the anterior table of the frontal sinus. The anterior table of the frontal sinus is then replaced and secured with plates and screws. In patients with type I foreheads, we perform burring alone without osteotomy. We then perform a temporal brow lift and/or hairline advancement. The galea and skin are reapproximated and attention is turned to the mandible.

## Gonial angle reduction

A gingivobuccal incision is made with electrocautery and the soft tissue and periosteum elevated off the angle of the mandible. Gonial angle reduction can be achieved through ostectomy or burring. A 3D cutting guide positioned based on custom-made mandibular splints can be used to guide ostectomy of the gonial angle. Alternatively, burring alone, with a protected oscillating power rasp, can be used. We find that burring of the gonial angle alone without significant reduction of the vertical mandibular height via ostectomy tends to preserve soft tissue draping and limit postoperative jowling.

## Reduction genioplasty

Depending on preoperative anatomy, reduction genioplasty may incorporate reduction or augmentation of chin height, chin advancement, and chin narrowing. Less severe phenotypes can be managed with burring alone.

A gingivobuccal incision is made, and the chin is exposed with a periosteal elevator, taking care to visualize and protect the mental nerves bilaterally. In patients with severe masculine features, we perform a reduction pattern osseous genioplasty, which entails a horizontal osteotomy with a central vertical wedge resection of the chin segment with a reciprocating saw based on prefabricated cutting guides as previously described. The bony segments are then secured with the custom titanium plate using predrilled holes. Burring with a power rasp may be required to smooth palpable step offs of the mandibular body created by chin advancement and narrowing. Alternatively, in less severe phenotypes, an L-shaped guide is seated, and the chin is drilled and marked with Bonny blue dye in a process similar to the forehead setback. Rasping with an oscillating power rasp as guided by the drilled and dye-stained holes is then performed until adequate reduction is achieved. The mentalis is resuspended, and the intraoral incision closed in a running-locking fashion.

Additional soft tissue maneuvers including reduction rhinoplasty, lip augmentation with dermal grafting, lip shortening, and tracheal shave may also be performed.

## Fidelity verification

There is a limited role for verification of CAD/CAM fidelity in FFS. Because there is no clinical indication for obtaining postoperative CT scans in these patients, no objective data are available for quantifying the accuracy of osseus maneuvers. In addition, the goal of the procedure is to alleviate dysphoria of perceived facial appearance, thus the gold standard metric for evaluating successful surgery is postoperative, validated, patient-reported quality of life outcomes measures rather than CAD/CAM fidelity.

## Pearls/pitfalls

- Complete cephalometric analysis, as one would perform for orthognathic surgery, is essential, and orthognathic skeletal discrepancies should be corrected before feminization surgery.
- Consultation with the patient after computer-assisted surgical planning with the use of CAD/CAM technology assists in shared decision-making about the magnitude in skeletal maneuvers.
- Dependence on CAD/CAM technology without comprehensive clinical facial analysis and a thorough understanding of the specific triggers of dysphoria for individual patients will result in errors in surgical decision-making.
- Burring, rather than ostectomy, of the gonial angle limits excessive periosteal denuding required to seat the large ostectomy guides and preserves the inferior aspect of the gonial/mandibular angle for optimal soft tissue draping and prevention of postoperative jowling.

## Outcomes/complications

A minority of studies have examined the use of CAD/CAM and cutting guides in facial feminization surgery,[17,20,21] especially in vivo.[17,21] Although small in number, or lacking control groups, these studies have consistently demonstrated improved safety, operative efficiency and accuracy with these techniques. Gray et al. demonstrated improved accuracy, decreased operative times and decreased rates of intradural violation and inferior alveolar nerve injury of FFS maneuvers on cadavers compared to the control group.[20] Accuracy was assessed by comparing planned movements and postsimulation 3D CT reconstructions of the cadavers. Guides seemed to be most effective in the forehead and least so in the gonial angle ostectomy, likely due to challenging visualization and access in this region.[20] Tawa et al. showed CAD/CAM to be both safe, though they had no control group, and accurate, with high rates of patient satisfaction.[17] Similar to prior work, our group has experienced no intraoperative or postoperative complications with our process of CAD/CAM and 3D cutting guides in a series of 70 patients. In regard to operative efficiency, no available studies provide in vivo comparisons with and without CAD/CAM. Assessing operative efficiency in FFS is especially challenging due to the variable nature and number of procedures performed on a case-by-case basis; however, operative times of up to 12 to 16 hours have been described.[2,13] We have found our average operative duration to be more in the 6- to 8-hour range, though this obviously varies based on the number of included maneuvers. Clearly, further studies are needed to evaluate the impact of CAD/CAM on operative efficiency and patient-reported outcomes in gender confirming surgery.

## Conclusions

CAD/CAM and cutting guides provide a safe and efficient method to transfer preoperative surgical plans to intraoperative maneuvers in facial feminization surgery. Computer-assisted planning using a reference female skull provides a standardized method to guide the magnitude of osseus maneuvers and enables simulation of multiple operative plans. Key areas for planning and cutting guides include forehead setback, brow recontouring, gonial angle reduction, and chin reduction/genioplasty. The use of these guides provides precise transfer of surgical plan to the operating theatre both through clear delineation of anatomical landmarks (frontal sinus outline) or real-time feedback about remaining osseus reduction (forehead contouring). Available evidence suggests that CAD/CAM improves safety in FFS; however, future studies are required to investigate the cost-benefit analysis and impact on patient reported outcomes in those who undergo CAD/CAM for gender confirming facial surgery.

## Take home points

- The key areas targeted by CAD/CAM in FFS include the brow, lateral orbit, mandibular angle, and chin.
- Utilization of 3D planning compared to a standardized female skull offers objective metrics for planning osseus movements.
- The brow and lateral orbital hooding can be addressed with a combination of both burring and anterior table setback, depending on the preoperative anatomy. Custom guides facilitate this process by demonstrating the appropriate depth of forehead reduction and anterior table setback as well as the outlines of osteotomy for elevation of the anterior table.
- Osseus genioplasty can be planned to include vertical and transverse ostectomies to both narrow and shorten the chin. Post movement burring of resulting prominences are key to shaping a smooth jawline and preventing palpable or visible step offs.
- CAD/CAM improves safety (decreased intradural and nerve injury) and operational efficiency. Future studies are needed comparing patient-reported outcomes in FFS with and without CAD/CAM.

## References

1. Ousterhout DK. Feminization of the forehead: contour changing to improve female aesthetics. *Plast Reconstr Surg*. 1987;79(5): 701-713. doi:10.1097/00006534-198705000-00003.
2. Ousterhout DK. *Facial Feminization Surgery: A Guide for the Transgendered Woman*. Omaha, Nebraska: Addicus Books; 2012.
3. Deschamps-Braly JC. FACS approach to feminization surgery and facial masculinization surgery: Aesthetic goals and principles of management. *J Craniofac Surg*. 2019;30(5): 1352-1358. doi:10.1097/SCS.0000000000005391.
4. Canner JK, Harfouch O, Kodadek LM, et al. Temporal trends in gender-affirming surgery among transgender patients in the United States. *JAMA Surg*. 2018;153(7):609-616. doi:10.1001/jamasurg. 2017.6231.

5. Dagi AF, Boskey ER, Nuzzi LC, et al. Legislation, market size, and access to gender-affirming genital surgery in the United States. *Plast Reconstr Surg Glob Open*. 2021;9(2):e3422. doi:10.1097/GOX.0000000000003422.
6. Gilde JE, Shih CW, Kleinberger AJ. Frontal sinus transillumination in cranioplasty for facial feminization surgery. *JAMA Facial Plast Surg*. 2019;21(6):566-567. doi:10.1001/jamafacial.2019.0606.
7. Cho SW, Jin HR. Feminization of the forehead in a transgender: Frontal sinus reshaping combined with brow lift and hairline lowering. *Aesthetic Plast Surg*. 2012;36(5):1207-1210. doi:10.1007/s00266-012.9939-5.
8. Altman K. Forehead reduction and orbital contouring in facial feminization surgery for transgender females. *Br J Oral Maxillofac Surg*. 2018;56(3):192-197. doi:10.1016/j.bjoms.2018.01.009.
9. Altman K. Facial feminization surgery: current state of the art. *Int J Oral Maxillofac Surg*. 2012;41(8):885-894.
10. Spiegel JH. Discussion: Osseous transformation with facial feminization surgery: improved anatomical accuracy with virtual planning. *Plast Reconstr Surg*. 2019;144(5):1169-1170. doi:10.1097/PRS.0000000000006195.
11. Spiegel JH. Gender affirming and aesthetic cranioplasty: What's new? *Curr Opin Otolaryngol Head Neck Surg*. 2020;28(4):201-205. doi:10.1097/MOO.0000000000000640.
12. Capitán L, Gutiérrez Santamaría J, Simon D, et al. Facial gender confirmation surgery: A protocol for diagnosis, surgical planning, and postoperative management. *Plast Reconstr Surg*. 2020;145(4):818e-828e. doi:10.1097/PRS.0000000000006686.
13. La Padula S, Hersant B, Chatel H, et al. One-step facial feminization surgery: The importance of a custom-made preoperative planning and patient satisfaction assessment. *J Plast Reconstr Aesthet Surg*. 2019;72(10):1694-1699. doi:10.1016/j.bjps.2019.06.014.
14. Kalmar CL, Xu W, Zimmerman CE, et al. Trends in utilization of virtual surgical planning in pediatric craniofacial surgery. *J Craniofac Surg*. 2020;31(7):1900-1905. doi:10.1097/SCS.0000000000006626.
15. Chen Z, Mo S, Fan X, You Y, Ye G, Zhou N. A meta-analysis and systematic review comparing the effectiveness of traditional and virtual surgical planning for orthognathic surgery: Based on randomized clinical trials. *J Oral Maxillofac Surg*. 2021;79(2):471.e1-471.e19. doi:10.1016/j.joms.2020.09.005.
16. World Professional Association for Transgender Health. *Standards of Care for the Health of Transsexual, Transgender, and Gender Nonconforming People [7th Version]*. 2012. Available at: https://www.wpath.org/publications/soc.
17. Tawa P, Brault N, Luca-Pozner V, et al. Three-dimensional custom-made surgical guides in facial feminization surgery: prospective study on safety and accuracy. *Aesthet Surg J*. 2021;41(11):NP1368-NP1378. doi:10.1093/asj/sjab032.
18. Hoang H, Bertrand AA, Hu AC, Lee JC. Simplifying facial feminization surgery using virtual modeling on the female skull. *Plast Reconstr Surg Glob Open*. 2020;8(3):e2618. doi:10.1097/GOX.0000000000002618.
19. Dang BN, Hu AC, Bertrand AA, et al. Evaluation and treatment of facial feminization surgery: part I. forehead, orbits, eyebrows, eyes, and nose. *Arch Plast Surg*. 2021;48(5):503-510. doi:10.5999/aps.2021.00199.
20. Gray R, Nguyen K, Lee J, et al. Osseous transformation with facial feminization surgery: Improved anatomical accuracy with virtual planning. *Plast Reconstr Surg*. 2019;144(5):1159-1168. doi:10.1097/PRS.0000000000006166.
21. Mandelbaum M, Lakhiani C, Chao JW. A novel application of virtual surgical planning to facial feminization surgery. *J Craniofac Surg*. 2019;30(5):1347-1348. doi:10.1097/SCS.0000000000005090.

Chapter | 24 |

# Virtual reality and augmented reality in surgery

*Lee WT Alkureishi, Chad Purnell*

CHAPTER OUTLINE



## Introduction

Presurgical planning is a broad term, encompassing everything from simple visualization of two-dimensional (2D) radiographic images to a true rehearsal of complex three-dimensional (3D) surgical movements based on computed tomographic (CT) or magnetic resonance imaging (MRI).[1] Over the last few decades, physical model surgery has given way to digital techniques, with 3D reconstruction of CT images now commonplace and the availability of complex software capable of simulating osteotomies and bony repositioning. These presurgical plans can then be accurately translated to the operating room via a variety of 3D-printed patient-specific guides, templates, and/or implants[2] (Fig. 24.1).

These techniques of presurgical planning have gained widespread acceptance and can be considered the gold-standard for many areas of craniomaxillofacial surgery, including orthognathic surgery[3] and microvascular jaw reconstruction.[4] However, there remain some challenges with the current techniques and workflows:

- **Software complexity.** Currently available software is multifunctional and quite powerful, but as a result, presents a complicated control interface with a steep learning curve. This is a "barrier to entry" for most surgeons, with most presurgical planning sessions therefore being driven by a software engineer rather than the surgeon.
- **Lack of depth perception and feel.** Digitally reconstructed 3D models of CT images provide a significantly improved means of visualizing the 3D anatomy of complex structures. However, when viewed on a typical flat-screen monitor these can best be described as a "pseudo-3D" image, lacking the depth perception of a physical object. As a result, fine manipulation or measurement of the object can be more difficult and/or imprecise.
- **Limited software tools.** The software tools used to create digital osteotomies share many features with those found in more traditional 3D engineering software. As a result, they work well for linear or geometric cuts, such as a Le Fort I osteotomy. However,

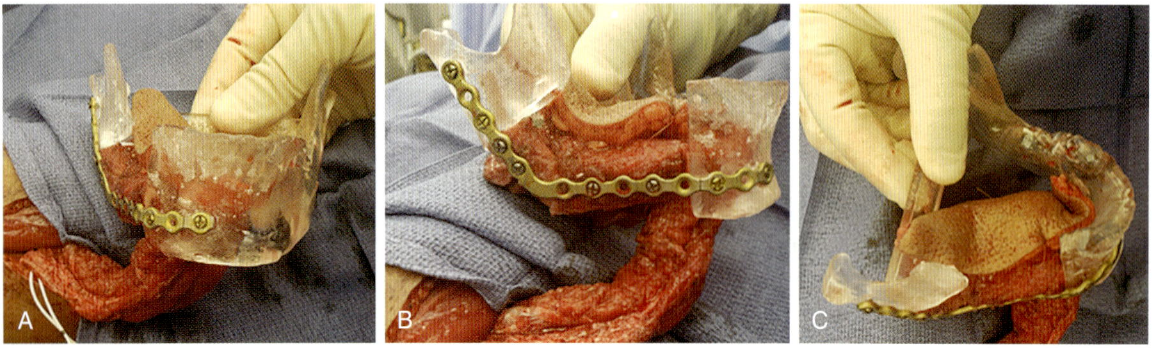


**Fig. 24.1** Prefabricated guides, implants, and templates. A three-dimensional printed model of the mandibular defect is used to prefabricate a reconstruction plate preoperatively, and for intraoperative contouring and plating of the fibula construct prior to ischemia time. (Reproduced with permission from © 2018 Intuitive Surgical, Inc. Used with permission.)

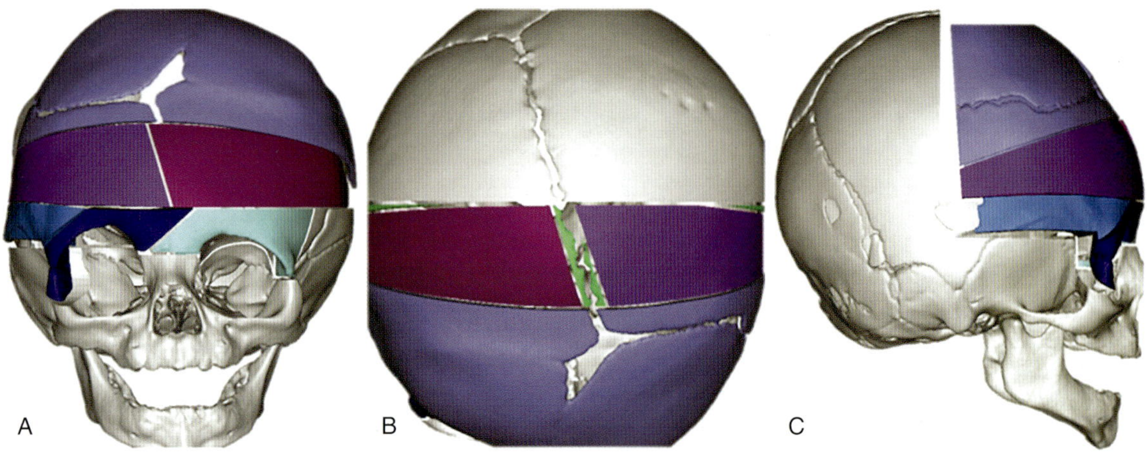


**Fig. 24.2** Complex and organic osteotomy patterns are labor-intensive and difficult to simulate using conventional medical modeling software. Owing to software and interface limitations, the end result still may not truly represent the surgeon's intent. (Reproduced with permission from © 2018 Intuitive Surgical, Inc. Used with permission.)

the limitations of these tools become quite apparent when attempting to simulate a more complex curved osteotomy, such as that required for a fronto-orbital advancement (Fig. 24.2).

- **Inability to adapt to intraoperative findings.** A variety of surgical splints, guides, templates, or custom implants can be manufactured based on the outputs of presurgical planning and can help to ensure the reproducibility of the plan on the day of surgery. However, the accuracy of surgery based on these guides assumes the patient's anatomy is unchanged from the preoperative imaging and, if intraoperative findings necessitate a change in the surgical plan, these pregenerated aids can therefore be rendered useless.

Since 2006, the Division of Plastic Surgery and the Department of Industrial and Mechanical Engineering at the University of Illinois, Chicago, have been working in collaboration to address the abovementioned limitations. The outcome of this collaboration is a purpose-built virtual-reality-based software platform named ImmersiveView (ImmersiveTouch, Inc, Chicago). ImmersiveView provides a solid foundation and comprehensive virtual toolkit, enabling surgeon-led presurgical visualization and true 3D-VR planning of a wide variety of surgical procedures. In addition, the digital outputs of VR-based planning have been designed according to industry standards, facilitating the production of familiar "gold-standard" surgical guides/splints, as well as integration with existing, new, and emerging technologies, such as intraoperative navigation[5] and the rapidly developing field of augmented reality (AR). These intraoperative guidance modalities can potentially provide an ideal complement to the state-of-the-art presurgical planning afforded by the VR environment, and the marrying of these technologies provides a completely digital workflow, from imaging and diagnosis to the completion of surgery.

## Clinical considerations

For an emerging technology such as VR or AR to be clinically useful, it must meet the following criteria:

- Tangible improvement in at least one aspect of surgical workflow
- Wide availability
- Cost-effective
- Can be utilized in timely fashion

The benefits of VR are well established and include improved visualization, environmental immersion, and, importantly, depth perception. These benefits have been realized in a wide variety of fields, including aviation, military training, video gaming, and entertainment.[6]

The concepts behind stereoscopic photography and animation can be traced back as far as 1832, and true head-mounted VR displays were first developed in 1960.[7] There were steady improvements over the next several decades, but the introduction of low-cost high-performance consumer devices, such as the Oculus Rift in 2012 (Meta Platforms Inc, Menlo Park CA, formerly OculusVR) marked a watershed in the popularity and availability of the technology. The rapid surge in the market for VR videogaming has helped to drive the cost of entry down, and the continual improvement in hardware performance now produces high-resolution images with a rapid refresh rate, which is well suited to the display of anatomical images.

Surgical applications for VR range from simple preoperative anatomical visualization, and resident and student education, to realistic simulation of complex osteotomies and bony movements, placement of implants, and reconstruction planning. In this chapter, we will describe these applications in detail.

The depth perception afforded by the virtual reality environment is one of the most important benefits of VR because it allows the user to reach out and touch or grab the virtual object as they would in real life. This, in turn, allows for simplification of the user interface, which is controlled by motion-controlled handpieces with minimal requirement for button presses. The end result of this is a very shallow learning curve, allowing the surgeon (or resident, or student) to control the simulation or planning session without the need for an intermediary technician. This puts the control of surgical planning back into the hands of the surgeon.

Another key requirement relates to the time required for preparation of images for surgical planning or simulation purposes. This is especially true for nonelective surgeries, such as facial trauma, where surgery often takes place within 24 hours after patient presentation. In such cases, the recently developed ability to work directly with raw digital imaging and communications in medicine (DICOM) data means that the surgeon can take images directly from the scanner and load into the VR space for manipulation and immediate planning with no unnecessary delays. This has important implications not only for the trauma setting, but also potentially in the setting of intraoperative changes to the surgical plan and the need to adapt to unexpected anatomy or pathology (ImmersiveView, ImmersiveTouch Inc, Chicago IL).

The variety of procedures that can benefit from VR and AR visualization and planning is broad, including trauma and elective bony reconstruction, both within the craniofacial skeleton and elsewhere in the body. However, the bony anatomy only tells part of the story, and for many procedures, the ability to visualize the soft tissues can be equally important. To that end, MRI image compatibility and the option to overlay images from different modalities potentially opens up VR-based planning for tumor resections, vascular surgeries, and more (ImmersiveTrauma 4.2, ImmersiveTouch, Inc).

AR provides the potential to take surgical planning (performed in VR or otherwise) into the operating room. AR, by definition, is the fusion of computer-generated data and the environment in real time.[8] This allows a surgeon to view information while simultaneously viewing the operative field. The pinnacle of AR potential is to provide patient-specific anatomic or imaging data, linked via anatomic points to the patient to allow a surgeon to "see through" the patient and identify deep anatomic structures and treatment targets. However, significant hurdles still remain in workflow, device availability, fidelity, and ease of use in order to extend immersive AR into a technology to be used routinely for a wide range of cases.

For workflow for VR see eFig. 24.1: Virtual reality workflow.ppt.

For workflow for AR see eFig. 24.2: Augmented reality workflow.ppt.

## Hardware considerations

### Virtual reality hardware

The hardware requirements for VR have remained fairly constant since its introduction, and include the following:

- A separate display device for each eye.
- Motion tracking of the user's head movements.
- A control mechanism.

Dual display devices provide separate images, which are then interpreted by the user's brain and "reconstructed" into a true 3D image with accurate depth perception. The motion tracking is used to adjust the user's viewpoint according to head position, providing the natural sensation of moving around a physical object.

Although VR headsets resembling current hardware have been commercially available for several decades, the constant improvement in computer processing power and graphic displays has resulted in high-resolution, high-refresh-rate images with extremely precise motion tracking of both the user's viewpoint and hand movements[9]. The latest generation of headsets have incorporated motion tracking sensors into the headset and controllers, negating the need for external sensors, and even functioning without the need for a separate computer (Oculus Quest, Meta Platforms Inc, Menlo Park CA). While currently available VR surgical planning solutions continue to use a high-performance laptop to drive the software, continued improvement in the performance of these stand-alone VR headsets is expected, and they are likely to become predominant in the near future.

Perhaps the most important aspect of the hardware for most surgeons relates to the control mechanism, since the means of physical interaction with the VR environment will dictate the achievable simplicity of the software interface. The most common controllers are deceptively simple handheld triggers with just a few buttons for each hand (Fig. 24.3). However, the handpieces also incorporate internal gyroscopes, magnetometers, and accelerometers, which are capable of translating the user's natural hand movements into the virtual environment, which limits the need for complex button use. The user can simply reach out toward the VR anatomy, "grab" it by squeezing the controller, and move it as they would a physical object (Video 24.1).

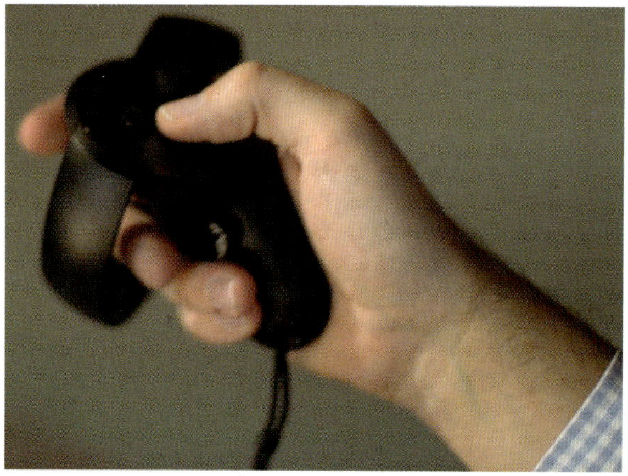

**Fig. 24.3** Handsets are used to control the virtual reality environment. Relatively few buttons help to keep the control simple and intuitive, but are supplemented by internal gyroscopes, magnetometers, and accelerometers for motion tracking.

### Augmented reality hardware

Unlike VR, AR can be experienced through several different mechanisms. At its core, AR requires a few critical elements:[10]

- A sensor to capture images in real time.
- Registration to link sensor images to computer-generated data.
- A display or display(s) to display the merged image.

At its simplest, all-in-one solutions are available, such as those on a smartphone, which utilize an onboard camera and light detection and ranging (LiDAR) scanner as sensors, combined with in-device registration computations, and display through the phones screen. Although this type of more rudimentary 2D display can have uses in the operating room, technology that allows stereoscopic vision has more clinical potential. Stereoscopic vision allows a surgeon to visualize deep structures in their correct anatomic position simultaneously with the operative field in three dimensions. This type of system is significantly more complex, requiring appropriate registration and visualization in three dimensions. The majority of these systems utilize an optical see-through head-mounted display (HMD) that allows the user to see the world around them directly, while images are projected into the users view. Only recently have all-in-one HMDs been widely available, such as HoloLens (Microsoft, Redmond, WA) and Magic Leap One (Magic Leap, Plantation, FL). These products have significantly improved the ability to access and utilize AR for surgeons as well as the general population. HoloLens has been more commonly utilized in surgery thus far.

The natural application of AR to the operating room provides additional challenges. Maintaining the surgeon's visualization of the operative field requires that the HMD does not obstruct vision and has a wide field of view. It must also be light enough to wear while operating, especially for extended periods of time. Both weight and field of view are improving with each successive generation of AR devices.

Further, registration presents an essential challenge in AR, especially in cases where the operative field is somewhat mobile and/or the targets are soft tissue and not bony. High levels of precision are required. There are several techniques that can be utilized based on the type of procedure being performed. For facial procedures, occlusion-based registration guides can be used, but are not practical to be in place during the entire surgery – instead these would be in place for critical portions of the operation to improve fidelity.[11-14] Fiducial registration via a bone-anchored skull post or a facemask may be used, as in standard intraoperative navigation. In cases where the operative field can be completely immobilized, such as in a pinned skull, registration is least complicated and can typically be accomplished through standard fiducial registration. Even more challenging is the utilization of AR for deformable soft structures, such as the liver. Registration in these organs is challenging because the structures themselves are soft and mobile, and change shape and location with respirations. Utilizing AR for these types of structures likely will require complex physics-based algorithms.[15]

## Software considerations

The Department of Engineering at the University of Illinois, Chicago, has a strong background in VR, and its application to a variety of surgical simulations.[16,17] In collaboration with the Division of Plastic Surgery, a suite of software tools have been developed with the intention of providing improved visualization of patient-specific anatomy, a simple interface with a shallow learning curve, and a more efficient workflow for surgical planning.

### ImmersiveView: a virtual reality toolkit

This basic suite of software tools, known as ImmersiveView, allows near instantaneous loading of patient-specific DICOM data for immediate visualization in the VR environment. This brings the benefits of improved visualization, rapid and precise viewpoint adjustment, and precise control over the displayed image to the realm of presurgical anatomical visualization (Fig. 24.4). Within ImmersiveView, the user can interact with the patient model much as they would a physical object, but with the added ability to "slice" the model to view internal anatomy in any orientation, not limited to standard axial, coronal and sagittal views. The reformatted slice data can be overlaid on the VR model, allowing simultaneous viewing of the CT or MRI images and the 3D-VR model. Measurements can also be made, with the ability to quickly "zoom" the image by simply pulling toward the user, and "snap" the points of measurement to the patient anatomy. This allows very precise anatomical measurements to be made without a large time commitment (Fig. 24.5).

The control interface for the software has been kept as simple as possible, in order to streamline the learning curve. Button presses are limited to squeezing the handle trigger to "grab" or hold and move objects, while instruments such as measuring tools, pens, or surgical instruments are actuated through a squeeze of the index finger trigger (Fig. 24.6). In this way, the vast majority of functions within the software can be accessed through these two simple button presses. Changing between tools is accomplished through the use of a virtual toolkit, which is opened through a button press.

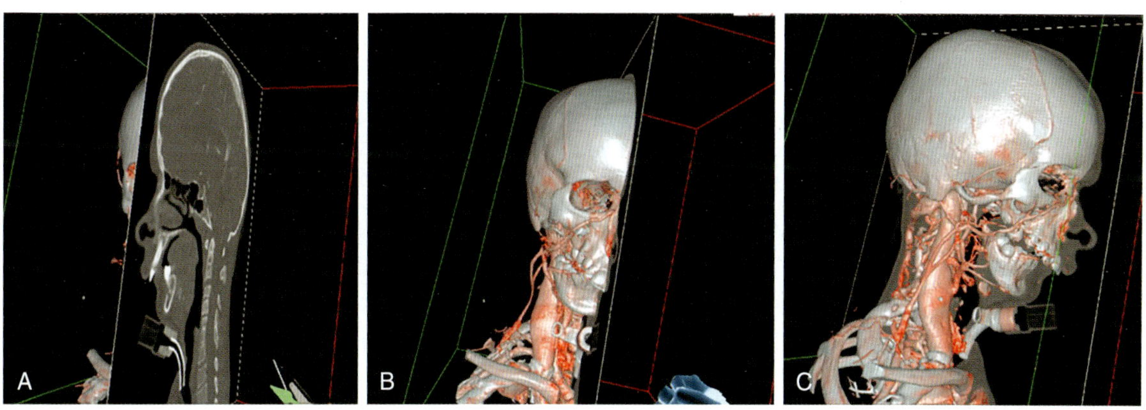


**Fig. 24.4** ImmersiveView software allows rapid three-dimensional virtual reality model generation from standard digital imaging and communications in medicine data.

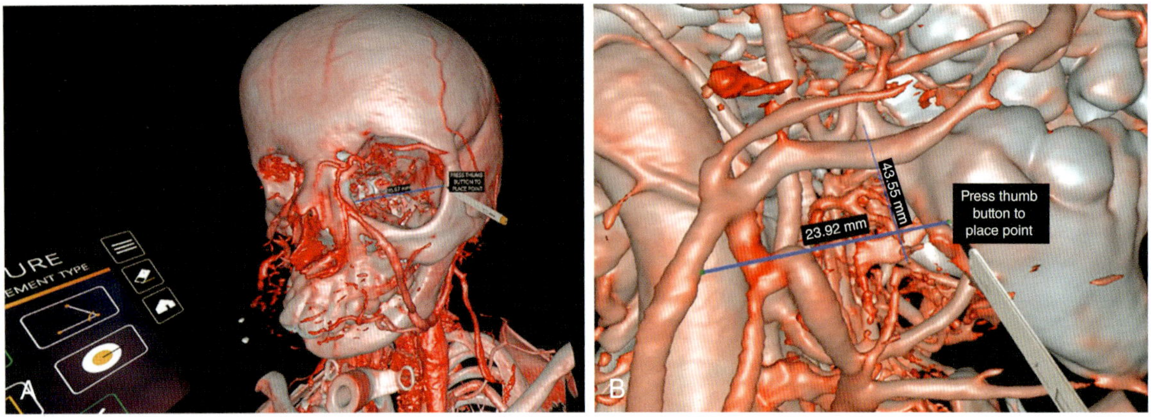


Fig. 24.5 Measurements made within the ImmersiveView software. Measured points can snap to anatomy or be free-floating and can be readjusted after placement.

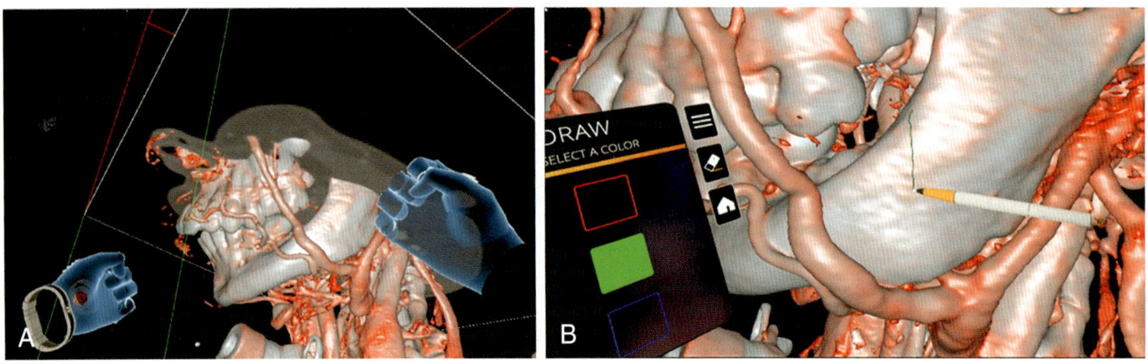


Fig. 24.6 Simple hand gestures and minimal button presses are used to control the virtual reality interface. (A) "Grabbing" the model to translate, rotate, or zoom. (B) A variety of instruments can be selected from a virtual toolbox and actuated with a single button press.

In addition, this platform of basic tools forms the foundation for a variety of specialty modules facilitating true surgical planning for a variety of complex procedures, ranging from craniofacial implant placement to microvascular jaw reconstruction, as well as applications outside of the craniofacial skeleton. These specialty applications are outlined in more detail later in this chapter and the accompanying files.

To date, there is no widely available AR software platform for surgery. This is for several reasons. Software utilized for AR must overcome all of the same challenges of VR software, including ease of use for input of DICOM files, windowing, and image manipulation. Software for AR specifically must deal with several challenges in addition to these. Control of basic software functions must be hands-free to allow a surgeon the ability to operate in a sterile field. The software must also be able to adjust for small position changes of the patient. The level of fidelity required depends on the type of surgery. Proprietary solutions are being developed for specific types of surgery, such as spine surgery.[18] However, a universal or semi-universal platform for AR during surgery will be much more complex to develop, given the myriad nuances of specific procedures and specialists' needs.[19]

## Applications

The most obvious benefit of viewing in the VR space is improved visualization, with the ability to quickly alter the viewpoint or magnification in an intuitive fashion. However, the full suite of tools available within the VR space provides the ability to interact with the anatomy,

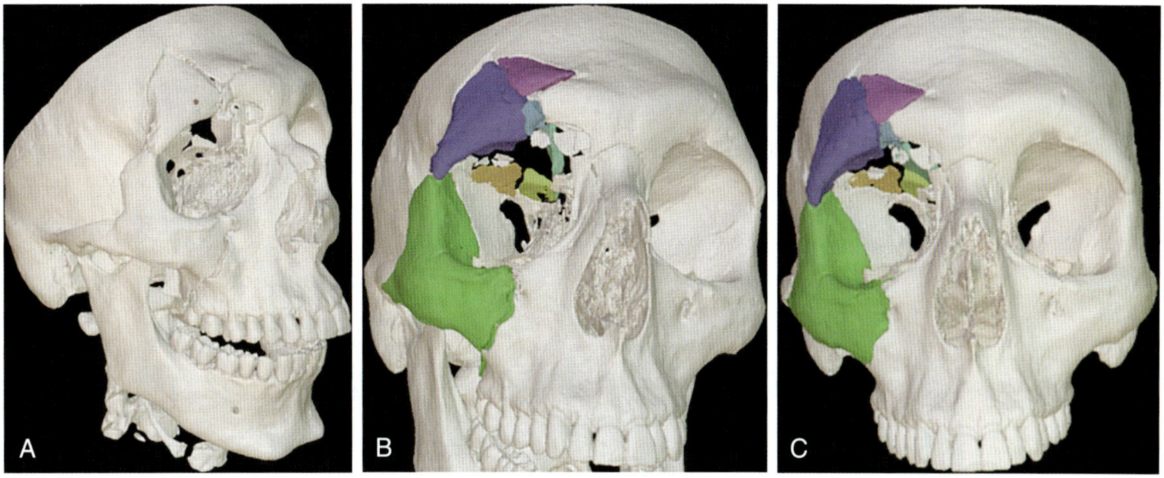


Fig. 24.7 Segmentation and reduction of a zygomaticomaxillary and orbital roof fracture. (A) Preoperative view. (B) Segmentation of the fracture segments is accomplished through a "paint" tool, followed by separation of the segmented fragments from the facial skeleton. (C) The fracture segments can be individually reduced by freehand moves or the use of precision sliders.

simulating a variety of procedures and providing a true surgical planning environment:

- Performing geometric, curvilinear, or freeform osteotomies.
- Segmenting the model.
- Altering the position of portions of the model.
- Altering the contour of the bone by addition or subtraction.
- Mirroring the anatomy.
- Combining multiple models or portions of models within the same space.
- Use of normative models to aid with reconstruction planning.
- Incorporating implants, osteosynthesis plates, or other devices.

Using this platform of tools, VR visualization of patient-specific anatomy has rapidly found utility for a wide variety of craniomaxillofacial procedures over the last few years, including:

- Maxillofacial trauma
- Orthognathic surgery
- Craniofacial implant planning
- Jaw reconstruction

## Maxillofacial trauma

In the setting of maxillofacial trauma, the time from injury to diagnosis and subsequent surgical management can be very short and, as a result, presurgical planning solutions are seldom used for these fractures. Rapid and automated processing of raw CT image data can provide a 3D-VR model within minutes of scan acquisition, and this has potentially important implications for the care of trauma patients. Viewing in VR provides an unprecedented degree of control over the viewpoint, but moreover, the tools within the VR platform allow rapid segmentation of bony anatomy, anatomical reduction of fracture segments, and data export of the simulated post-operative anatomy within a very short time frame (Fig. 24.7). This potentially allows the use of surgical aides, such as positioning guides (Fig. 24.8) or intraoperative navigation (Fig. 24.9) as adjuncts to the operative procedure, without incurring unnecessary delays in care. Similarly, this near instantaneous image processing can be applied to intraoperative CT scan data, allowing rapid

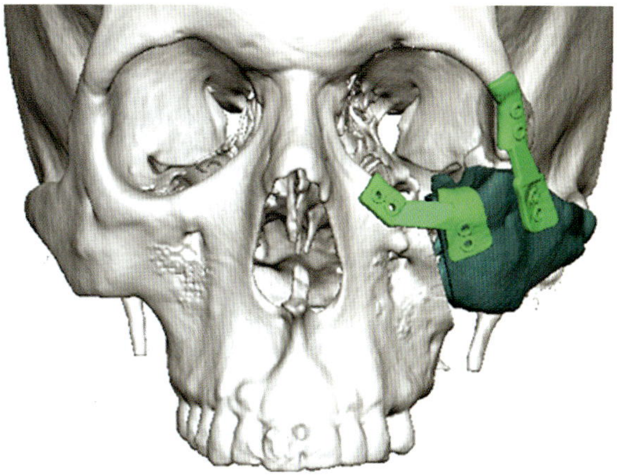

Fig. 24.8 Positioning guides for fracture reduction.

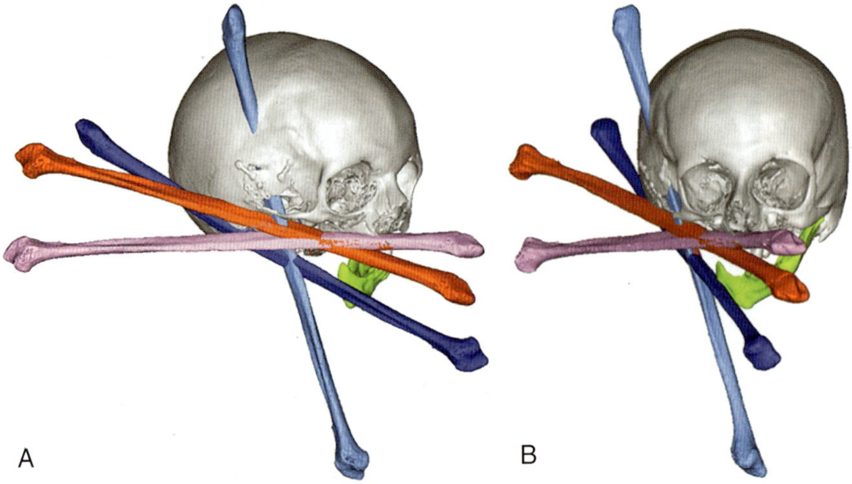


**Fig. 24.15** Microvascular jaw reconstruction planning using conventional medical modeling software.

software is designed to allow for these combined requirements and can adapt to the continuous evolution of surgical techniques and innovations.

## Augmented reality

The potential clinical applications for AR are broad. Almost any type of surgery would benefit from an intraoperative anatomic guide or the ability to simultaneously view patient imaging or data. The earliest uses of AR have been neurosurgical, such as spine surgery, cranial tumor resection, or separation of craniopagus twins, all of which allow relative immobility of the operative field with cranial pins.[20] As technology improves, the ability to overlay more complex data with more patient motion will become available.

We anticipate that as AR becomes more powerful and universal, it will be applied to all but the simplest of surgeries. AR has immense potential to make surgeries more efficient and decrease complications related to "surgical misadventures" or losing one's bearings in a challenging 3D space. The potential for surgical education is also quite large for both VR and AR. Multiple studies have shown that these types of platforms provide faster and more effective surgical skill acquisition than more traditional methods.[21]

## Fidelity/verification

As with all CT viewing software, windowing of the CT image can be adjusted according to the tissue of interest. This adjustment is achieved through the use of simple sliders and gives the surgeon the ability to optimize the balance between display of the anatomy and minimization of scatter, noise, or metal artifact (Fig. 24.17).

Before relying on any medical imaging software, it is necessary to ensure the accuracy of the displayed anatomy, measured distances, and/or planned movements. In the paper by Anik et al,[22] a comparative study was performed evaluating linear and angular measurements on both physical models, using a coordinate measuring machine, and within the VR environment on CT-scanned versions of the same models. The authors found no significant difference between the physical and VR measurements ($p = 0.413$, $p = 0.533$), while VR measurements showed both high intra-rater and inter-rater reproducibility (inter-class coefficients of 0.99–1.00). The magnitude of any observed errors was felt to be well within the acceptable limits for intended use, and comparable to existing software workflows.

## Conclusion

The incorporation of state-of-the-art technology, such as VR and AR has the potential to improve many aspects of presurgical visualization and planning, intraoperative execution and postoperative verification/monitoring. The pace of development of these technologies is rapid and continues to progress. VR represents a natural evolution of our currently utilized techniques and provides the opportunity to expand our indications for presurgical planning and patient-specific guided surgery. The

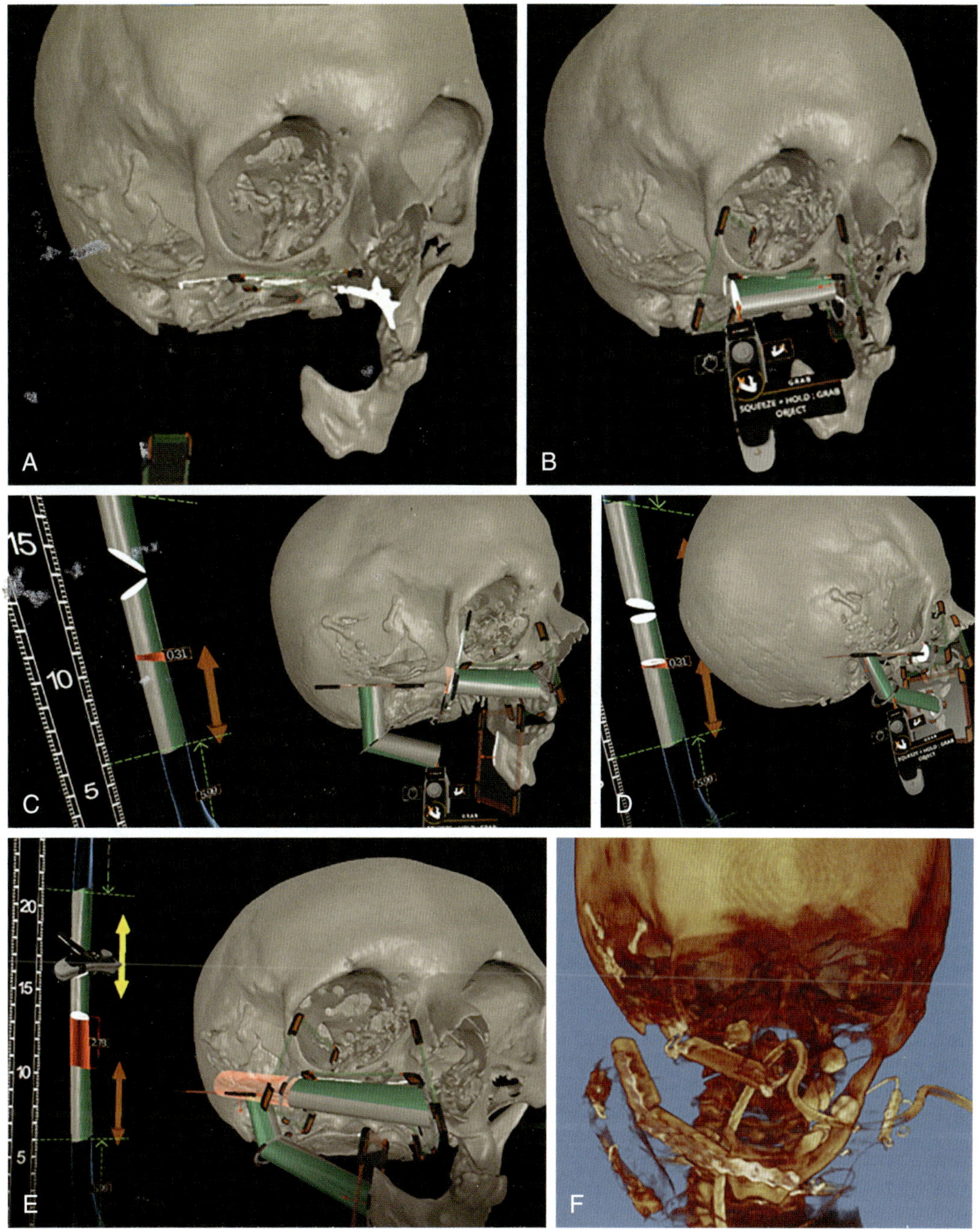


Fig. 24.16 Complex maxilla and mandible reconstruction planning can be accomplished in much shorter time-frame compared with conventional planning software. (A) Complex maxillary and mandibular defect after tumor resection in childhood. (B,C) Drawing the path for a single fibula neomaxilla-neomandible construct. (D) Adjustments to number, length, rotation, and axial position of individual segments can be performed on-the-fly using adjustment handles. (E) Gap segments can be created, further expanding the possibilities for complex reconstruction or double-barreling. (F) The completed reconstruction.

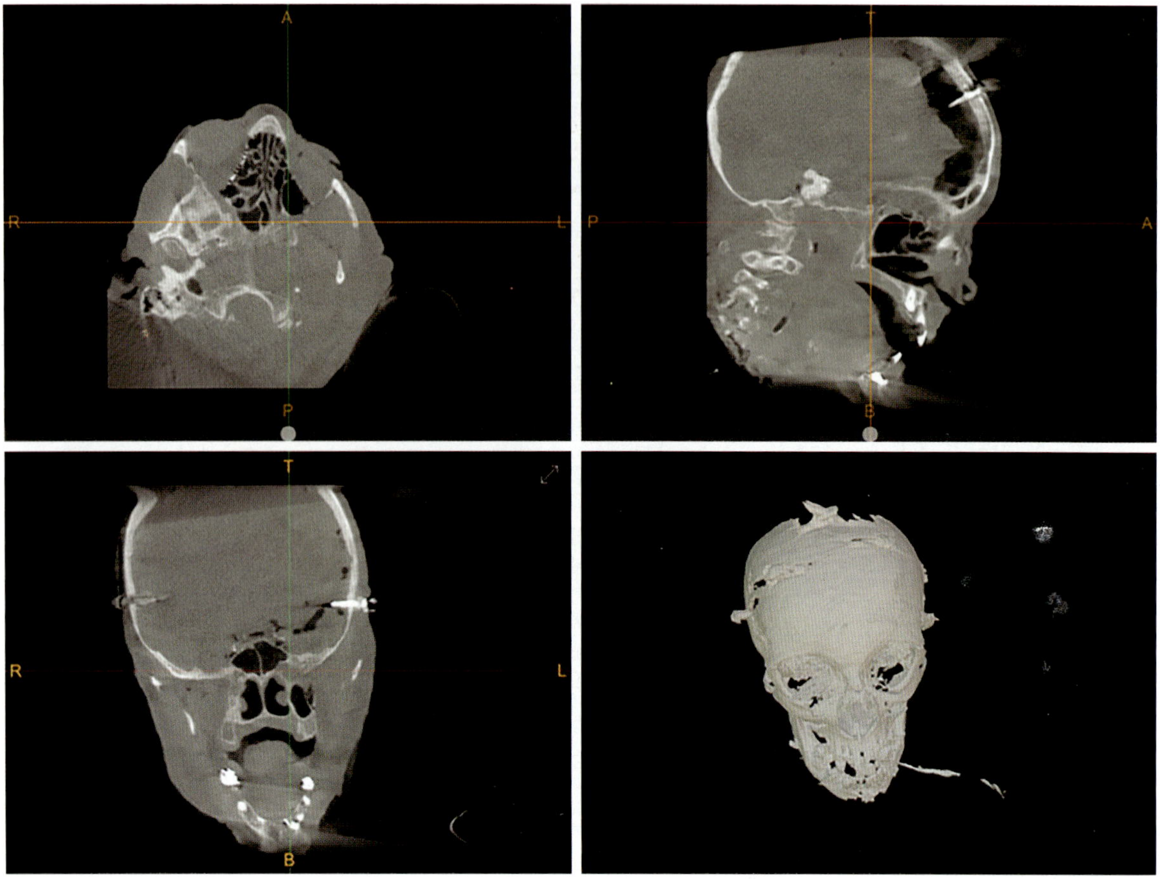


**Fig. 24.17** Thresholding, or windowing, of the image is achieved through simple sliders.

addition of AR techniques, intraoperative image overlays, and image-guided surgery is a hugely promising area of research that will undoubtedly continue to find new applications as the hardware progressively improves. It is feasible that, as AR techniques improve, the need for conventional intraoperative navigation technologies may diminish. The interplay between preoperative VR and intraoperative AR is an interesting area of study, and we are excited to see the developments to come over the next few years.

## Take-home points

- The VR environment provides an unprecedented level of detail and control over the viewing of 3D reconstruction patient anatomy models.
- The simplified control interface provides an intuitive method of interaction and a shallow learning curve, facilitating ease of use.
- The software tools provided within the VR platform allow viewing, marking, cutting, moving, and measuring of the patient anatomy, allowing the realistic and accurate simulation of a variety of surgical procedures.
- AR can project digital images as an overlay onto real-life objects or patients, with a variety of potential surgical applications.
- AR guidance offers an exciting future alternative to conventional surgical navigation techniques.
- Accurate patient registration and motion tracking are key to the success and accuracy of AR techniques.
- As AR headsets and hardware/software continues to improve, we anticipate their application will gain more widespread use.

## References


1. Altobelli DE, Kikinis R, Mulliken JB, et al. Computer-assisted three-dimensional planning in craniofacial surgery. *Plastic Reconstr Surg*. 1993;92:576-587.
2. Zhao L, Patel PK, Cohen M. Application of virtual surgical planning with computer assisted design and manufacturing technology to cranio-maxillofacial surgery. *Arch Plast Surg*. 2012;39: 309-316.
3. Farrell BB, Franco PB, Tucker MR. Virtual surgical planning in orthognathic surgery. *Oral Maxillofac Surg Clin North Am*. 2014;26:459-473.
4. Pucci R, Weyh A, Smotherman C, Valentini V, Bunnell A, Fernandes R. Accuracy of virtual planned surgery versus conventional free-hand surgery for reconstruction of the mandible with osteocutaneous free flaps. *Int J Oral Maxillofac Surg*. 2020;49(9):1153-1161.
5. Mathis SA, Arias E, Zhao LP, Purnell CA, Patel PK, Alkureishi LWT. Same-day virtual reality surgical planning and intraoperative navigation: A new surgical workflow for craniofacial trauma and reconstruction. Presented at the Plastic Surgery Meeting, *American Society of Plastic Surgeons Annual Meeting*, Atlanta GA, October 2021.
6. Cipresso P, Giglioli IAC, Raya MA, Riva G. The past, present, and future of virtual and augmented reality research: a network and cluster analysis of the literature. *Front Psychol*. 2018;9:2086.
7. Sutherland IE. *The Ultimate Display. Multimedia: From Wagner to Virtual Reality*. Norton: New York USA; 1965.
8. Vávra P, Roman J, Zonča P, et al. Recent development of augmented reality in surgery: a review. *J Healthc Eng*. 2017;2017:4574172.
9. Thompson C. Stereographs were the original virtual reality. *Smithsonian Magazine*. October 2017.
10. Shuhaiber JH. Augmented reality in surgery. *Arch Surg*. 2004;139(2):170-174. doi:10.1001/archsurg.139.2.170.
11. Zhu M, Liu F, Zhou C, et al. Does intraoperative navigation improve the accuracy of mandibular angle osteotomy: Comparison between augmented reality navigation, individualised templates and free-hand techniques. *J Plast Reconstr Aesthet Surg*. 2018;71(8):1188-1195.
12. Zhu M, Chai G, Lin L, et al. Effectiveness of a novel augmented reality-based navigation system in treatment of orbital hypertelorism. *Ann Plast Surg*. 2016;77(6):662-668.
13. Han W, Yang X, Wu S, et al. A new method for cranial vault reconstruction: augmented reality in synostotic plagiocephaly surgery. *J Craniomaxillofac Surg*. 2019;47(8):1280-1284.
14. Qu M, Hou Y, Xu Y, et al. Precise positioning of an intraoral distractor using augmented reality in patients with hemifacial microsomia. *J Craniomaxillofac Surg*. 2015;43(1):106-112.
15. Haouchine N, Dequidt J, Berger MO, Cotin S. Deformation-based augmented reality for hepatic surgery. *Stud Health Technol Inform*. 2013;184:182-188.
16. Luciano CJ, Banerjee PP, Sorenson JM, et al. Percutaneous spinal fixation simulation with virtual reality and haptics. *Neurosurgery*. 2013;72(suppl 1):89-96.
17. Alaraj A, Luciano CJ, Bailey DP, et al. Virtual reality cerebral aneurysm clipping simulation with real-time haptic feedback. *Neurosurgery*. 2015;11 suppl 2(0 2):52-58.
18. Dennler C, Jaberg L, Spirig J, et al. Augmented reality-based navigation increases precision of pedicle screw insertion. *J Orthop Surg Res*. 2020;15(1):174.
19. Vles MD, Terng NCO, Zijlstra K, Mureau MAM, Corten EML. Virtual and augmented reality for preoperative planning in plastic surgical procedures: a systematic review. *J Plast Reconstr Aesthet Surg*. 2020;73(11):1951-1959.
20. Meola A, Cutolo F, Carbone M, Cagnazzo F, Ferrari M, Ferrari V. Augmented reality in neurosurgery: a systematic review. *Neurosurg Rev*. 2017;40(4):537-548.
21. Sheik-Ali S, Edgcombe H, Paton C. Next-generation virtual and augmented reality in surgical education: a narrative review. *Surg Technol Int*. 2019;35:27-35.
22. Anik AA, Xavier BA, Hansmann J, et al. Accuracy and reproducibility of linear and angular measurements in virtual reality: a validation study. *J Digit Imaging*. 2020;33(1):111-120.

Chapter 25

# Robots in craniofacial surgery

*Dale J Podolsky, Christopher R Forrest*

CHAPTER OUTLINE



## Introduction

Surgical approaches in craniofacial surgery follow specific principles due to the complex anatomy of the head and neck and the aesthetic sensitivity of the region. The approaches can be categorized into two domains as a result of these factors, which are summarized in Table 25.1. The first domain includes limited approaches to avoid significant soft tissue disruption that minimizes or avoids incisions within aesthetically sensitive areas.[1] The disadvantages of these limited approaches include reduced visualization and manipulability of instruments, which can impact the precision and ability to successfully perform the procedure as well as the ability to perform more complex maneuvers. The second domain includes larger degloving approaches to access more distant sites or when more extensive soft tissue or bony manipulation and fixation is required. These approaches provide excellent visualization at the expense of increased morbidity.[2]

Surgical robots offer improved visualization, access, and dexterity[3] and are well suited for craniofacial surgery where access is limited, and precision is required to perform precise dissections and bone cuts while avoiding critical structures. The technical capabilities of a robot may allow performance of more extensive procedures using more limited approaches.

## Surgical robotics

### The da Vinci surgical system

The da Vinci surgical system is the most utilized surgical robot platform worldwide. The system is a master-slave teleoperated robot, where the surgeon sits at a surgeon console and remotely controls the robotic arms (Fig. 25.1). The latest multi-port version of the da Vinci is the Xi and the newest system is the da Vinci SP (single-port) (Fig. 25.2). The Xi contains four robotic arms with one arm acting as the endoscope. Each arm couples to an

**Table 25.1 Examples, advantages and disadvantages comparing limited and degloving approaches to the craniofacial skeleton**

| Examples | Advantages | Disadvantages |
|---|---|---|
| **Limited approaches** | | |
| Eyelid incisions<br>Lynch incision<br>Brow incision<br>Closed rhinoplasty | Smaller incisions<br>Less blood loss<br>Less soft tissue disruption | Reduced visualization<br>Reduced manipulability of instruments<br>More difficult to perform complex maneuvers |
| **Large degloving approaches** | | |
| Bicoronal incision<br>Temporal incision<br>Upper buccal sulcus<br>Submandibular<br>Retromandibular<br>Rhytidectomy | Improved visualization<br>Better access<br>Well-hidden incision | More soft tissue disruption<br>Larger incisions and subsequent scarring<br>Increased blood loss<br>More soft tissue disruption<br>Long-term effects with aging |

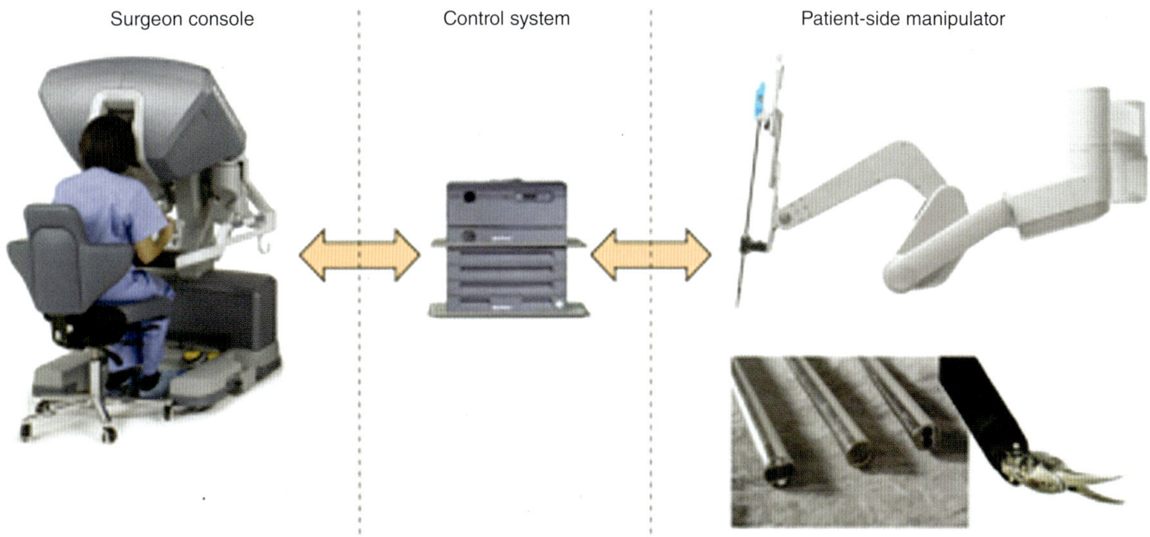


**Fig. 25.1** The overall design of the da Vinci system, which is teleoperated controlled by the surgeon at the surgeon console. The console controls the robotic arms of the patient-side manipulator. Each patient-side manipulator contains a wristed instrument that can be interchanged for different tool tips. (Image from Azizian M, Liu M, Khajali I, Sorger J, Oh D, Daimios S. The da Vinci Surgical System. In: Abedin-Nasab MH, E. *Handbook of Robotic and Image-Guided Surgery*: Elsevier; 2020:39–55.

EndoWrist instrument that contains the specific surgical instrument or tool that articulates at a distal "wrist", providing a total of 7 degrees of freedom (Fig. 25.3 and Table 25.2).[4] The SP system has the same number of arms (one binocular camera and three instrument arms) that all traverse through a single tube 2.5 cm in diameter. Both the SP[5] and previous generation systems[6] have been utilized for transoral robotic surgery (TORS).

## The limitations of the da Vinci for craniofacial surgery

The da Vinci system is only suitable for soft tissue procedures with the system lacking the capability to cut bone. The SP system is more compact and is a significant step forward in single-port access. However, the instruments are large and may be suboptimal for the curvatures and

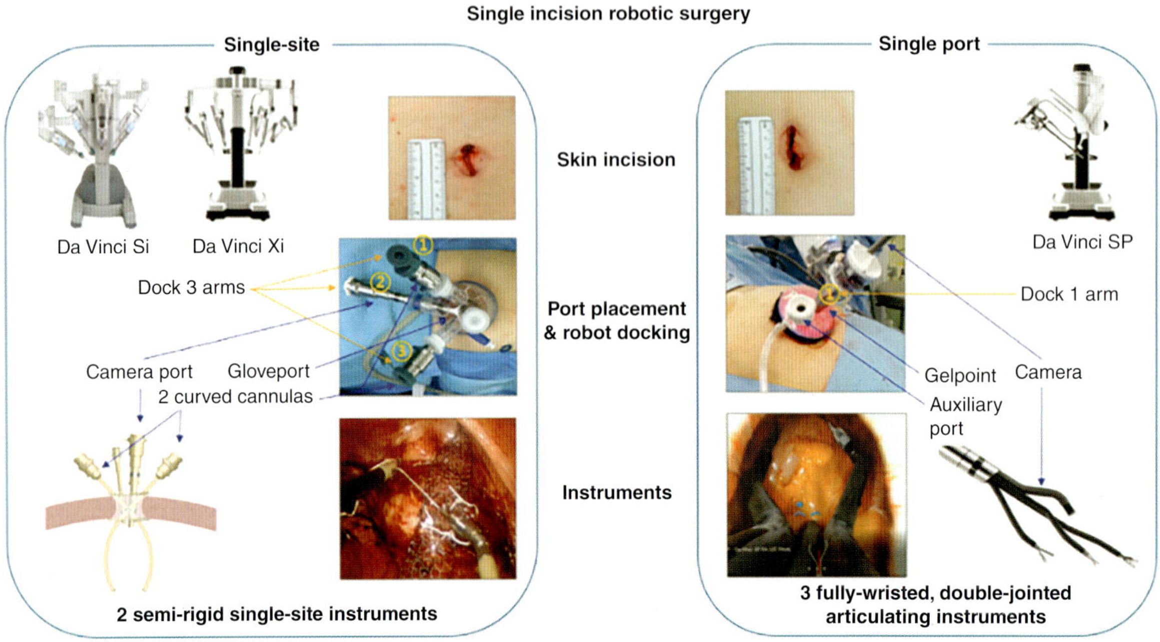


**Fig. 25.2** Comparison between the da Vinci single-site and single-port system designs. Single-site uses the multi-port da Vinci Si or Xi in comparison to the da Vinci single port (SP). (Image from Lee SR, Roh AM, Jeong K, Kim SH, Chae HD, Moon HS. First report comparing the two types of single-incision robotic sacrocolpopexy: Single site using the da Vinci Xi or Si system and single port using the da Vinci SP system. *Taiwan J Obstet Gynecol*. 2021;60(1):60–5.)

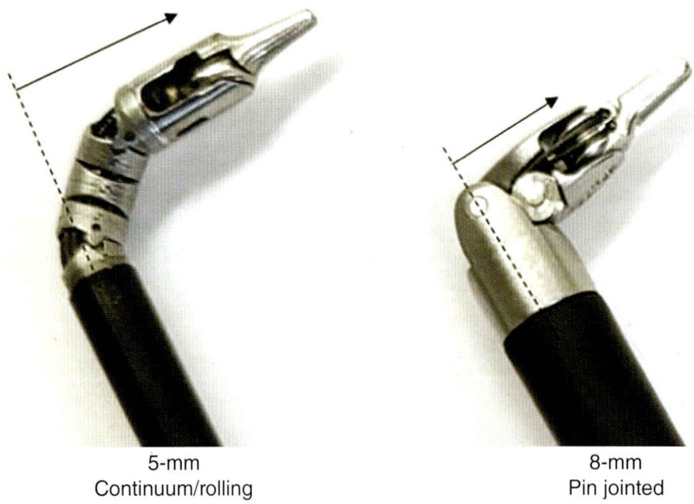


**Fig. 25.3** Comparison of the 8-mm to 5-mm EndoWrist instruments. The 8-mm instruments utilize a pin jointed mechanism compared to the 5-mm multilink snake arm mechanism. Although larger, the 8-mm instruments have a more compact articulating mechanism and, counterintuitively, perform better in confined areas, in comparison to the 5-mm instruments.

**Table 25.2 Advantages and disadvantages comparing the 5- and 8-mm da Vinci EndoWrist instruments**

| | Design | Advantages | Disadvantages |
|---|---|---|---|
| 5-mm EndoWrist instruments | Multilink backbone design | Smaller diameter<br>Lower profile | Less compact articulation<br>Impaired performance within smaller workspace |
| 8-mm EndoWrist instruments | Pin joint design | More compact articulation<br>Improved performance within smaller workspace | Larger diameter |

tight crevices of the facial bones and calvarium. In addition, a bone-cutting robot should take advantage of navigation to ensure cutting paths are accurately executed, and the da Vinci lacks this capability. Nonetheless, an understanding of the da Vinci system's design, capabilities, and limitations, especially given its significant widespread use, can help formulate the design of future systems that are optimized for specific types of surgical procedures.

## Clinical considerations

The field of craniofacial robotics can be classified into soft tissue- and bone-related procedures.

Research and development of robotic systems for craniofacial applications is scarce. A review of robotics in oral, craniofacial, and head and neck surgery in 2012 revealed only two studies investigating craniofacial robotic systems, with the majority of studies conducted in the field of transoral robotic surgery (TORS) and robotic-assisted (para) thyroidectomy.[7] The first of these two studies investigated the use of a hexapod robot for trepanation of the skull in patients with calvarial tumor.[8] The second study presented a robot with an attached bone mill that performs autonomous bone cuts of the calvarium for patients with craniosynostosis using path-planning and navigation.[9]

## Soft tissue procedures

Transoral robotic surgical (TORS) procedures involving resection and reconstruction of oropharyngeal lesions is the most common soft tissue application of robotics in the head and neck region.[6] An extension of TORS is transoral robotic cleft surgery (TORCS), which has been trialed in a series of 10 patients using the da Vinci surgical system demonstrating feasibility.[10] Khan et al. demonstrated the feasibility of using the da Vinci Si for cleft palate and pharyngeal wall surgery in a cadaver.[11] Podolsky et al. tested the da Vinci Si and Xi for cleft palate surgery using a high-fidelity cleft palate simulator.[12] Both studies demonstrated that using the da Vinci for cleft palate surgery has specific advantages compared to traditional approaches, such as improved visualization, access, and precision. However, challenges included frequent instrument-instrument and instrument-oral cavity collisions as a result of the close proximity of each robotic arm while accessing through the single orifice of the oral cavity.[12]

## Bone-related procedures

Literature on craniofacial bone cutting robots has been increasing. The two main classifications of craniofacial specific robots are for performing craniotomies and orthognathic surgery.

### Robotic craniotomies

A group from Germany developed a robotic system that can perform craniotomies with application for craniosynostosis procedures. The system comprises a CASPER robot system, optical tracking, and a craniotome to perform the osteotomies. After testing on phantoms and animals, the system was successfully trialed in a single patient.[9] A different system intended for use in craniosynostosis surgery utilized a registration method without physical fiducials using a three-dimensional (3D) scanner. The system then used a robot to draw paths on a phantom skull model with excellent accuracy.[13]

### Robotic orthognathic surgery

Orthognathic surgery represents an opportunity for robotics to improve the precision, accuracy, and safety of osteotomies and repositioning of the maxilla and mandible and several systems have been described. A group from South Korea described the use of a robot to more accurately reposition the maxilla using navigation in phantom models.[14,15]

Several groups have developed systems that involve an industrial-style robot with a bone cutting instrument in conjunction with navigation localization. One particular system utilized a C8L robotic arm with an attached reciprocating saw and optical tracker. A comparison was made

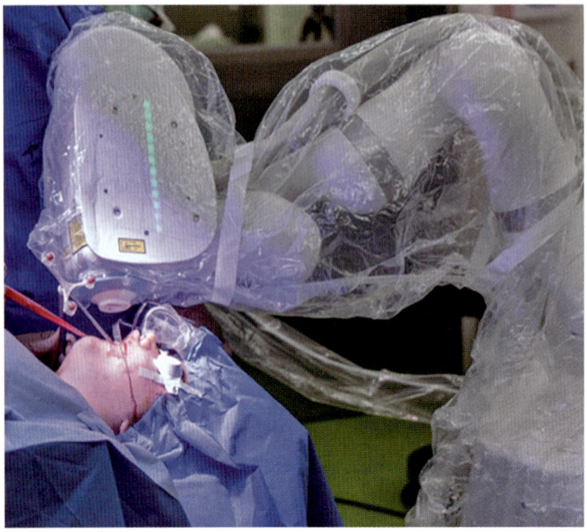

**Fig. 25.4** Cold Ablation Robot-guided Laser Osteotome (CARLO®) performing a midface osteotomy on a patient. (Image from Holzinger D, Ureel M, Wilken T, et al. First-in-man application of a cold ablation robot guided laser osteotome in midface osteotomies. *J Craniomaxillofac Surg*. 2021;49(7):531–7.)

between the robot and surgeons for Le Fort I osteotomies and genioplasty using phantom models and no difference was found between the two groups.[16] Sun et al. described an industrial KUKA robot with a drill to perform mandibular angle osteotomies on animals with reasonable accuracy.[17] Hara et al. described a novel robotic system with a workspace limitation safety mechanism to prevent injury to surrounding soft tissue. The system was tested in phantom models for drilling holes in the mandible and performing vertical ramus osteotomies.[18]

A recently developed robot called Cold Ablation Robot-guided Osteotome (CARLO®) represents a unique and exciting advancement in orthognathic surgery. The robot comprises a KUKA industrial robot with an Er: YAG laser, and a recent study utilized the system to perform osteotomies on the mandibles in pigs.[19] The same system also successfully performed a Le Fort I osteotomy in patients[20,21] (Fig. 25.4). CARLO® has also been investigated for the feasibility of its use for osteotomies of the mandible using cadavers.[22]

## Methods and considerations for a craniofacial-specific robot

### Intraoperative navigation

Surgical navigation involves the utilization of imaging registered to the patient as well as intraoperative tracking to direct tools and to provide a 3D roadmap of anatomy. Surgical navigation has been utilized extensively by neurosurgeons and is being increasingly used in craniofacial surgery.[23] A recent review found that the most common utilization of navigation in craniofacial surgery was for orbital surgery, procedures for defects of the maxilla and zygoma, temporomandibular joint surgery, orthognathic surgery, tumor ablation with reconstruction, and within pediatric craniofacial surgery.[24] A craniofacial surgical robot capable of reducing the invasiveness of procedures will almost certainly benefit from the use of navigation. With more minimal-access techniques and reduced visualization, navigation will ensure that osteotomies and tool paths are accurate and avoid critical structures.

### Ultrasonic bone-cutting devices

Ultrasonic saws are the most promising instruments for use in minimally invasive bone-cutting instruments due to their tissue selectivity. Ultrasonic saws use piezoelectric materials that oscillate at very high frequencies (>20 kHz) with very small strokes. The lower stroke distance of piezoelectric saws results in tissue selectivity and protection from injuring the surrounding soft tissue.[25] As a result of this, ultrasonic saws have become increasingly utilized in craniofacial surgery and have been shown to reduce blood loss, improve precision, and lower the incidence of postoperative swelling, hematoma, and nerve damage.[26] Piezoelectric saws have been shown to minimize injury to the dura as well as reduce the need to retract the brain in pediatric craniofacial procedures.[25] Disadvantages of ultrasonic saws are the slower cutting speeds, cost, and the different cutting characteristics requiring a longer learning curve.

Ultrasonic bone-cutting devices have been used in craniosynostosis surgery. A study investigated its use in 13 patients for endoscopic strip craniectomy for patients with sagittal and metopic craniosynostosis. The authors reported less blood loss while maintaining shorter operative times. Three patients had durotomies, which the authors attributed to earlier use of the device and that this can be avoided by using cottonoids on the dura for protection.[27]

## Robotic arm design

Although the da Vinci robot is a significant advancement as a result of the articulating tool tip wrists, the bulk of the arms are also rigid and less conducive to procedures within the craniofacial skeleton. The overall architecture of robotic arms can be grouped based on the commonalities of designs. Generally speaking, there are multiport and single-port robotic systems. Single-port systems are further classified as "X-type" or "Y-type" systems[28] and the advantages and disadvantages of each are summarized in Table 25.3 and illustrated in Fig. 25.5.

**Table 25.3 Comparison of the advantages and disadvantages of multi- and single-port robotic systems**

| | Advantages | Disadvantages |
|---|---|---|
| Multiport systems | Each port has a smaller diameter<br>Fewer instrument collisions if arms can be placed far apart | Larger footprint over the patient<br>Challenging to triangulate through a single orifice or port |
| Single-port systems | Requires a single incision<br>Instrument collisions are minimized<br>Smaller footprint over the patient | Instruments deploy distal to the port, which can make working in confined areas difficult<br>Instruments may have less degrees-of-freedom and articulation given the more compact design of the system |

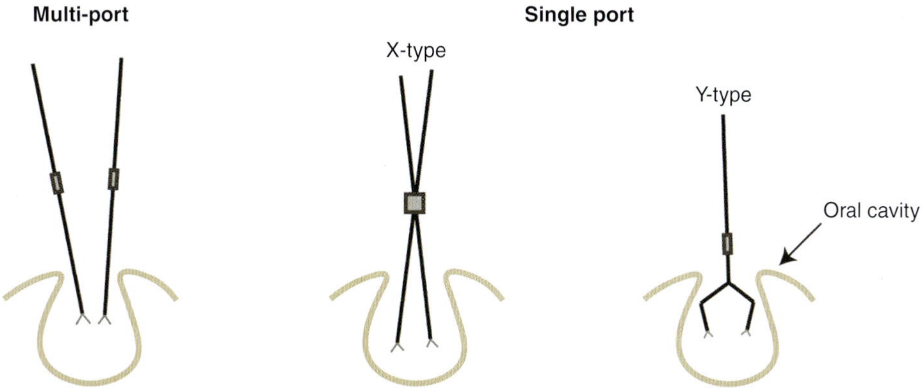


Fig. 25.5 Illustration of multiport and single-port robotic system architecture for oral cavity surgery.

## Multiport robotic systems

The da Vinci S, Si and Xi robotic systems fit into this category. However, several other systems have been developed that have a similar architecture, such as the RAVEN surgical system.[29] This type of robotic arm architecture is well suited for large body cavity surgery, such as procedures involving the abdomen and thorax where the arms can be positioned far away from each other to minimize instrument-instrument collisions. These types of systems have been adapted for TORS; however, they were never developed for single-access procedures through the oral cavity and therefore have limitations within this application. Single-access surgery requires positioning the arms closer together in parallel, which can result in reduced manipulability and instrument-instrument collisions.

## Single-port robotic systems

Significant advancements have been made in the development of robotic surgical systems that can access body cavities through a single incision. The da Vinci SP was developed for this purpose, and numerous additional systems have been developed with this capability.[30] The obvious advantage of single-port systems is the more compact nature of the design allowing multiple arms to traverse through a single incision to access a body cavity. Each robotic arm comprises an elbow joint in addition to the articulating tool tips allowing the arms to span and access larger workspaces. An evolution of TORS would likely benefit from the use of single-port systems and there are significant developments in this arena using the da Vinci SP.[31]

In 2015, Medrobotics received US Food and Drug Administration approval to use their Flex® system for transoral procedures. The Flex® system uses a multilink flexible endoscope that can more readily navigate through the curvatures required to access the oropharynx. The system uses manual instruments that traverse through the multilink endoscopic platform.[32,33]

A new system currently being developed is the adaptive and compliant transoral robotic surgery (ACTORS) system (Fig. 25.6). This system combines elements of the SP and Flex® systems where the slave side of the robot contains flexible parallel manipulators with articulating mechanisms comprising five degrees-of-freedom (DOF). The

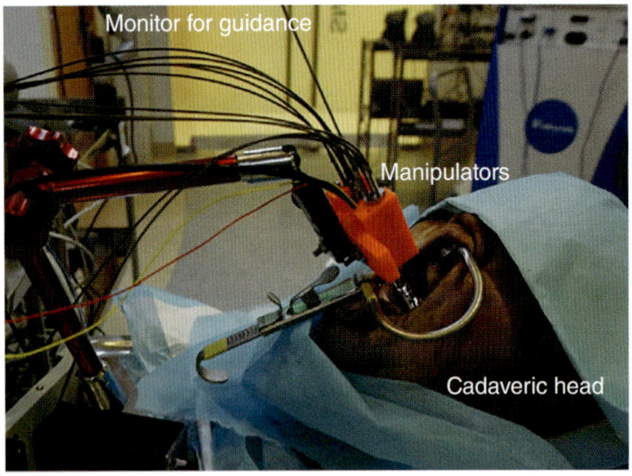


**Fig. 25.6** The adaptive and compliant transoral robotic surgery (ACTORS) system tested in a cadaver for a transoral approach. (Image from Ren H, Li C, Qiu L, Lim CM. ACTORS: Adaptive and Compliant Transoral Robotic Surgery with flexible manipulators and intelligent guidance. In: Abedin-Nasab MH, ed. *Handbook of Robotic and Image-Guided Surgery*. Elsevier; 2020:693–701.)

robot takes advantage of super-elastic nickel-titanium rods as well as a navigation system using patient imaging.[34]

The da Vinci SP, Flex®, and ACTORS systems represent significantly different designs. However, each system takes advantage of all working elements being contained within a single port or single mechanism. Conceptually, this would be advantageous for many of the surgical procedures used in craniofacial surgery given the confinements of the approaches and anatomy. However, significant technical challenges arise and the systems currently available are too large or lack the specific requirements of a craniofacial robot capable of cutting bone.

## Wrist designs

In addition to overall robotic system architecture, there are numerous different types of wrist mechanisms with specific advantages and disadvantages. A full review of these mechanisms is beyond the scope of this chapter. However, two review articles[35,36] provide an excellent overview of the various types of designs. Each type of wrist actuation and mechanism has specific advantages and disadvantages and the optimal design for a craniofacial robot would consider these factors.

# Future techniques

Development of a system capable of performing minimally invasive craniofacial surgery will require combining technology in robotics and bone cutting as well as navigation. Robotic capability will be necessary to traverse under soft tissue following the contours of the bony anatomy. The robot will be required to have an articulating mechanism where the tool tip can orient relative to bone to perform optimal bone cuts. Intraoperative navigation will be necessary to ensure the tool tips are directed appropriately with or without the aid of endoscopes for direct visualization. This will require planning the path of the robot preoperatively that will be implemented at the time of surgery. An ultrasonic saw will be used, taking advantage of its tissue selectivity. The robot will also require tool tip exchanges during surgery specifically between different soft and bone tissue cutting instruments. The requirements of a craniofacial robotic system can be seen in Table 25.4.

## Robotic craniosynostosis surgery

A robotic system for craniosynostosis surgery will ideally comprise of multiple arms and bone-cutting instruments, as well as direct visualization using endoscopes and/or navigation. Any new system will be an advancement of the endoscopic approaches currently being utilized.[37]

The system will operate within soft tissue pockets under the scalp walking along the bony contours of the calvarium and orbits. A flexible arm that can follow bony anatomy would be advantageous. Ideally, all instruments should be within a single mechanism requiring a single incision. However, multiple ports may be required to simultaneously visualize and manipulate bone under soft tissue. In addition to bone-cutting capability, the tool tips require soft tissue manipulation to create the paths necessary to access the relevant bony anatomy. Bone

**Table 25.4 Requirements of a craniofacial robotic surgical system**

1. Bone cutting capability
2. Minimize injury to surrounding structures
3. Manipulate soft tissue to create paths and pockets
4. Traverse within these soft tissue pockets
5. Traverse over, under, or within complex bony anatomy
6. Contain an articulating tool tip
7. Contain at least seven degrees of freedom
8. Require either direct visualization with an endoscope and/or navigation
9. Comprise of interchangeable tool tips
10. Comprise of multiple arms within a single mechanism or use a multiport design
11. Have the capability to move bone
12. Have the ability to fixate bone

remodeling will result from underlying brain growth in young infants primarily in the middle and posterior vault and therefore fixation will not be required in these circumstances. However, for later-presenting children and procedures involving the anterior vault and periorbital region, reshaping of bone and fixation may be necessary to obtain optimal results. This latter group presents a considerable challenge, and unique methods of moving and fixating bone will need to be developed and may involve a combination of robotics, navigation, and percutaneous fixation.

## Robotic orthognathic surgery

A robot for orthognathic surgery that is an advancement from traditional approaches may involve either traditional open techniques using novel bone-cutting instruments, such as the CARLO® system, or minimal access incisions on the face and within the oral cavity. For example, a Le Fort I osteotomy can be performed using a keyhole upper gingiva buccal sulcus incision creating a soft tissue pocket in a subperiosteal plane. Endoscopic assistance[38] and smaller upper gingival incisions[39] have been utilized in Le Fort I osteotomies to minimize invasiveness and improve visualization. As earlier described, robotic systems for mandibular osteotomies have already been investigated.[17,18] Further testing is required to ensure the safety of these systems as well as comparison studies determining the advantages compared to traditional approaches. Future advancements may involve novel bone-cutting instruments and automation using navigation through smaller keyhole incisions as well as unique mechanisms to perform fixation within more minimally invasive approaches.

## Robotic Le Fort II and Le Fort III surgery

Attempts have been made to reduce the invasiveness of Le Fort II and Le Fort III osteotomies using endoscopes and piezoelectric saws. Hara et al. utilized an endoscope with a piezoelectric saw to perform a Le Fort II osteotomy with fixation without the need for a bicoronal incision in seven patients. The procedure required a modified osteotomy pattern with the superior nasofrontal and vertical pyriform osteotomies more anteriorly positioned compared to a traditional Le Fort II as these were accessed from an upper gingivobuccal sulcus incision.[40] Taylor et al. demonstrated the feasibility of performing a more minimally invasive Le Fort III osteotomy in cadavers using a piezoelectric saw through periorbital and keyhole upper gingivobuccal sulcus incisions.[41] Hollier et al. demonstrated the feasibility of performing a Le Fort III osteotomy without a bicoronal incision for patients undergoing distraction using periorbital and oral incisions using a reciprocating saw in three patients. The authors reported less blood loss and operative time compared to a bicoronal approach.[42] These examples represent an attempt to minimize morbidity using bone-cutting and vision technology. The addition of robotic technology will further improve these minimally invasive approaches enhancing accuracy, capability, and safety.

## Robotic cleft palate surgery

As already described, the da Vinci system has been used to perform cleft palate repair in infants in a pilot study in 10 children[10] and has been characterized with respect to its feasibility.[4,11] However, these studies highlight some of the limitations of this system. Furthermore, newer systems such as the Flex® and ACTOR systems are unlikely to have the dexterity capable of advancing cleft palate surgery. The feasibility study investigated by Podolsky et al.[4] determined that the da Vinci 8-mm EndoWrist instruments using the Xi system are superior to the 5-mm instruments using the Si system due to the more compact wrist mechanism, despite their larger size (Fig. 25.7). However, the 8-mm instruments are too large for the infant oral cavity workspace. As a result, the same group developed a novel wristed instrument using a more compact articulating mechanism that is 5 mm in diameter (Fig. 25.8 and Fig. 25.9)[43] and further miniaturized to 3 mm in diameter (Fig. 25.10).[44] These new wrist designs provide 7-DOF utilizing cable guide channels as opposed to pulleys which reduces the length of the mechanism. The instruments utilize a deported actuation system using cams (rotary mechanisms that transfer rotational to linear movement) to account for cable length changes during articulation of the wrist (Fig. 25.9). The smaller profile of the mechanism while maintaining its dexterity is optimal for cleft palate repair and reduces the number of instrument-instrument and instrument-oral cavity collisions (Fig. 25.10). These instruments have been extensively characterized and tested and are ready for in vivo animal testing prior to human trials.

## Conclusions

The application of robotics in craniofacial surgery is in its infancy. Several challenges exist with respect to more widespread implementation and adoption. Beyond the technical challenges of developing a suitable system for specific applications, the cost of the technology will need to be offset by improvements in patient outcomes and safety. Robotic surgery is an accelerating field that is finding novel applications in surgery. Craniofacial

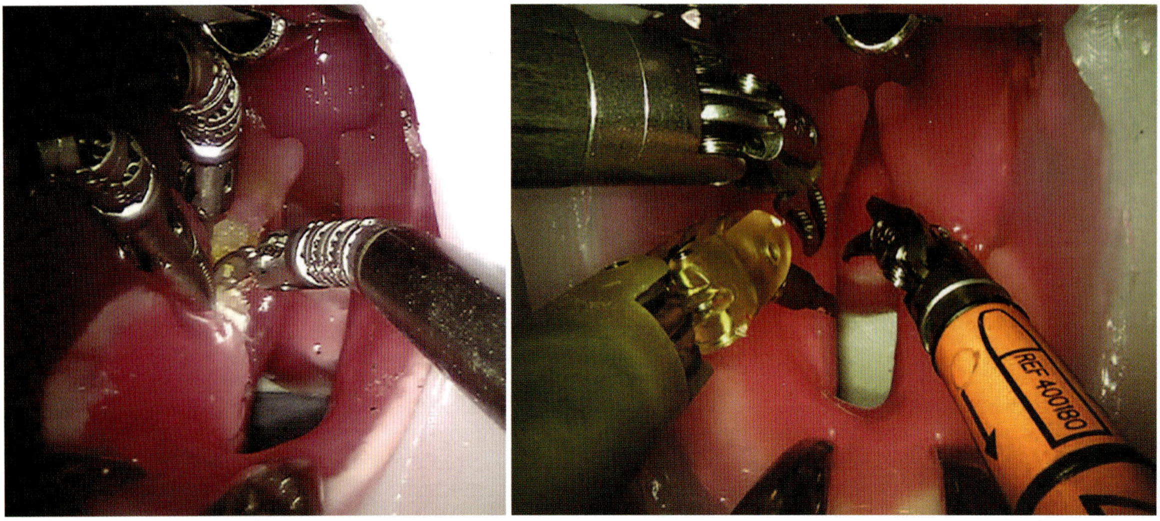


**Fig. 25.7** Testing the da Vinci surgical system for cleft palate repair using a high-fidelity cleft palate simulator. (Left) 5-mm EndoWrist instruments compared to the; (Right) 8-mm EndoWrist instruments.

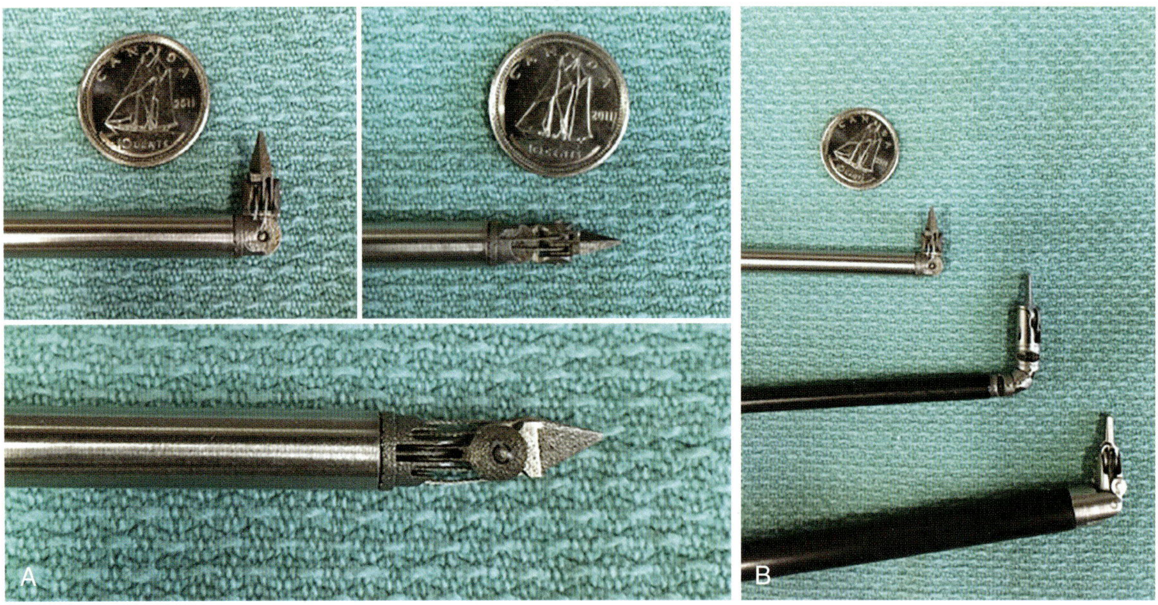


**Fig. 25.8** (A) New wrist design three-dimensionally printed in 17-4PH stainless steel. (B) New wrist shown in comparison to the da Vinci® EndoWrist® 5-mm and 8-mm instruments.

surgery is a field that should take advantage of robotic capability to develop novel approaches that allow performance of more complex maneuvers within more minimally invasive approaches. Future applications within craniofacial surgery will continue to evolve as technological advancements are made and we should take advantage of robotics to improve the care of patients with craniofacial presentations.

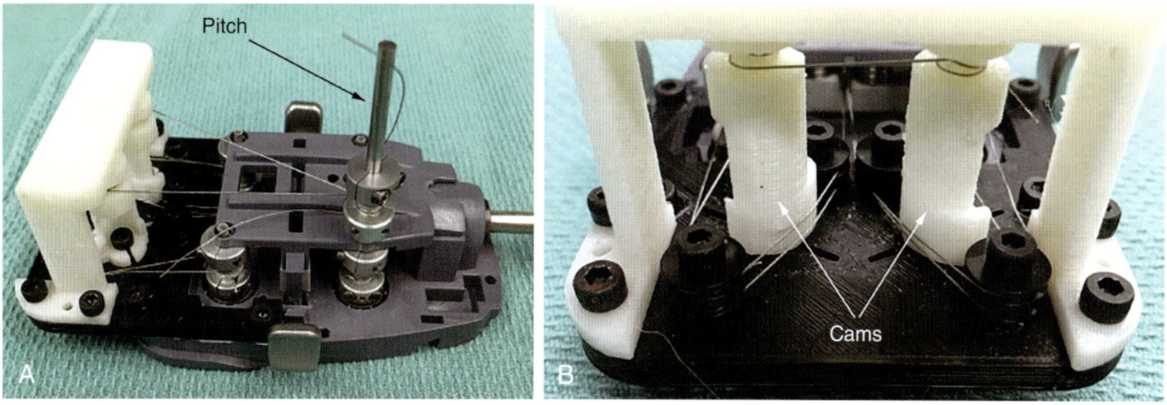


**Fig. 25.9** (A) Side view of cam mechanism (rotary mechanisms that transfer rotational to linear movement) coupled to wrist pitch. (B) Close-up view showing the cams contacting the gripper actuation cables.

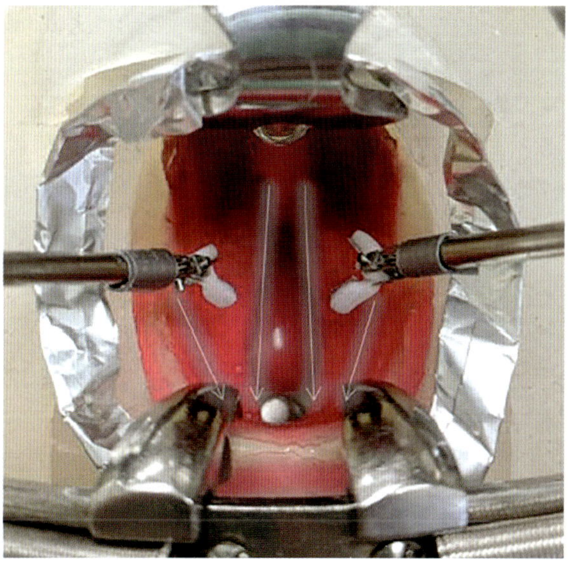

**Fig. 25.10** The novel 3-mm diameter instruments within the cleft palate simulator oral cavity workspace demonstrating the optimized size and performance within this specific workspace.

## Take-home points

- Craniofacial surgery may benefit from the enhanced capabilities of a surgical robot.
- The most widely used surgical robotic systems have a limited ability to perform craniofacial surgery.
- Craniofacial-specific robotic surgical systems have been developed for certain applications, but widespread use has been limited.
- A craniofacial robot will require safe bone-cutting technology, navigation, and unique robotic arm design to perform craniofacial surgery.
- Areas within craniofacial surgery that may readily take advantage of robotic technology include orthognathic surgery, craniosynostosis, complex midface surgery, and cleft palate repair.

## References


1. Jin HR, Yeon JY, Shin SO, Choi YS, Lee DW. Endoscopic versus external repair of orbital blowout fractures. *Otolaryngol Head Neck Surg*. 2007;136(1):38-44.
2. Sakamoto Y, Tamada I, Sakamoto T, Ishii T, Kishi K. Le Fort III distraction osteogenesis without bicoronal incision. *J Craniofac Surg*. 2020;31(6):1753-1755.
3. Kazanzides P, Fichtinger G, Hager GD, Okamura AM, Whitcomb LL, Taylor RH. Surgical and interventional robotics: core concepts, technology, and design. *IEEE Robot Autom Mag*. 2008;15(2):122-130.

4. Podolsky DJ, Fisher DM, Wong Riff KWY, Looi T, Drake JM, Forrest CR. Infant robotic cleft palate surgery: a feasibility assessment using a realistic cleft palate simulator. *Plast Reconstr Surg*. 2017;139(2):455e-465e.
5. Chan JYK, Wong EWY, Tsang RK, et al. Early results of a safety and feasibility clinical trial of a novel single-port flexible robot for transoral robotic surgery. *Eur Arch Otorhinolaryngol*. 2017;274(11):3993-3996.
6. Selber JC, Sarhane KA, Ibrahim AE, Holsinger FC. Transoral robotic reconstructive surgery. *Semin Plast Surg*. 2014;28(1):35-38.
7. De Ceulaer J, De Clercq C, Swennen GR. Robotic surgery in oral and maxillofacial, craniofacial and head and neck surgery: a systematic review of the literature. *Int J Oral Maxillofac Surg*. 2012;41(11):1311-1324.
8. Engelhardt M, Bast P, Jeblink N, et al. Analysis of surgical management of calvarial tumours and first results of a newly designed robotic trepanation system. *Minim Invasive Neurosurg*. 2006;49(2):98-103.
9. Eggers G, Wirtz C, Korb W, et al. Robot-assisted craniotomy. *Minim Invasive Neurosurg*. 2005;48(3):154-158.
10. Nadjmi N. Transoral robotic cleft palate surgery. *Cleft Palate Craniofac J*. 2016;53(3):326-331.
11. Khan K, Dobbs T, Swan MC, Weinstein GS, Goodacre TE. Trans-oral robotic cleft surgery (TORCS) for palate and posterior pharyngeal wall reconstruction: a feasibility study. *J Plast Reconstr Aesthet Surg*. 2016;69(1):97-100.
12. Podolsky DJ, Fisher DM, Wong Riff KW, Looi T, Drake JM, Forrest CR. Infant robotic cleft palate surgery: a feasibility assessment using a realistic cleft palate simulator. *Plast Reconstr Surg*. 2017;139(2):455e-465e.
13. Lu S, Luo Y, Xie D, Wang W, Zheng W, Gong J. Spatial mapping method of craniosynostosis surgical robot based on point cloud registration. In: *2021 6th Asia-Pacific Conference on Intelligent Robot Systems (ACIRS)*. Tokyo, Japan: 2021:1-6. doi:10.1109/ACIRS52449.2021.9519346.
14. Han JJ, Woo SY, Yi WJ, Hwang SJ. Robot-assisted maxillary positioning in orthognathic surgery: a feasibility and accuracy evaluation. *J Clin Med*. 2021;10(12):2596.
15. Woo SY, Lee SJ, Yoo JY, et al. Autonomous bone reposition around anatomical landmark for robot-assisted orthognathic surgery. *J Craniomaxillofac Surg*. 2017;45(12):1980-1988.
16. Wu J, Hui W, Chen S, et al. Error analysis of robot-assisted orthognathic surgery. *J Craniofac Surg*. 2020;31(8):2324-2328.
17. Sun M, Chai Y, Chai G, Zheng X. Fully automatic robot-assisted surgery for mandibular angle split osteotomy. *J Craniofac Surg*. 2020;31(2):336-339.
18. Hara K, Ma Q, Suenaga H, Kobayashi E, Sakuma I, Masamune K. Orthognathic surgical robot with a workspace limitation mechanism. *IEEE ASME Trans Mechatron*. 2019; 24(6):2652-2660.
19. Baek KW, Deibel W, Marinov D, et al. Clinical applicability of robot-guided contact-free laser osteotomy in cranio-maxillo-facial surgery: in-vitro simulation and in-vivo surgery in minipig mandibles. *Br J Oral Maxillofac Surg*. 2015;53(10):976-981.
20. Ureel M, Augello M, Holzinger D, et al. Cold ablation robot-guided laser osteotome (CARLO®): From bench to bedside. *J Clin Med*. 2021;10(3):450.
21. Holzinger D, Ureel M, Wilken T, et al. First-in-man application of a cold ablation robot guided laser osteotome in midface osteotomies. *J Craniomaxillofac Surg*. 2021;49(7):531-537.
22. Augello M, Baetscher C, Segesser M, Zeilhofer HF, Cattin P, Juergens P. Performing partial mandibular resection, fibula free flap reconstruction and midfacial osteotomies with a cold ablation and robot-guided Er:YAG laser osteotome (CARLO®): A study on applicability and effectiveness in human cadavers. *J Craniomaxillofac Surg*. 2018;46(10):1850-1855.
23. Tel A, Bagatto D, Tuniz F, et al. The evolution of craniofacial resection: a new workflow for virtual planning in complex craniofacial procedures. *J Craniomaxillofac Surg*. 2019; 47(9):1475-1483.
24. DeLong MR, Gandolfi BM, Barr ML, Datta N, Willson TD, Jarrahy R. Intraoperative image-guided navigation in craniofacial surgery: review and grading of the current literature. *J Craniofac Surg*. 2019;30(2):465-472.
25. Ramieri V, Saponaro G, Lenzi J, et al. The use of piezosurgery in cranial surgery in children. *J Craniofac Surg*. 2015;26(3):840-842.
26. Spinelli G, Mannelli G, Zhang YX, et al. Complex craniofacial advancement in paediatric patients: piezoelectric and traditional technique evaluation. *J Craniomaxillofac Surg*. 2015; 43(8):1422-1427.
27. Chaichana KL, Jallo GI, Dorafshar AH, Ahn ES. Novel use of an ultrasonic bone-cutting device for endoscopic-assisted craniosynostosis surgery. *Childs Nerv Syst*. 2013;29(7):1163-1168.
28. Cheon B, Gezgin E, Ji DK, et al. A single port laparoscopic surgery robot with high force transmission and a large workspace. *Surg Endosc*. 2014; 28(9):2719-2729.
29. Hannaford B, Rosen J, Friedman DW, et al. Raven-II: an open platform for surgical robotics research. *IEEE Trans Biomed Eng*. 2013;60(4):954-959.
30. Petroni G, Niccolini M, Caccavaro S, et al. A novel robotic system for single-port laparoscopic surgery: preliminary experience. *Surg Endosc*. 2013;27(6):1932-1937.

31. Van Abel KM, Yin LX, Price DL, Janus JR, Kasperbauer JL, Moore EJ. One-year outcomes for da Vinci single port robot for transoral robotic surgery. *Head Neck*. 2020;42(8):2077-2087.
32. Poon H, Li C, Gao W, Ren H, Lim CM. Evolution of robotic systems for transoral head and neck surgery. *Oral Oncol*. 2018; 87:82-88.
33. Tan Wen Sheng B, Wong P, Teo Ee Hoon C. Transoral robotic excision of laryngeal papillomas with Flex® Robotic System – A novel surgical approach. *Am J Otolaryngol*. 2018;39(3):355-358.
34. Ren H, Li C, Qiu L, Lim CM. ACTORS: Adaptive and Compliant Transoral Robotic Surgery with flexible manipulators and intelligent guidance. In: Abedin-Nasab MH, ed. *Handbook of Robotic and Image-Guided Surgery*. Elsevier; 2020:693-701.
35. Catherine J, Rotinal-Libersa C, Micaelli A. Comparative review of endoscopic devices articulations technologies developed for minimally invasive medical procedures. *Appl Bionics Biomech*. 2011;8:151-171.
36. Jelinek F, Arkenbout EA, Henselmans PWJ, Pessers R, Breedveld P. Classification of joints used in steerable instruments for minimally invasive surgery—A review of the state of the art. *J Med Device*. 2015;9(1):010801.
37. Jimenez DF, Barone CM. Endoscopic technique for sagittal synostosis. *Childs Nerv Syst*. 2012;28(9):1333-1339.
38. Rohner D, Yeow V, Hammer B. Endoscopically assisted Le Fort I osteotomy. *J Craniomaxillofac Surg*. 2001;29(6):360-365.
39. Seblain D, Bourlet J, Sigaux N, Khonsari RH, Chauvel Picard J, Gleizal A. Minimally invasive versus standard approach in LeFort 1 osteotomy in patients with history of cleft lip and palate. *J Stomatol Oral Maxillofac Surg*. 2018;119(3):187-191.
40. Hara S, Mitsugi M, Kanno T, Nomachi A, Kawakami S, Tatemoto Y. Endoscopically assisted intraoral modified Le Fort II type midfacial advancement using piezoelectric surgery and an intraoperative RED system. *J Oral Maxillofac Surg*. 2013;71(2):e93-e103.
41. Taylor JA, Maercks RA, Runyan CM, Jones DC, Gordon CB. Endoscopically assisted Le Fort III osteotomy using an ultrasonic scalpel: a feasibility study in cadavers. *J Craniofac Surg*. 2009;20(6):2211-2214.
42. Hollier L, Kelly P, Babigumira E, Potochny J, Taylor T. Minimally invasive Le Fort III distraction. *J Craniofac Surg*. 2002;13(1): 44-48.
43. Podolsky DJ, Diller E, Fisher DM, et al. Utilization of cable guide channels for compact articulation within a dexterous three degrees-of-freedom surgical wrist design. *J Med Device*. 2019;13(1):011003.
44. Wu GCY, Podolsky DJ, Looi T, Kahrs LA, Drake JM, Forrest CR. A 3 mm wristed instrument for the da Vinci robot: Setup, characterization, and phantom tests for cleft palate repair. *IEEE Trans Med Robot Bionics*. 2020;2(2):130-139.

Chapter 26

# Computer-assisted design and manufacturing of tissue engineering craniofacial scaffolds

Yuxiao Zhou, Srujan Singh, Warren Grayson

CHAPTER OUTLINE



## Introduction

Critical-sized craniofacial defects (defects that cannot heal spontaneously within a patient's lifetime without surgical intervention) occur due to trauma, craniotomy (surgical removal of part of the craniofacial bone to expose the brain for tumor resection), and congenital malformations. They present major challenges to facial reconstruction. These defects can cause a series of complications, including infection, vision impairment, headache, neurological deficits, and soft tissue infection.[1-5] The contemporary gold standard for repairing large craniofacial defects is autologous bone graft,[6] which very often involves secondary surgeries in patients for bone harvest and is sometimes susceptible to bone resorption after transplantation.[7] Additionally, carving anatomical shapes from harvested bone further complicates the procedure.

The computer-assisted design/computed-assisted manufacturing (CAD/CAM) craniofacial reconstruction based on medical imaging techniques, such as cone-beam computed tomography (CBCT) and magnetic resonance imaging (MRI), provides useful information for pretreatment surgery plans and can generate anatomically shaped scaffolds that fit patient-specific defects. Compared to conventional manufacturing, which requires space to store large inventories of standard scaffolds, the CAD/CAM-based on-demand printing saves storage space. The key component in the workflow includes (1) identifying the defect region and mechanical constraints, (2) designing scaffold geometry and installing fixation tabs, (3) choosing the print method and parameters, (4) printing the scaffold, and (5) performing quality assurance assessments. Conventional scaffold materials used to treat craniofacial defects in clinical trials include titanium, bioceramics, and bioactive glasses and polymers.[5,8-12] With the advancement of three-dimensional (3D) bioprinting technology, the osteogenic performance of scaffolds can be enhanced significantly by combining living cells and biological molecules during printing.

Tissue engineering scaffolds are porous structures that facilitate vascularization and tissue ingrowth in contrast to solid structures. However, with increasing porosity, the mechanical robustness of scaffolds is weakened.[13] For biodegradable scaffolds, maintaining the mechanical stiffness in the transient period where bone formation and scaffold degradation occur simultaneously in the defect is challenging and needs to be taken special care of during the scaffold design to avoid scaffold failure after transplantation.

## Clinical considerations

Due to the unique structure and function of craniofacial bones, the clinical considerations while treating craniofacial defects are different from those for other bone defects. Specifically, for facial defects, aesthetics is an important consideration while making treatment plans. Reconstructing symmetric craniofacial structures relative to the undamaged side and minimizing postoperative scars are among patients' primary needs.

The nerves in the craniofacial region have complex architectures that emanate from the brain stem and run throughout the face. The facial nerves control the muscles that enable facial expressions. As a result of craniofacial injury, there is a high risk of acute craniofacial pain (pain that lasts less than six months). If not managed properly, the acute pain can evolve into chronic pain[14] which requires special management.[15] Inflammation of sinus (sinusitis) and soft tissues can also cause facial pain. Craniofacial pain is not limited to the site of the injury and can possibly cause pain in other craniofacial structures as well and is an important clinical consideration during craniofacial scaffold transplantation.

For fractures with significant soft tissue damage that exhibit less regenerative capacity, osteogenic factors are necessary to enhance the bioactivity of transplanted bone scaffolds. In this case, autologous cells may need to be isolated intraoperatively from the patient's bone marrow or adipose tissue.

The patient's medical history also needs to be addressed during craniofacial scaffold transplantation. Factors such as infections associated with trauma, radiation and drug therapy, and allergies, need to be considered while choosing scaffold materials. For example, radiation therapy is commonly used for head and neck malignancy treatment. However, overexposure to radiation can disturb bone growth in pediatric patients,[16] retard bone regeneration in craniofacial defects,[17,18] and even cause fatal complications.[19]

## Workflow for computer-assisted design/computed-assisted manufacturing

Please see Fig. 26.1.

## Computer-assisted design

Pease see Fig. 26.2 and Video 26.1.

## Computer-assisted manufacturing

Please see Fig. 26.3 and Video 26.2.

## Operative technique

Currently, there is no patient data for 3D-printed, porous, biodegradable craniofacial scaffolds in clinical trials. The porcine craniofacial bone defect model is used as a surrogate for human patients in many preclinical studies.[20-22] In the study performed by Singh et al.,[22] a clinically translatable point-of-care (POC) cell-based reconstruction strategy was proposed to treat 2-cm, full-thickness, critical-sized defects in the zygomatic arches of Yucatan minipigs (Fig. 26.4). Pretreatment computed tomography (CT) images of minipig skulls were collected and used to design

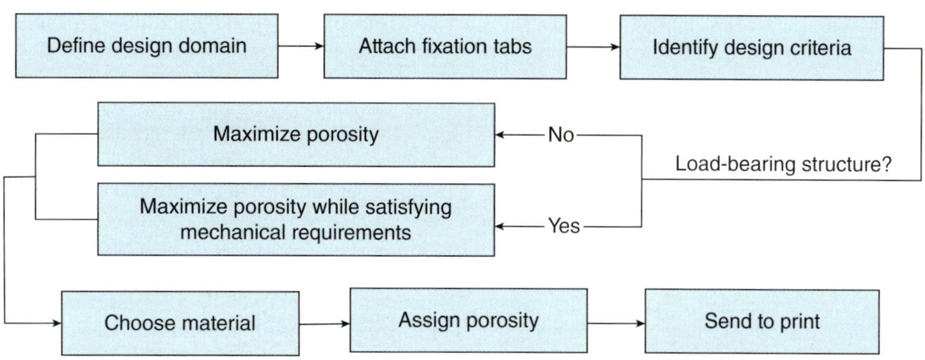


**Fig. 26.1** Computer-assisted design/computed-assisted manufacturing workflow.

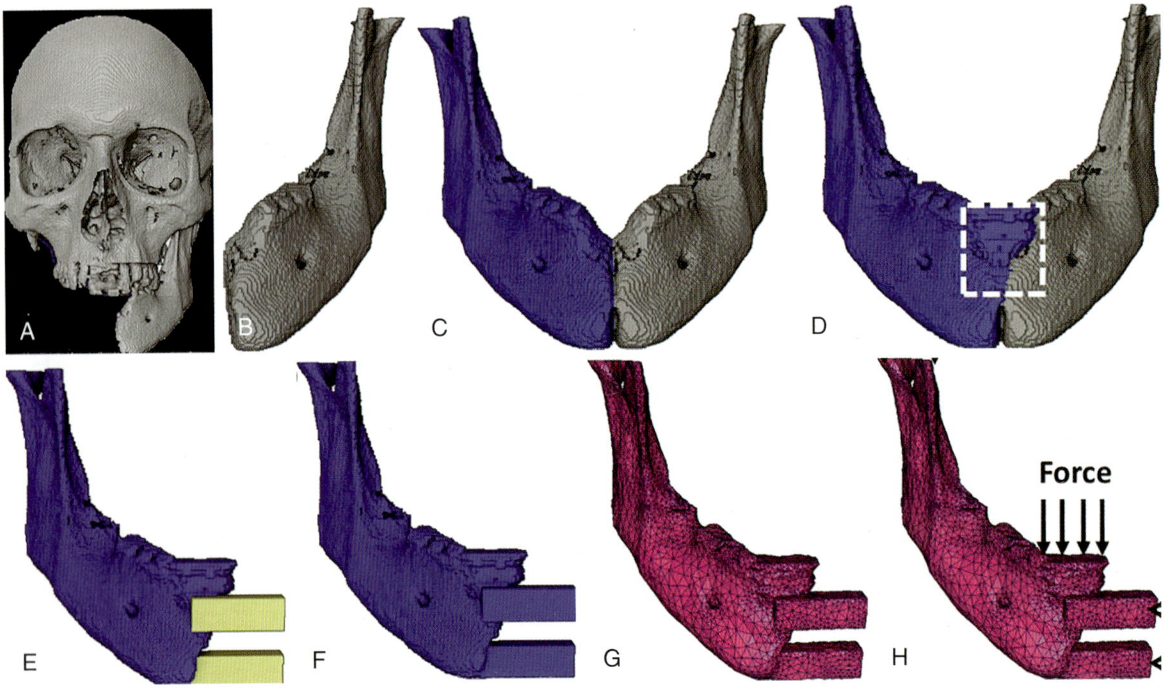


**Fig. 26.2** Example of a patient with hemimandibular injury. (A) Reconstruct craniofacial structure from clinical computed tomography data. (B) Identify and extract defect region. (C) Create scaffold geometry by flipping contralateral intact side mandible. (D) Fill empty region between flipped side and intact side (indicated by *white dashed box*). (E) Add fixation tab to desired location on scaffold. The fixation tabs are used to install screws connecting scaffold and local mandible bone. (F) Combine scaffold and fixation tabs to form a single volume. This step is taken to prepare the scaffold volume for finite element meshing procedure. (G) Mesh scaffold geometry for finite element analysis. (H) Apply physiologically realistic loading conditions (masticatory force in this mandibular scaffold case) and proper boundary constraints (here we assume the region indicated by triangles is fixed during loading). The results help identify regions that need high mechanical stiffness, and these regions need to be assigned lower porosities for better mechanical performance.

customized poly-ε-caprolactone-decellularized bone (PCL-DCB) scaffolds, augmented with autologous porcine stromal vascular fraction (SVF) harvested during surgery to promote robust bone regeneration. During the surgery, defects were created following animal-specific cutting guides and treated with defect-specific PCL-DCB scaffolds (Fig. 26.5A). After surgery, the *in vivo* bone healing was investigated during a 52-week period. *In vivo* CT images were collected, and significant bone formation around the scaffold was observed in most defects (Fig. 26.5B).

## Fidelity/verification

For favorable regenerative outcomes, it is generally believed that the physical dimensions and porosity of 3D-printed scaffolds closely match the desired design parameters of the custom scaffold. To date, no robust strategy exists to perform print quality assurance (QA) tests on tissue-engineered bone scaffolds. Taking inspiration from a well-established registration technique for 3D volumes, namely iterative closest points (ICP),[23] Zhang et al. developed an independent iterative closest point script (I-$ICP_{10}$) which facilitates objective and quantitative print quality assessment of bone custom scaffolds with complex geometry and (both homogeneous and heterogeneous) pore architecture.[24] Briefly, CBCT scans of the 3D-printed scaffolds were acquired. Using I-$ICP_{10}$, the reconstructed volumes of the printed scaffolds were registered with the initial design volume. Thereafter, voxel-to-voxel comparisons were performed between the two volumes to identify areas of mismatch and quantify the amount of deviation of the intended design. The whole workflow is shown in Fig. 26.6. Such a method can be incorporated as a QA checkpoint into the fabrication pipeline of custom scaffolds. Based on the tolerance limit, it can be determined whether a 3D-printed scaffold qualifies for subsequent clinical use.

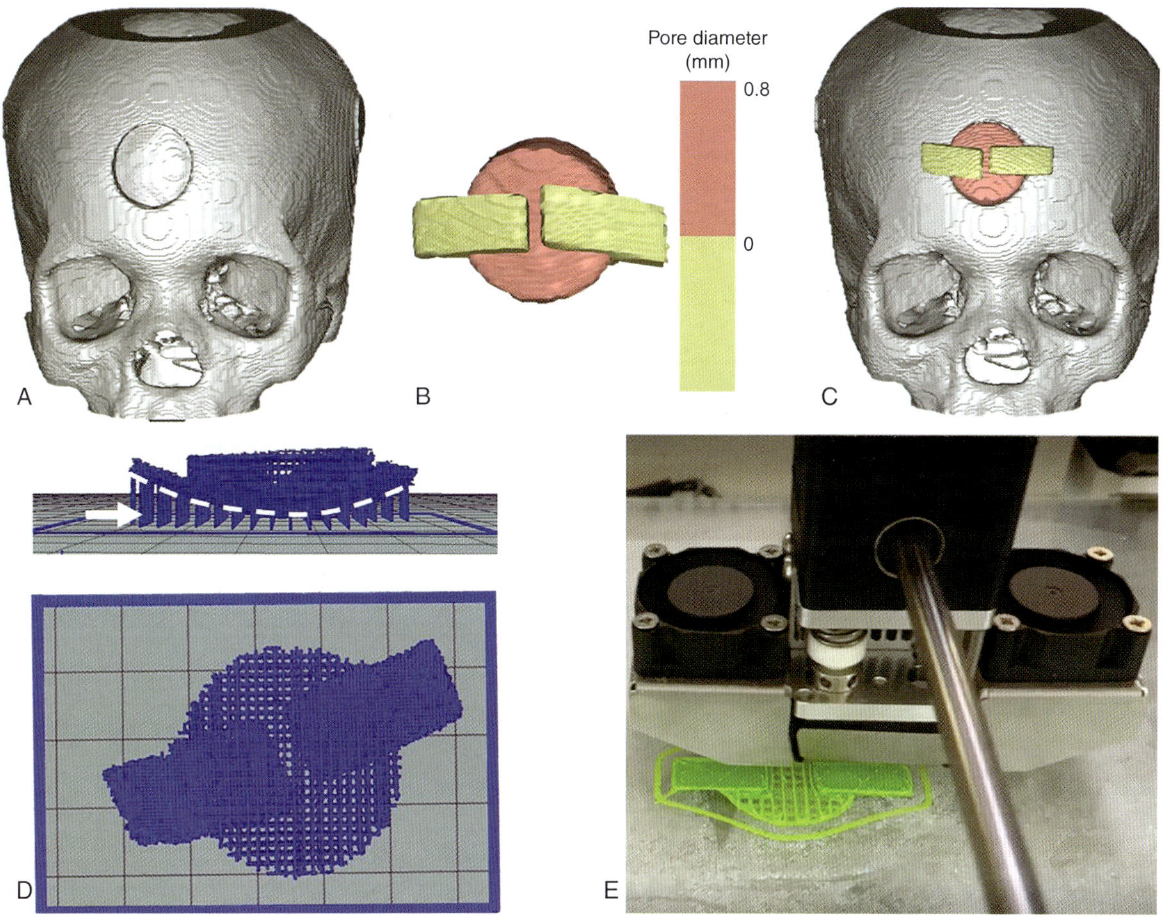


**Fig. 26.3** Computer-assisted manufacturing procedure. (A) Reconstruct craniofacial geometry from patient clinical computed tomography data and identify defect region. (B) Extract defect geometry, generate anatomically shaped scaffold and attach fixation tabs. Scaffold is porous for better vascularization after transplantation, and fixation tabs are solid for higher mechanical stiffness. (C) Assemble designed scaffold into cranial defect. (D) Generate G-code for scaffold with desired porosity and microarchitecture using in-house slicer program called scafSLICR[26] (E) (Top) Side view of the scaffold sent to 3D printing. This scaffold includes supporting structures (indicated by *white arrow*), which is the region between scaffold boundary (*white dashed line*) and print bed. (Bottom) Frontal view of the scaffold, showing porous scaffold and solid fixation tabs.

## Pearls/pitfalls

- The application of CAD/CAM provides a promising solution for critical-sized craniofacial defect reconstruction by restoring function and facial aesthetics for the defect region.
- For load-bearing scaffolds, mechanical requirements are important considerations during design to avoid unexpected fractures after craniofacial reconstruction surgery.
- For midfacial defects, clinical CT data need to have enough resolution to capture thin structures with bone thickness less than 1 mm in midfacial and maxillomandibular regions.
- Currently, the application of CAD/CAM technology in facial reconstruction is limited to bone structure only. The restoration of other accompanying structures (such as teeth and tongue) is currently fulfilled via transplantation in clinical trials.[25]

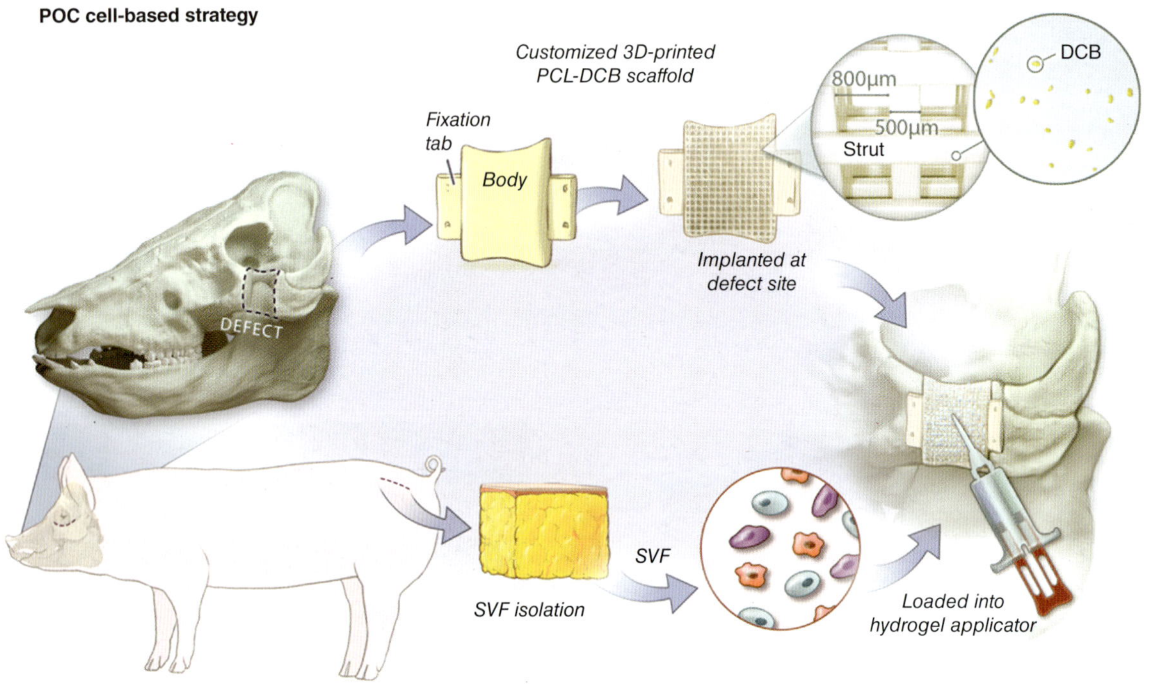


**Fig. 26.4** Point-of-care (POC) cell-based strategy for treating critical-sized midfacial bone defects. Pretreatment computed tomography images of skulls were collected. Defect-specific scaffolds with solid fixation tabs were designed. Scaffolds were printed with clinical-grade poly-ε-caprolactone-decellularized bone via fused deposition modeling with isotropic, interconnected pores, to promote vascularization and osteogenesis after transplantation. At the time of surgery, 2-cm bilateral full-thickness defects in zygomatic arches were created following animal-specific cutting guides at preselected locations and treated with scaffolds. Concurrently, stromal vascular fraction was isolated from subcutaneous adipose tissue, resuspended in fibrinogen solution, loaded into a double-barreled hydrogel applicator with thrombin in the second barrel, and infused into defect site without precultivation. (From Singh S, Nyberg EL, O'Sullivan AN, et al. Point-of-care treatment of geometrically complex midfacial critical-sized bone defects with 3D-Printed scaffolds and autologous stromal vascular fraction. *Biomaterials*. 2022;82:121392. https://doi.org/10.1016/J.BIOMATERIALS.2022.121392).

## Outcomes/complications

The CAD/CAM technology improves the accuracy of preoperative computer-assisted surgical planning (CaSP), including scaffold design and manufacturing. The combination of CaSP and point-of-care procedures can help reduce intraoperative error and enhance overall treatment outcomes.

Potential complications of CAD/CAM-assisted craniofacial reconstruction include infection, bone resorption, vascular compromise, delayed healing due to poor soft tissue envelope (especially for facial reconstruction after segmental fracture where the soft-tissue envelope is not intact), vision impairment for periorbital trauma, headache, neurological deficits, soft tissue infection,[1-4] and tissue-associated scaffold mismatch with skeletal bone development for adolescent patients.

## Conclusion

The success of craniofacial reconstruction includes restoration of facial aesthetics and delicate functions (such as respiration, facial expression, and mastication). The advancement of CAD/CAM has lifted constraints on the shape and structure of scaffolds and has provided more controllable mechanical performance and a higher possibility of predictable treatment outcomes in the short and long term.

In order to realize the application of CAD/CAM in clinical trials, it is necessary to standardize the design and

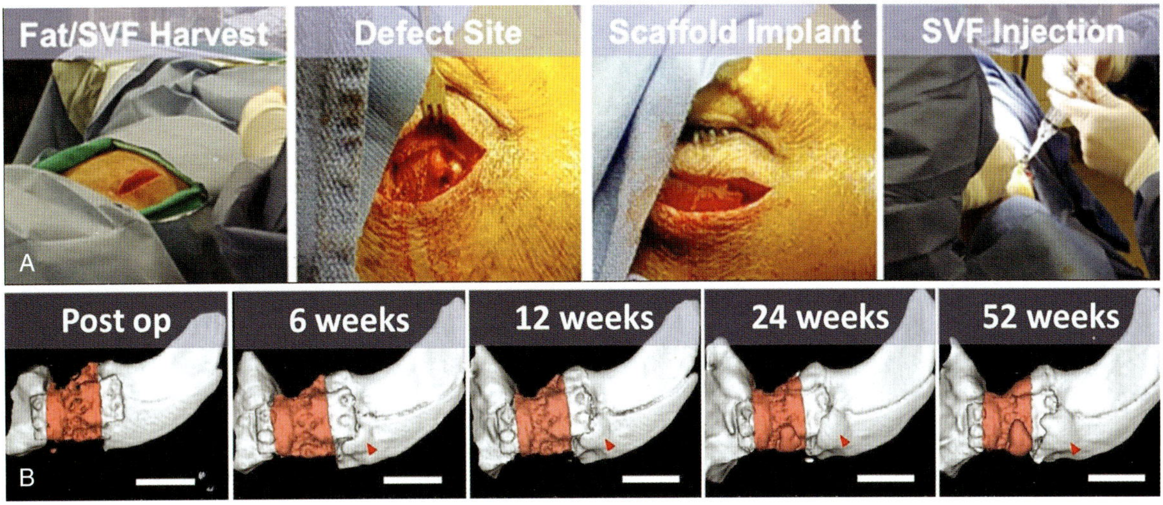


**Fig. 26.5** Surgery procedure and defect healing in Yucatan minipig zygomatic defect model. (A) Point-of-care surgery procedure, including fat harvest, defect site creation, scaffold implant transplantation, and stromal vascular fraction injection. (B) Bone regeneration in zygomatic defect evaluated from *in vivo* follow-up computed tomography scans collected at multiple time points during the 52 weeks after transplantation. Scale bar = 2 cm. (From Singh S, Nyberg EL, O'Sullivan AN, et al. Point-of-care treatment of geometrically complex midfacial critical-sized bone defects with 3D-Printed scaffolds and autologous stromal vascular fraction. *Biomaterials*. 2022;82:121392.)

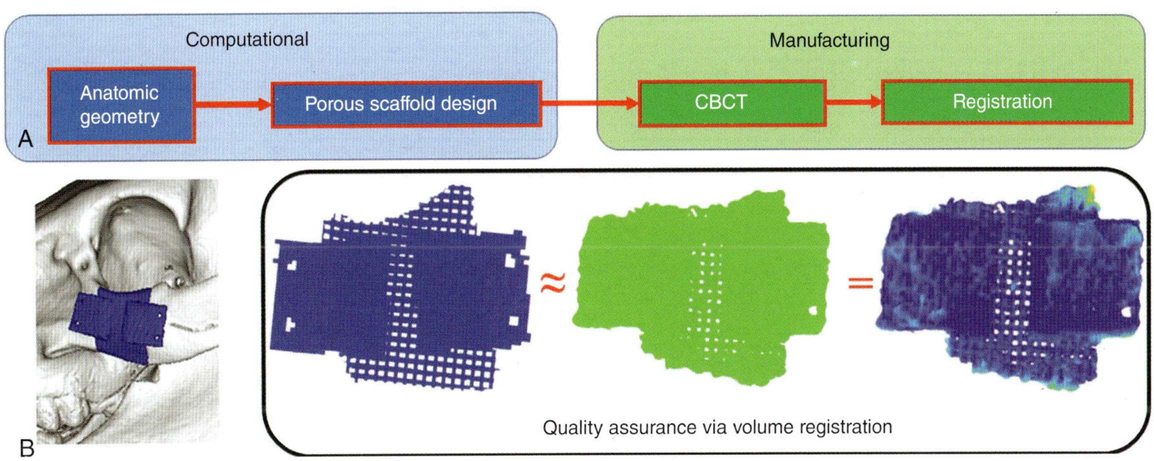


**Fig. 26.6** Defect-specific tissue engineering scaffolds require robust quality assurance metrics. (A) General workflow for design and manufacture of custom, porous bone scaffolds. Solid scaffold geometry is generated from the anatomic geometry of defect site. (B) Custom design and manufacture of 2-cm porcine zygomatic porous scaffold to treat the shown defect. A solid scaffold is assigned a custom porous pattern (*blue*). The design is three-dimensional (3D) printed and scanned. Cone-beam computed tomography scan (*green*) of manufactured scaffold provides its digital representation. Subsequent quality assurance (QA) involves a voxel-to-voxel comparison between the manufactured scaffold and design intent to produce a quality readout in the form of a heatmap of print mismatch within the 3D printed scaffold. (From Zhang N, Singh S, Liu S, Zbijewski W, Grayson WL. A robust, autonomous, volumetric quality assurance method for 3D printed porous scaffolds. *3D Print. Med*. 2022;81(8):1–9. https://doi.org/10.1186/S41205-022-00135-X.)

surgery procedures, generate implants with mechanical and biological properties similar to the native bone around the defects, enhance bioactivity by combining with regenerative medicine, and regulate the degradation profile of the scaffolds more precisely.

## Take-home points

- CAD/CAM can generate anatomically shaped scaffolds to satisfy patients' specific requirements and guide surgery planning.
- Mechanical constraints added to scaffolds need to be considered while designing load-bearing scaffolds, such as mandibular and maxillary scaffolds.
- Larger porosity increases the bioactivity of scaffolds but compromises the mechanical strength of scaffolds. Porosity and mechanical strength need to be considered simultaneously during scaffold design.
- Finite element analysis is a powerful computational tool for assessing the mechanical strength of scaffolds for preoperative treatment planning.
- Print quality assurance assessment is essential in establishing standards for the scaffold manufacturing process in future clinical trials.

## References


1. Geisler FH, Rodriguez E, Manson PN. Chapter 22: Traumatic skull and facial fractures. In: Ellenbogen RG, Abdulrauf, SI, Sekhar, LN, eds. *Principles of Neuroogical. Surgery*. Elsevier; 2012:365-393. Available at: https://doi.org/10.1016/B978-1-4377-0701-4.00022-1.
2. Edvinsson JCA, Viganò A, Alekseeva A, et al. The fifth cranial nerve in headaches. *J Headache Pain*. 2020;21:65. Available at: https://doi.org/10.1186/s10194-020-01134-1.
3. Lonjaret L, Guyonnet M, Berard E, et al. Postoperative complications after craniotomy for brain tumor surgery. *Anaesth Crit Care Pain Med*. 2017;36:213-218. Available at: https://doi.org/10.1016/J.ACCPM.2016.06.012.
4. Kim SH, Lee SJ, Lee JW, Jeong HS, Suh IS. Staged reconstruction of large skull defects with soft tissue infection after craniectomy using free flap and cranioplasty with a custom-made titanium mesh constructed by 3D-CT-guided 3D printing technology: two case reports. *Medicine*. 2019;98(6):e13864. Available at: https://doi.org/10.1097/MD.0000000000013864.
5. Champeaux C, Froelich S, Caudron Y. Titanium three-dimensional printed cranioplasty for fronto-nasal bone defect. *J Craniofac Surg*. 2019;30:1802-1805. Available at: https://doi.org/10.1097/SCS.0000000000005493.
6. Schmidt AH. Autologous bone graft: Is it still the gold standard? *Injury*. 2021;52:S18-S22. Available at: https://doi.org/10.1016/j.injury.2021.01.043.
7. Klijn RJ, van den Beucken JJJP, Bronkhorst EM, Berge SJ, Meijer GJ, Jansen JA. Predictive value of ridge dimensions on autologous bone graft resorption in staged maxillary sinus augmentation surgery using Cone-Beam CT. *Clin Oral Implants Res*. 2012;3:409-415. Available at: https://doi.org/10.1111/J.1600-0501.2011.02342.X.
8. Sumida T, Otawa N, Kamata Y, et al. Custom-made titanium devices as membranes for bone augmentation in implant treatment: clinical application and the comparison with conventional titanium mesh. *J Cranio-Maxillofacial Surg*. 2015;3:2183-2188. Available at: https://doi.org/10.1016/j.jcms.2015.10.020.
9. Park EK, Lim JY, Yun IS, et al. Cranioplasty enhanced by three-dimensional printing. *J Craniofac Surg*. 2016;27:943-949. Available at: https://doi.org/10.1097/SCS.0000000000002656.
10. Saijo H, Igawa K, Kanno Y, et al. Maxillofacial reconstruction using custom-made artificial bones fabricated by inkjet printing technology. *J Artif Organs*. 2009;12:200-205. Available at: https://doi.org/10.1007/s10047-009-0462-7.
11. Brie J, Chartier T, Chaput C, et al. A new custom made bioceramic implant for the repair of large and complex craniofacial bone defects. *J Craniomaxillofac Surg*. 2013;41:4037. Available at: https://doi.org/10.1016/j.jcms.2012.11.005.
12. Goh BT, Teh LY, Tan DPB, Zhang Z, Teoh SH. Novel 3D polycaprolactone scaffold for ridge preservation – a pilot randomised controlled clinical trial. *Clin Oral Implants Res*. 2015;26:271-277. Available at: https://doi.org/10.1111/clr.12486.
13. Nyberg Y, O'Sullivan A, Grayson W. scafSLICR: A MATLAB-based slicing algorithm to enable 3D-printing of tissue engineering scaffolds with heterogeneous porous microarchitecture. *PLoS One*. 2019;14(11):e0225007. Available at: https://doi.org/10.1371/journal.pone.0225007.
14. Khan J, Zusman T, Wang Q, Eliav E. Acute and chronic pain in orofacial trauma patients. *J. Endod*. 2019;45:S28-S38. Available

at: https://doi.org/10.1016/J.JOEN.2019.05.010.

15. Gordin E, Lee TS, Ducic Y, Arnaoutakis D. Facial nerve trauma: Evaluation and considerations in management. *Craniomaxillofac Trauma Reconstr.* 2015;8:1. Available at: https://doi.org/10.1055/S-0034-1372522.
16. Gevorgyan A, La Scala GC, Neligan PC, Pang CY, Forrest CR. Radiation-induced craniofacial bone growth disturbances. *J Craniofac Surg.* 2007;18(5):1001-1007. Available at: https://doi.org/10.1097/scs.0b013e31812f7584.
17. Hu WW, Ward BB, Wang Z, Krebsbach PH. Bone regeneration in defects compromised by radiotherapy. *J Dent Res.* 2010;89:77-81. Available at: https://doi.org/10.1177/0022034509352151.
18. Jung HM, Lee JE, Lee SJ, Lee JT, Kwon TY, Kwon TG. Development of an experimental model for radiation-induced inhibition of cranial bone regeneration. *Maxillofac Plast Reconstr Surg.* 2018;40:34. Available at: https://doi.org/10.1186/s40902-018-0173-1.
19. Nguyen MT, Billington A, Habal MB. Osteoradionecrosis of the skull after radiation therapy for invasive carcinoma. *J Craniofac Surg.* 2011;22(5):1677-1681. Available at: https://doi.org/10.1097/SCS.0b013e31822e5f83.
20. Chen D, Wu JY, Kennedy KM, et al. Tissue engineered autologous cartilage-bone grafts for temporomandibular joint regeneration. *Sci Transl Med.* 2020;12(565):62-77. Available at: https://doi.org/10.1126/scitranslmed.abb6683.
21. Dewey MJ, Milner DJ, Weisgerber D, et al. Repair of critical-size porcine craniofacial bone defects using a collagen-polycaprolactone composite biomaterial. *Biofabrication.* 2021;14:10.1088/1758-5090/ac30d5. Available at: https://doi.org/10.1088/1758-5090/AC30D5.
22. Singh S, Nyberg EL, O'Sullivan AN, et al. Point-of-care treatment of geometrically complex midfacial critical-sized bone defects with 3D-printed scaffolds and autologous stromal vascular fraction. *Biomaterials.* 2022;282:121392. Available at: https://doi.org/10.1016/J.BIOMATERIALS.2022.121392.
23. He Y, Liang B, Yang J, Li S, He J. An iterative closest points algorithm for registration of 3D laser scanner point clouds with geometric features. *Sensors.* 2017;17:1862. Available at: https://doi.org/10.3390/s17081862.
24. Zhang N, Singh S, Liu S, Zbijewski W, Grayson WL. A robust, autonomous, volumetric quality assurance method for 3D printed porous scaffolds. *3D Print Med.* 2022;81(8):1-9. Available at: https://doi.org/10.1186/S41205-022-00135-X.
25. Khalifian S, Brazio PS, Mohan R, et al. Facial transplantation: the first 9 years. *Lancet.* 2014;384:2153-2163. Available at: https://doi.org/10.1016/S0140-6736(13)62632-X.
26. Nyberg E, O'Sullivan A, Grayson W. scafSLICR: A MATLAB-based slicing algorithm to enable 3D-printing of tissue engineering scaffolds with heterogeneous porous microarchitecture. *PLoS One.* 2019;14(11):e0225007. doi:10.1371/journal.pone.0225007.

Chapter 27

# Computer-assisted planning in maxillofacial prosthetics

*David J. Reisberg, Eduardo Arias, Akanksha Srivastava, Nikesh Regmi*

**CHAPTER OUTLINE**



## Introduction

Six separate procedures will be described in this chapter. Each demonstrates the value of computer-assisted planning and the interaction between the craniofacial surgeon and other members of the prosthetics and design team. In each case, the definitive outcome is first visualized and then planning for the actual procedure commences with an eye toward this goal. This is restorative-driven care.[4-6] This is analogous to the construction of a new home where one first selects the appearance of the desired structure, then goes about planning and designing to achieve this outcome. Fig. 27.1 depicts the digital workflow common to all procedures described.

1. **Single tooth replacement with an osseointegrated implant.** In cases of cleft lip and palate it is common for a tooth to be congenitally missing in the line of the clefted alveolus. The placement of an osseointegrated implant in the edentulous site of a congenitally missing tooth has become a standard in cleft care.[7] It allows for an aesthetic and functional restoration while avoiding the need to unnecessarily restore adjacent teeth or connect teeth together, creating a more hygienic oral environment. It may require hard and/or soft tissue grafting of the site prior to implant placement.

2 and 3. **Complex oral rehabilitation: reconstruction of maxilla/mandible with microvascular free flap/osseointegrated implants/fixed prosthesis.** The same basic principles, protocol, and workflow for computer-assisted surgery and restoration of a single missing tooth apply to more complex craniofacial cases that involve multiple missing teeth and often, segments of the jaw and soft tissues. These situations arise most commonly in connection with a tumor resection but may be the result of craniofacial trauma or a congenital condition. In addition to replacing missing teeth, the restorative process may require the addition of bone with or without soft tissue. The cases demonstrated in Videos 27.2 and 27.3 required microvascular flap reconstruction following oncologic resection. In each situation, computer-assisted surgical planning (CaSP) and prosthesis design and fabrication yielded a predictable outcome that is both aesthetic and functional.

4. **Soft tissue augmentation.** When surgery is performed to augment deficient soft tissue facial contours, computer-assisted planning and computer-generated surgical guides assist the surgeon to achieve a more symmetrical, predictable appearance.
5. **Autologous ear construction.** When craniofacial reconstruction with autologous tissue is possible, the prosthetics team provides computer-assisted planning and surgical guides that enable the surgeon to achieve ideal position and form of the reconstruction.

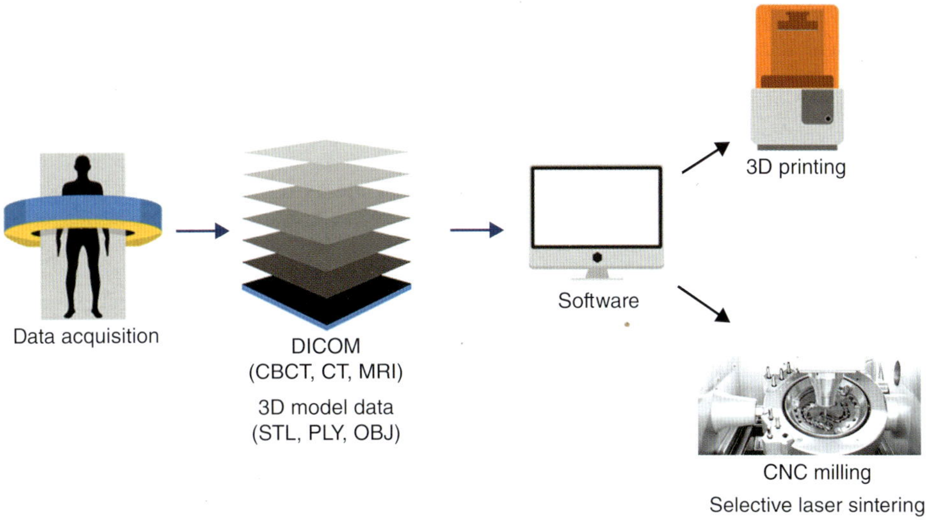


**Fig. 27.1** Digital workflow in maxillofacial prosthetics.

6. **Implant-retained facial prosthesis.** In congenital or acquired situations where an ear, nose, or orbit is missing or deformed, surgical correction using autologous tissues is the most natural means of restoring form and function. However, the nature and location of the defect, the lack of available soft tissue, the patient's medical condition, or their preference may preclude a reconstruction that is purely autologous. In such cases, prosthetic rehabilitation with osseointegrated craniofacial implants is a preferred option. An implant-retained facial prosthesis utilizing a computer-assisted surgical plan and prosthetic design and fabrication offers improved aesthetics, retention, and patient comfort over an adhesive retained one.

## Clinical considerations

1. **Single tooth replacement with an osseointegrated implant.** The edentulous site must be of appropriate clinical and radiographic width to allow for an aesthetic restoration without interfering with the roots of adjacent teeth. In a cleft-related edentulous space, the maxillofacial prosthodontist must work closely with the orthodontist to establish and maintain proper tooth spacing and root alignment of adjacent teeth so as not to impose on the ideal implant position. A cone-beam computed tomography (CBCT) scan will detect root position and bone volume (height and width) at the site. If there is inadequate bone volume at the implant site and a bone graft is required, computer-assisted planning helps to guide proper positioning of the bone graft to allow for later ideal implant placement.

2 and 3. **Complex oral rehabilitation: reconstruction of maxilla/mandible with microvascular free flap/osseointegrated implants/fixed prosthesis.** When placing osseointegrated implants and a fixed dental restoration as part of an extensive oral rehabilitation, there are many more considerations than with a single tooth replacement. Intricate planning sessions with the surgeon, maxillofacial prosthodontist, and the biomedical technologist are required for such complex surgeries. When an autogenous microvascular free flap and osseointegrated implants will be part of the reconstruction, three-dimensional (3D) spiral and CBCTs, a comprehensive oral examination, and an intraoral scan are necessary data. Anatomical and clinical considerations for this procedure include location of the defect, dimensions of the bony replacement, occlusal relationships, donor site selection, perfusion of the planned flap, and orientation of the bone segment relative to pedicle position. The location of nerves and vessels and position of the reconstruction plate and screws must be identified so the planned position of each implant will not interfere. The additional use of virtual reality software provides unique visualization capabilities at both the donor and host sites and enhance the surgeon's ability to evaluate the anatomy and plan the surgery along with the other members of the rehabilitation team.[8–12]

4. **Soft tissue augmentation.** The goal of this procedure is to achieve facial symmetry and aesthetic improvement

that can provide the patient with a sense of psychological well-being and confidence in both a social or work-related environment and improve their quality of life. The surgeon, working with the maxillofacial prosthetics team, can develop a computer-assisted plan to achieve the desired augmentation and then a computer-generated surgical guide to be used during the surgery to insure the desired outcome.[13]

5. **Autologous ear construction.** Autologous reconstruction is one of the most difficult tasks for the reconstructive surgeon. The goal of this procedure is to create an external ear that mimics the contralateral side in size, shape, position, and orientation. This becomes a challenge during the procedure when the unaffected ear is draped and inaccessible for reference. Computer-assisted planning and surgical guides provided by the maxillofacial prosthetics team assist the surgeon in all stages of the reconstruction.
6. **Implant-retained facial prosthesis.** The use of osseointegrated craniofacial implants to retain a facial prosthesis significantly improves the overall success of the restoration. The most common application sites are the auricular, nasal, and orbital areas. Depending on skin quality and contour at the defect site, and the visual acuity and manual dexterity of the patient or caregiver, adhesive-retained facial prostheses may be difficult to properly position and retain. There is also additional time and maintenance required due to the daily required application and removal of skin adhesive as well as potential skin irritation from the adhesive. An implant-retained facial prosthesis overcomes all of these problems. It is a more retentive and aesthetic restoration that is easier to position and remove. It is easier to maintain as the daily preparation and cleaning regimen is less cumbersome and there is no skin irritation from adhesives.

Considerations in planning for such a prosthesis are the presence of adequate bone and the condition of the skin through which the implants will pass. Digital information including a CT scan, a facial scan, and computerized imaging of the planned prosthesis will assist in determining the location of the implants to avoid anatomical structures, such as the mastoid air cells (auricular), frontal and maxillary sinuses (nasal), infraorbital nerve, and frontal sinus (orbital).

## Workflow for computer-assisted design/computer-assisted manufacturing

For all procedures, the workflow for data collection, computer-assisted design/planning, and surgical/prosthetic procedures are similar. As you view these videos, these will be described in detail for each procedure. Video 27.1 illustrates placement and restoration of a single implant supported tooth utilizing computer-assisted technologies, which allowed for a minimally invasive surgical procedure, shorter surgical time, reduced postoperative healing, and increased patient satisfaction with an immediate tooth restoration. Video 27.2 explains the basic principles of integrating surgical and prosthetic planning using virtual reality, computer-assisted design (CAD), computer numerical control (CNC) milling, and 3D printing. Video 27.3 details the workflow for prosthetically driven surgical planning and procedure implementation, including computer-assisted data collection, designing, and manufacturing. Videos 27.4, 27.5, and 27.6 describe extraoral surgical and prosthetic procedures.

## Fidelity/verification

Today, there is extensive evidence supporting improved surgical precision, prosthetic predictability, and patient outcomes with utilization of CAD/ computer-assisted manufacturing (CAM) in dentistry and prosthodontics when compared to analog techniques. Although, the level of precision achieved is only as accurate as the data entered into the system. Using an advanced planning software that allows predictable integration of data from several sources, such as digital imaging and communications in medicine (DICOM) and STL data, is essential.

In complex craniofacial rehabilitation cases, team collaboration is key in minimizing planning errors. Additionally, presurgical simulation with analog or printed models for verification of manufactured osteotomy guides, reconstruction plates, and custom-made prostheses ensures a seamless and predictable operating room procedure and minimizes unforeseen circumstances. Intraoperatively, fidelity of the CAD/CAM process is verified by the position of the interim prosthesis over the planned implants and by its occlusal relationship to the opposing dental arch for intraoral rehabilitation cases. Postoperatively, CBCTs may also be compared to verify fidelity of the computer-assisted procedure.

## Pearls/pitfalls

Although computer-assisted planning adds precision and accuracy to surgical and prosthetic outcomes, this process does add cost to the procedure. Computer software and equipment must be purchased and maintained, there is a need for trained individuals to perform the planning, and there are laboratory costs associated with fabrication of surgical guides and prostheses.

## Outcomes/complications

Surgical success and complications are most notable in a few days to a few months after a procedure has been carried out. In contrast, prosthetic complications are pertinent over the patient's remaining life. For instance, implant screw and abutment loosening/fractures are the most frequently occurring prosthetic complication that affect over 40% of implants, and can further lead to bone loss, implant fracture, or implant failure. A common reason for this is malpositioned implants that overexert forces on abutment screws. Managing such complications tend to be time-consuming, expensive, and frustrating for the patient and the maxillofacial prosthodontist. Restorative driven surgical planning is critical in avoiding such prosthetic complications.

## Conclusion

Computer assistance has improved the quality of the outcomes for simple and complex prosthetic and surgical/prosthetic craniofacial procedures. While added costs are of concern, the authors hope that, over time, these will be reduced and recognized as standard of care. All healthcare parties need to recognize that the ultimate goal of care is the improved quality of life for our patients.

## References


1. Izet M. The most influential scientists in the development of medical informatics. *Acta Inform Med*. 2016;24(6):422-423. doi:10.5455/aim.2016.24.422-423.
2. Christopher A. The role of computers in dentistry. *J Am Dent Assoc*. 1967;74(3):720-724.
3. Blatz MB, Conejo J. The current state of chairside digital dentistry and materials. *DCNA*. 2018;63(2):720-724. doi:10.1016/j.cden.2018.11.002.
4. Wang F, Wu Y, Zou D, Wang G, Kaigler D. Clinical outcomes of dental implant therapy in alveolar cleft patients: a systematic review. *Int J Oral Maxillofa Implants*. 2014;29(5):1098-1105.
5. Jaquiery C, Rohner D, Kunz C, et al. Reconstruction of maxillary and mandibular defects using prefabricated microvascular fibular grafts and osseointegrated dental implants – A prospective study. *Clin Oral Implants Res*. 2004;15(5):598-606. doi:10.1111/j.1600-0501.2004.01065.x.
6. Runyan CM, Sharma V, Staffenberg DA, et al. Jaw In A Day™ – State of the art in maxillary reconstruction. *J Craniofac Surg*. 2016;27(8):2101-2104. doi:10.1097/SCS.0000000000003139.
7. Seikaly H, Idris S, Chuka R, et al. The Alberta Reconstructive Technique: An occlusion-driven and digitally based jaw reconstruction. *Laryngoscope*. 2019;129(suppl 4):S1-S14. doi:10.1002/lary.28064.
8. Alkureishi L, Patel PK, Cohen MN, Zhao L, Banerjee P. Immersive-Touch virtual-reality surgical platform for craniofacial surgery by craniofacial surgeons: taking back the control. *Plast Reconstr Surg – Glob Open*. 2019;7(8S-2):175-176. doi:10.1097/01.GOX.0000583848.46832.e5.
9. Anik AA, Xavier BA, Hansmann J, et al. Accuracy and reproducibility of linear and angular measurements in virtual reality: a validation study. *J Digit Imaging*. 2019;33(1):111-120. doi:10.1007/s10278-019-00259-3.
10. Saini D, Williams Jr QL, Alkureishi L, et al. A systematic review of the latest technologies in cranial vault remodeling and its outcomes for correction of craniosynostosis. *Surg Res J*. 2021;1(2):1-12.
11. Sureshkumar H, Xu R, Erukulla N, Wadhwa A, Zhao L. "Snap on" or not? A validation on the measurement tool in a virtual reality application. *J Digit Imaging*. 2022;35:692-703. doi:10.1007/s10278-022-00582-2.
12. Mathis SBS, Cataneo JL. Zhao MD, et al. Same-day virtual reality surgical planning and intraoperative navigation: a new surgical workflow for craniofacial trauma and reconstruction, plastic and reconstructive surgery. *Glob Open*. 2021;9(suppl 10):141-142. doi:10.1097/01.GOX.0000799828.32968.fc.
13. Arias E, Huang Y-H, Zhao L, Seelaus R, Patel P, Cohen M. Virtual surgical planning and three-dimensional printed guide for soft tissue correction in facial asymmetry. *J Craniofac Surg*. 2019;30:846-850.

# Index

## D



## E



## F